PRECANCEROUS LESIONS
OF THE
GASTROINTESTINAL TRACT

Precancerous Lesions of the Gastrointestinal Tract

Editors

Paul Sherlock, M.D.
Department of Medicine
Memorial Sloan-Kettering
Cancer Center
New York, New York

Basil C. Morson, M.D.
Pathology Department
St. Mark's Hospital
London, England

Luigi Barbara, M.D.
Department of Gastroenterology
University of Bologna
S. Orsola Hospital
Bologna, Italy

Umberto Veronesi, M.D.
Istituto Nazionale
Per 10 Studio la Cura
dei Tumori
Milan, Italy

Raven Press ■ New York

Raven Press, 1140 Avenue of the Americas, New York, New York 10036

Library of Congress Cataloging in Publication Data
Main entry under title:

Precancerous lesions of the gastrointestinal tract.

"International Symposium on Precancerous Lesions of the Gastrointestinal Tract in October 1981 . . . Bologna, Italy"—Acknowledgments.
Includes bibliographies and index.
1. Gastrointestinal system—Cancer—Congresses.
2. Precancerous conditions—Congresses. I. Sherlock, Paul. II. International Symposium on Precancerous Lesions of the Gastrointestinal Tract (1981 : Bologna, Italy) [DNLM: 1. Gastrointestinal neoplasms—Congresses. 2. Precancerous conditions—Congresses. WI 149 P923 1981]
RC280.D5P74   1983   616.99′433   82-24011
ISBN 0-89004-883-5

Made in the United States of America

Preface

Cancer of the gastrointestinal tract is a major problem worldwide. Gastric cancer still represents a major illness in Japan and in certain parts of Europe, Asia, and South America. Cancer of the esophagus and primary cancer of the liver primarily tend to be diseases of underdeveloped countries but continue to account for a substantial number of cancer deaths in industrialized countries as well. Cancer of the colon is an important health problem in the United States and many of the Western European countries, and it appears to be increasing in the less industrialized nations of the world.

It is unfortunate that the majority of patients found to have cancer of the gastrointestinal tract will be beyond cure by the time the diagnosis is made and will die from their disease. We must do much better. This dismal record of survival signals the need for the identification of etiologic and risk factors, pathogenesis, and more effective diagnostic techniques to be used in the incipient stage of disease as well as more effective treatment modalities.

The gastrointestinal tract is the site of clearly identifiable premalignant lesions that progress to cancer after varying periods of time. This allows us the unique opportunity to study the pathogenesis of cancer and to practice secondary cancer prevention by identifying the premalignant lesion and either removing it or applying various surveillance techniques to detect the developing cancer at an early stage.

The first section of this book discusses some general etiologic factors in the pathogenesis of gastrointestinal cancer, such as the environmental and genetic aspects. The second section discusses precancerous lesions of the esophagus and stomach including experimental studies in pathogenesis, markers of high risk, and surveillance techniques. The third section considers precancerous lesions of the small intestine and colon with regard to pathogenesis, experimental carcinogenesis, markers for increased risk, and surveillance techniques. The final section consists of chapters on principles of screening and the value of endoscopy in the surveillance of high-risk groups.

The editors hope that this volume will provide information useful in the understanding of premalignant conditions of the gastrointestinal tract. It marks the increasing interest in gastrointestinal tract cancer and the universal concern for the patient with this cancer transcending most boundaries of language, custom, commerce, and politics. It is hoped that we will all be encouraged to join forces in continuing the study of gastrointestinal cancer and its precursor lesions.

This book will be of interest to clinicians, researchers, specialists in gastrointestinal disease and gastrointestinal cancer, as well as general and family practitioners.

Paul Sherlock, M.D.
Basil C. Morson, M.D.
Luigi Barbara, M.D.
Umberto Veronesi, M.D.

Acknowledgments

The International Symposium on Precancerous Lesions of the Gastrointestinal Tract was held in October 1981, in the lovely city of Bologna, Italy. This symposium was made possible by the generosity of the Menarini Foundation and Dr. Sergio Gorini, President of this Foundation.

The sponsors of the symposium were the World Health Organization, International Union Against Cancer, International Academy of Pathology, European Society of Gastrointestinal Endoscopy, and the Italian Society of Gastroenterology.

Contents

SMALL INTESTINE AND COLON

GENERAL CONSIDERATIONS REGARDING SCREENING

Contributors

R. N. Allan
The General Hospital and
University of Birmingham
Steel House Lane
Birmingham B4 6NH, United Kingdom

Luigi Barbara
Department of Gastroenterology
University of Bologna
S. Orsola Hospital
40138 Bologna, Italy

Guido Biasco
Department of Gastroenterology
University of Bologna
S. Orsola Hospital
40138 Bologna, Italy

H. J. R. Bussey
Research Department
St. Mark's Hospital
City Road
London EC1V 2PS, England

A. Caignard
Research Group on Immunology of
  Digestive Tumors
CNRS-ERA 628, INSERM U-45
Laboratory of Immunology
Faculté de Médecine
21033 Dijon, France

R. Cheli
Department of Gastroenterology
Ospedale S. Martino
16132 Genova, Italy

M. Classen
Department of Gastroenterology
Johann-Wolfgang-Goethe-Universität
Franfurt am Main
Federal Republic of Germany

Pelayo Correa
Professor of Pathology
Louisiana State University
Medical Center
1901 Perdido Street
New Orleans, Louisiana 70112

Massimo Crespi
The Service of Environmental
  Carcinogenesis, Epidemiology and
  Prevention
Istituto Regina Elena
Viale Regina Elena 291
00121 Rome, Italy

Andrea Dalaiti
Department of Gastroenterology
University of Bologna
S. Orsola Hospital
40138 Bologna, Italy

Eleanor E. Deschner
Memorial Sloan-Kettering Cancer
  Center
1275 York Avenue
New York, New York 10021

Giulio Di Febo
Department of Gastroenterology
University of Bologna
S. Orsola Hospital
40138 Bologna, Italy

Jef Geboers
Division of Epidemiology
School of Public Health
University of Leuven
Capucijnenvoer, 33
B-3000 Leuven, Belgium

A. Giacosa
Department of Gastroenterology
Ospedale S. Martino
16132 Genova, Italy

Giuseppe Gizzi
Department of Gastroenterology
University of Bologna
S. Orsola Hospital
40138 Bologna, Italy

Walter Grigioni
Department of Histopathology
University of Bologna
Policlinico S. Orsola
Via Massarenti 9
40138 Bologna, Italy

S. Gyde
General Hospital and
University of Birmingham
Steel House Lane
Birmingham B4 6NH, United Kingdom

P. Hermanek
Department of Internal Medicine
University of Erlangen-Nürnberg
Krankenhausstrasse 12
D-8520 Erlangen
Federal Republic of Germany

Michael J. Hill
Research Department
St. Mark's Hospital
City Road
London EC1V 2PS, England

J. F. Jeannin
Research Group on Immunology of
Digestive Tumors
CNRS-ERA 628, INSERM U-45
Laboratory of Immunology
Faculté de Médecine
21033 Dijon, France

K. Jessen
Department of Gastroenterology
Johann-Wolfgang-Goethe-Universität
Frankfurt am Main
Federal Republic of Germany

Aage Johansen
Institute of Pathology
Bispebjerg Hospital
DK-2400 Copenhagen NV, Denmark

Jozef Victor Joossens
Division of Epidemiology
School of Public Health
University of Leuven
Capucijnenvoer, 33
B-3000 Leuven, Belgium

R. Lambert
Centre D'Epidemiologie
C.N.R.S.L.P. 5440
Faculté de Médecine de Lyon
Av. Rockefeller
69003 Lyon, France

Martin Lipkin
Memorial Sloan-Kettering Cancer
Center
1275 York Avenue
New York, New York 10021

Cesare Maltoni
Istituto Di Oncologia "Felice Addarii"
Ospedale S. Orsola-Malpighi
Viale Ercolani, 4/2
40138 Bologna, Italy

F. Martin
Research Group on Immunology of
Digestive Tumors
CNRS-ERA 628, INSERM U-45
Laboratory of Immunology
Faculté de Médecine
21033 Dijon, France

M. S. Martin
Research Group on Immunology of
Digestive Tumors
CNRS-ERA 628, INSERM U-45
Laboratory of Immunology
Faculté de Médecine
21033 Dijon, France

Alain P. Maskens
Avenue Lambeau, 62
B-1200 Brussels, Belgium

E. M. H. Mathus-Vliegen
Division of Gastroenterology
University of Amsterdam
Academic Medical Center
Amsterdam, The Netherlands

Richard B. McConnell
Department of Medicine
University of Liverpool
Gastroenterology Unit
Broadgreen Hospital
Liverpool L14 3LB, England

Mario Miglioli
Department of Gastroenterology
University of Bologna
S. Orsola Hospital
40138 Bologna, Italy

Andrea Minarini
Department of Gastroenterology
University of Bologna
S. Orsola Hospital
40138 Bologna, Italy

A. Montori
Via di Villa Ada, 10
00199 Rome, Italy

B. C. Morson
Department of Pathology
St. Mark's Hospital
City Road
London EC1V 2PS, England

Nubia Muñoz
Division of Epidemiology and
    Biostatistics
International Agency for Research on
    Cancer
150 Cours Albert Thomas
69372 Lyon Cedex 08, France

J. Myren
Department of Gastroenterology
Department of Medicine 9
Ullevål Hospital
Oslo 1, Norway

Kinichi Nabeya
Second Surgical Department
Kyorin University
School of Medicine
6–20–2 Shinkawa, Mitaka City
Tokyo 181, Japan

Takeo Nagayo
Aichi Cancer Center
Research Institute
81–1159, Kankoden Tashiro-cho
Chikusa-ku, Nagoya, Japan 464

J. Offerhaus
Division of Gastroenterology
University of Amsterdam
Academic Medical Center
Amsterdam, The Netherlands

O. Olsson
Research Group on Immunology of
    Digestive Tumors
CNRS-ERA 628, INSERM U-45
Laboratory of Immunology
Faculté de Médecine
21033 Dijon, France

P. Paolucci
Department of Surgery
Johann-Wolfgang-Goethe-Universität
Frankfurt am Main
Federal Republic of Germany

Alessandro Piccaluga
Department of Histopathology
University of Bologna
Policlinico S. Orsola
Via Massarenti 9
40138 Bologna, Italy

Robert H. Riddell
Department of Pathology
Laboratory of Surgical Pathology
University of Chicago
950 East 59th Street
Chicago, Illinois 60637

J. F. Riemann
Department of Internal Medicine
University of Erlangen-Nürnberg
Krankenhausstrasse 12
D-8520 Erlangen
Federal Republic of Germany

L. Risa
Via C. Lorenzini, 11
00137 Rome, Italy

Donatella Santini
Department of Histopathology
University of Bologna
Policlinico S. Orsola
Via Massarenti 9
40138 Bologna, Italy

H. Schmidt
Department of Internal Medicine
University of Erlangen-Nürnberg
Krankenhausstrasse 12
D-8520 Erlangen
Federal Republic of Germany

Henry Thompson
The General Hospital
Steel House Lane
Birmingham B4 6NH, United Kingdom

G. N. J. Tytgat
Division of Gastroenterology
University of Amsterdam
Academic Medical Center
Amsterdam, The Netherlands

Michele Vanzo
Department of Histopathology
University of Bologna
Policlinico S. Orsola
Via Massarenti 9
40138 Bologna, Italy

Kalle Varis
Second Department of Medicine
University of Helsinki
00290 Helsinki 29, Finland

Precancerous Lesions of the Gastrointestinal Tract, edited by P. Sherlock, B.C. Morson, L. Barbara, and U. Veronesi. Raven Press, New York © 1983.

Environmental and Genetic Factors in Gastrointestinal Cancer

Michael J. Hill

Bacterial Metabolism Research Laboratory, Salisbury, Wilts; and St. Marks Hospital Research Department, London EC1V 2PS, England

It has been estimated that 80% of human cancers are due to environmental factors and it is undoubtedly true that the environment plays an important part in determining the risk of a person developing a malignancy. However, it is becoming increasingly clear that most cancers have a mixed etiology involving both genetic and environmental factors. Our ultimate aim must be cancer prevention, and this will more likely be achieved if we have a better understanding of these interactions.

Any hypothesis regarding the causation of a disease should be compatible with as much of the available data as possible, and so we (25) at St. Mark's Hospital, London, have been attempting to combine the observations of histopathologists with those of the descriptive epidemiologists and of the metabolic epidemiologists to give an integrated picture of the etiology of colorectal cancer. Similar work in the field of gastric cancer has been carried out by Correa et al. (11).

In this chapter the evidence for and against the incrimination of genetic and environmental factors in the causation of gastric and of colorectal cancer is summarised. The efforts that have been made to rationalise this evidence are also discussed.

GASTRIC CANCER

Epidemiology

Gastric cancer is common in Japan, China, and much of the rest of Eastern Asia, and the Andean countries of South and Central America, and Eastern Europe (Table 1) but is less common in Western Europe, North America, and Australia (14). Throughout the world incidence rates are falling (Table 2) and gastric cancer is becoming relatively less important; in the United States less than 50 years ago gastric cancer was the most common form of cancer, whereas today it is only the 12th most common. Migrants from areas where the incidence of the disease is high (such as Japan and Eastern Europe) to areas of low incidence (such as the United States) experience only a small decrease in risk of the disease, but the children of the migrants have an incidence similar to that of the native-born Americans; this is interpreted as indicating that genetic factors do not determine the risk of gastric cancer in a population (since otherwise the children of the migrants should retain the high incidence of the disease experienced by their parents) but that the important environmental factors act in childhood or in adolescence.

TABLE 1. *The incidence of gastric, colonic, and rectal cancer in various countries*[a]

	Stomach	Colon	Rectum
Asia			
Japan	158.3	5.0	8.1
Taiwan	42.8	9.2	5.6
India	17.3	6.6	8.0
South America			
Uraguay	55.0	26.9	18.7
Chile	85.2	5.8	6.0
Colombia	81.6	5.7	3.9
Venezuela	53.5	7.3	4.4
Central America			
Puerto Rico	42.8	6.2	6.9
Jamaica	40.2	8.7	7.0
North America			
U.S. (white)	14.8	26.6	15.6
Canada (Alberta)	24.5	20.3	12.4
Australasia			
Australia	22.7	23.5	13.7
New Zealand	29.5	30.6	20.8
Western Europe			
England (S. Met. region)	30.7	15.8	16.2
Scotland	43.0	28.2	23.3
Denmark	37.4	17.1	20.8
France	33.0	20.2	16.8
Iceland	102.3	9.3	7.5
Eastern Europe			
Hungary	68.2	14.2	15.2
Romania	64.2	8.9	7.9
Poland	74.8	8.2	7.5
Southern Europe			
Italy	52.9	16.0	11.6
Yugoslavia	38.6	6.2	13.9
Africa			
Nigeria	21.9	2.8	3.1
Uganda	6.6	0	3.5
South Africa (white)	36.2	17.9	10.8
black	19.4	4.0	2.4

[a]Incidence ratios per 100,000 males per annum, age adjusted 35–64 years.
Data from Doll (14).

Since the stomach is the first resting place of the diet, it has been suggested by many epidemiologists that diet should be causally related to gastric cancer incidence. The results of attempts to support this have been inconclusive (Table 3) and it is clear that there is no simple relationship between diet and gastric carcinogenesis.

Histopathology

There have been many attempts to classify gastric cancers, largely with the aim of determining the prognosis of malignant lesions and the nature of early lesions. The Japanese

TABLE 2. *The change in incidence of gastric cancer with time in Japan and in Sweden[a]*

Year	Japan		Sweden	
	Males	Females	Males	Females
1955	211	105		
1956	206	104		
1957	221	101		
1959	218	98	67	32
1960	206	97	58	28
1961	207	100	62	25
1962	195	94	56	28
1963	194	94	50	26
1964	195	89	46	23
1965	190	89	46	23
1966	181	85		
1967	182	85		
1968	182	88		
1969	171	84		
1970	159	83		
1971	156	80		
1972	154	80		
1973	150	73		

[a]Data per 100,000 persons, ages 55–59.
Data for Japan is from Hirayama (26); data for Sweden is from Swedish Cancer Registry (45).

TABLE 3. *The relationship between diet and gastric cancer in various studies*

Location of population studied	Dietary items implicated in gastric carcinogenesis
Japan	Rice
Wales	Fried foods
Slovenia	Potatoes
Finland	Grain products
Iceland	Smoked fish
U.S.	Starchy foods and vegetables (fresh salad vegetables protective) Fried foods Fresh fruit and vegetables protective
Holland	Bacon

have had considerable success in this. The classification that appears to be most helpful to those interested in causation, however, is that devised by Lauren (32). On this classification carcinomas are described as diffuse, intestinal, or intermediate; it is a classification that requires much experience and judgement because no tumours are purely diffuse or purely intestinal. In Table 4 some of the nonhistopathological characteristics of the two types of tumour are listed (33). Diffuse tumours tend to predominate in young cases, whereas in older patients the intestinal form is more common; diffuse tumours tend to be ulcerous, intestinal cancers tend to be polypoid; tumours in the cardia or body of the stomach are more likely to be diffuse, those in the antrum are more likely to be intestinal. Intestinal metaplasia is an essential precursor lesion of the intestinal type but much less commonly precedes the diffuse type. The prognosis of the intestinal type is better than that of the diffuse type. The diffuse type is as common in women as in men, but the intestinal type is more commonly found in men than in women. In comparisons between Japanese living in Japan (a high incidence area) and those living in Hawaii (a low incidence area), the whole of the difference in gastric cancer incidence is due to differences in the intestinal form; there is no difference in the incidence of the diffuse form (12). Similarly, the temporal changes in the incidence of gastric cancer have been due to a decrease in incidence of the intestinal type, with no change in the incidence of the diffuse type of gastric cancer (40) in Norway. This indicates that the intestinal form of the disease is likely to be caused by environmental factors.

Genetic Factors

The role of genetic factors in gastric carcinogenesis is dealt with in detail by R. B. McConnell (*this volume*), but it is necessary to introduce the subject here also. There are few disease states known to predispose to gastric cancer, but three of the more important are blood group, pernicious anemia (PA), and hypogammaglobulinemia (HGG).

In 1953 Aird and Bentall (1) noted that patients with gastric cancer belonged to blood group O significantly less often than the average population in Britain. This has now been confirmed many times, although there have been a number of contrary results. A confusing factor may be the existence of the two Laurens types; Correa and co-workers showed that in Japan and Hawaii (12) and in Colombia (8) blood group A is associated with the diffuse type of gastric cancer but not with the intestinal type.

PA is the best-documented disease predisposing to gastric carcinogenesis and is itself genetically determined (6). Like the diffuse type of gastric cancer, PA is associated with blood group A (5,27,31). The risk of gastric cancer in patients with PA is three- to sixfold in excess of that in the normal population (4,39), the latency between diagnosis of PA and the diagnosis of the subsequent malignancy being on occasion only a few years.

TABLE 4. *Some properties of the two Lauren types of gastric cancer*

	Diffuse	Intestinal
Age at onset	Younger	Older
Male to female ratio	~1	>1
Gross morphology	Tend to be ulcerous	Tend to be polypoid
Location	Often in the cardia	Mainly antral
Blood group association	Group A	None
Prognosis	Poor	Relatively better ran for diffuse
Familial association	Strong	None
Association with environmental factors	None	Strong

HGG has recently been added to the list of predisposing diseases (17), patients having the disease having a 50-fold excess risk of gastric cancer in comparison with the normal population. Like PA, HGG is usually associated with gastric achlorhydria and atrophic gastritis.

There have been many studies of the risk of gastric cancer in relatives of index cases with the disease compared with control persons, most of which have been inconclusive. In more recent studies the results have been interpreted in terms of the Lauren types and this has been more fruitful. For example, Lehtola (33) found no excess risk of gastric cancer in relatives of patients with intestinal type or intermediate type gastric cancer but a sevenfold excess in those with diffuse type (Table 5). This indicates that genetic factors are important in the causation of diffuse type gastric cancer but not of intestinal type. Interestingly, relatives of PA patients are also more likely to develop gastric cancer (39) and gastric achlorhydria (34).

Histopathogenesis of Gastric Cancer

Correa (11), in a key paper, postulated a histopathological pathway of gastric carcinogenesis (Fig. 1) on the basis of their detailed studies of the disease in Colombia and supporting evidence from elsewhere. It is clearly a postulate for the etiology of the intestinal type. The

TABLE 5. *Relative risk of gastric cancer in relatives of patients with gastric cancer compared with relatives of age- and sex-matched control persons*

Histological type	Relative risk	Stat. signif.[a]
All gastric cancers	1.50	ns
Intestinal type	1.41	ns
Intermediate type	0.86	ns
Diffuse type	7.00	$p < 0.005$

[a]ns = not significant.
From Lehtola (33), with permission.

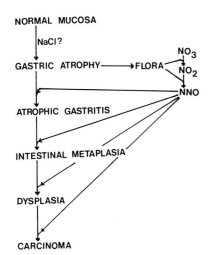

FIG. 1. The histopathological sequence in gastric carcinogenesis as proposed by Correa et al. (11).

first stage is the development of gastric atrophy, which is very common even in young adults in Colombia and Chile (Table 6) and has a high prevalence in many other countries with a high incidence of gastric cancer; the causation of this may be high salt intake (30) or malnutrition or wrong nutrition (46). This results in gastric achlorhydria and consequently bacterial overgrowth of the stomach. Bacteria reduce dietary nitrate to nitrite and also catalyze the subsequent N-nitrosation of suitable secondary amino groups by that nitrite; these N-nitroso compounds are then responsible for the intestinalisation of the gastric mucosa and subsequently for the development of increasingly severe dysplasia and, ultimately, malignancy.

The hypothesis has a wide measure of support among workers in the field of gastric carcinogenesis, and it pinpoints the key stage—the development of gastric atrophy and consequently achlorhydria. Gastric achlorhydria of iatrogenic origin (e.g., as a result of surgery for peptic ulcer) is also clearly associated with an excess risk of gastric cancer with a latency period of 15 to 20 years (44); the development of increasing dysplasia in the gastric remnant of such patients correlates with the gastric nitrite concentration (29). Evidence has also been put forward to support a role for N-nitroso compounds in gastric carcinogenesis associated with PA (41). Although the latency period has been reported to be short, the important time interval is that between diagnosis of gastric cancer and the initial development of bacterial overgrowth (almost impossible to deduce from patients notes) rather than the (much later) diagnosis of PA. We need, therefore, to try again to determine the latency period for this second stage of gastric carcinogenesis from PA patients. Interestingly, the latency from studies of partial gastrectomy patients is very similar to that which might be deduced from the studies of Armijo and Coulson (3) comparing Chilean provinces with respect to total nitrate exposure and gastric cancer risk.

It is likely that other factors are important in this second stage as well as N-nitroso compounds. Bile reflux has been cited by some as a possible source of agents causing epithelial dysplasia, and in particular the bile salts have received some attention. It is clear, however, that the hypothesis of Correa has already generated a lot of research into this stage of gastric carcinogenesis.

In contrast, the first stage, the generating of gastric atrophy and consequent bacterial overgrowth, is poorly understood. The most important cause of gastric achlorhydria in much of the world may simply be malnutrition, since many of the populations known to have a high prevalence of achlorhydria are malnourished (e.g., South India and the mountain regions of Narino in Colombia), but it is unlikely to be the cause in such relatively affluent countries as Japan, Finland, and Iceland. Joossens and Geboers (30) have hypothesised that dietary

TABLE 6. *Prevalence in two areas in Colombia of the gastric lesions that predispose to gastric cancer[a]*

	Narino	Cali
Estimated incidence of gastric cancer	150	23
No. of gastric biopsies	286	57
Histology normal	24.5%	45.6%
Superficial gastritis	19.2%	28.1%
Atrophic gastritis	53.3%	26.3%

[a]Incidence per 100,000 persons, ages 35–64, adjusted to the world standard population.
Data from Correa et al. (9).

salt is the major cause of gastric atrophy because of the resultant very high osmotic strength of the gastric contents. The basis for this hypothesis is that both gastric cancer and hypertension are highly correlated with each other geographically and temporally (both are decreasing in incidence at the same rate). In addition, genetic factors such as PA, HGG, and blood group A are associated with gastric atrophy, as are iatrogenic factors such as gastric surgery.

If the Correa hypothesis is correct, then it is possible to rationalise many of the epidemiological observations. Fresh fruit and vegetables are good sources of vitamin C, which is a potent scavenger (below pH4) of proximate carcinogens, nitrite, and other nucleophiles and so would inhibit the second stage of carcinogenesis. In addition, fresh foods do not, of course, contain preservatives such as salt (and indeed would replace preserved foods) and so would be expected to be "protective" against gastric atrophy. High intakes of cereals and potatoes are associated with poor nutrition; high intakes of preserved foods are associated with high salt intakes and both of these would be associated with gastric atrophy and achlorhydria. The association between gastric cancer and "dusty" work (such as coal mining, pottery work, etc.) may be the result of the gastritis caused by the irritant effect of the ingested dust.

LARGE BOWEL CANCER

Epidemiology

The epidemiology of large bowel cancer has been reviewed in detail recently by Correa and Haenszel (10). The disease is common in North America, North-West Europe, Australasia, and the River Plate area of South America and is relatively rare in South and East Asia, Eastern Europe, and the Andean countries of South and Central America (Table 1); there appears to be an inverse relation between the incidence of gastric cancer and large bowel cancer (Fig. 2). This is not evident, however, when the various regions of the United Kingdom are considered, since the incidence of both cancers increases from south to north and from east to west (7). The incidence of large bowel cancer increases with social class (Table 7), in contrast to gastric cancer.

Studies of migrants from Japan to the United States or from Eastern and Southern Europe to United States or Australia show that migrants achieve the incidence of bowel cancer of their new homeland within their lifetime. This indicates that the incidence of the disease in a population is determined by environmental factors and that racial genetic factors are of only minor importance in this respect. Environmental factors can be divided into those associated with the physical environment (the "shared environment," such as climate, geography, and air pollution) and the cultural environment (the "chosen environment," such as smoking, diet, and personal hygiene). Studies of racial groups in South Africa, religious groups in Bombay, groups of Chinese in Singapore, etc., all indicate that it is the cultural environment rather than the physical environment that is important in determining the risk of colorectal carcinogenesis. Most epidemiologists agree that the diet is the most important environmental factor, but there is little agreement on the component of the diet that is most closely correlated (Table 8).

There are two major types of study relating diet to the risk of colorectal cancer. These are case-control studies and population studies. Since the presence of a carcinoma in the large bowel almost certainly affects the diet (particularly, for example, causing loss of appetite), it is necessary to attempt to determine the diet prior to the formation of the tumour;

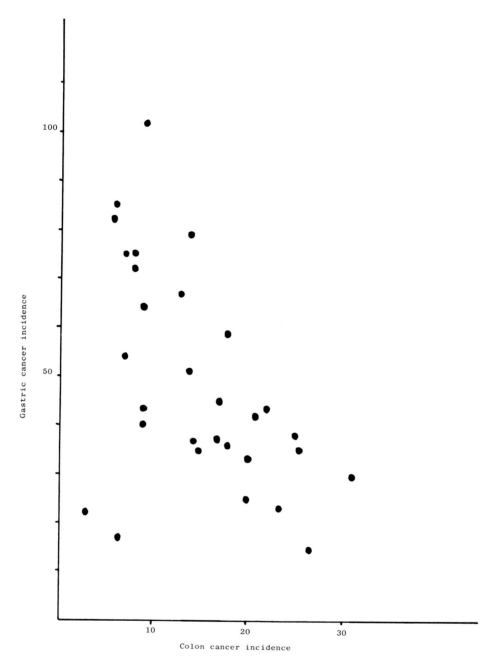

FIG. 2. The relationship between the incidence of gastric and that of colon cancer. (Data from Doll, ref. 14.)

this involves the use of diet recall, which is notoriously unreliable, and it is not surprising, therefore, that case-control studies have given widely variable results. In population studies the diet of a population is determined from, for example, FAO tables, whereas the cancer incidence in the population is obtained from various compilations (e.g., 14,15,43). These studies suffer from the drawback that the diet data are unreliable (e.g., they take no account of homegrown vegetables and do not allow for wastage of food); however, the inaccuracies

TABLE 7. *The relationship between social class and cancer of the large bowel and of the stomach*[a]

	Standardised mortality rates	
	Gastric Cancer	Colon cancer
U.K. population	(1.0)	(1.0)
Social class		
I (professional/managerial)	0.49	1.20
II	0.63	0.99
III (skilled workers)	1.01	1.05
IV (partly skilled)	1.14	0.92
V (unskilled workers)	1.63	1.09

[a]Data based on Registrar General's Reports covering the period 1959–1963.
From Hill (18), with permission.

TABLE 8. *The relation between diet and the incidence of large bowel cancer*[a]

Type of study	Dietary items strongly correlated
Comparison of 37 populations	Bound fat, animal fat, animal protein
Comparison of 32 populations	Meat, fat, animal protein
Comparison of 23 populations	Animal protein
Comparison of 41 populations	Meat, fat, cholesterol, fibre (inverse)
Comparison of 28 populations	Beer
Case-control	Meat, string beans
Case-control	No correlations
Case-control	No correlations
Case-control	Fat
Comparison 3 income groups	Fat, meat, fibre
Comparison of Finns and Danes	Fibre (inverse), meat
Case-control	Vitamins C and A (both inverse)

[a]See Hill (22) for references.

are, to some extent, consistent and the tables give a reasonable estimate of the relative intakes of various foods. These studies are, therefore, more reliable than those based on diet recall and those population studies involving large numbers of populations are unanimous in implicating dietary meat or its component animal protein and fat and in showing no correlation with dietary fibre. Figure 3 shows the relationship between the incidence of large bowel cancer and the amount of dietary fat. Note the points for Finland and Denmark on the figure; recent confirmation of the relative intakes of fat and fibre in these two countries

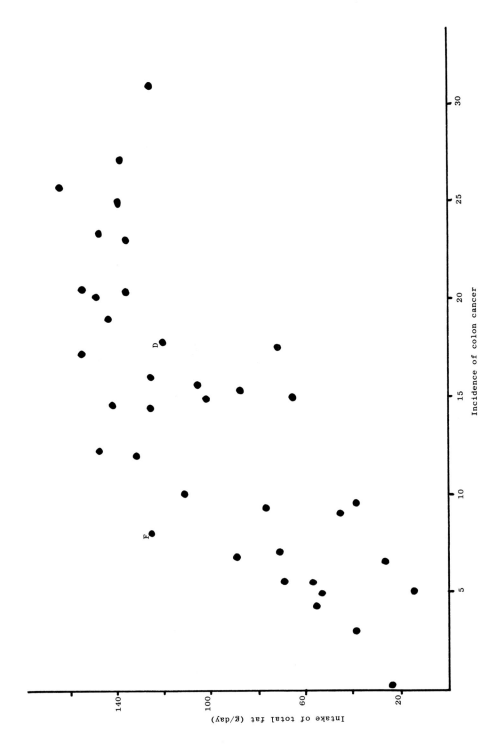

FIG. 3. The relation between total fat intake and colon cancer incidence. (Data from B. S. Drasar and J. Irving, 1973, *personal communication.*)

TABLE 9. *The relationship between selected food items and the risk of colorectal and of gastric cancer*

	Gastric cancer	Colorectal cancer
Meat	Protective	Causal
Fat	Protective	Causal
Starchy vegetables	Causal	Protective
Cereal foods	Causal	Protective?

(28) in no way invalidates the trends shown by the rest of the data. However, they indicate that the relationship between diet and bowel carcinogenesis is not directly causal; high intakes of fat or meat do not alone "cause" colorectal cancer and high intakes of fibre do not "protect" against colorectal carcinogenesis. Clearly the relationship is mediated in some way. Note that many of the factors correlated with large bowel cancer are inversely related to gastric cancer incidence and vice versa (Table 9).

There have been many investigations of the carcinogens present in the diet. These have been successful in that a wide range of carcinogens has been detected in food (Table 10). However, none of the carcinogens can be correlated with the risk of colorectal cancer; most are present in maximal amounts in the diets of populations at low risk of colorectal cancer. Although there is a good correlation between total calorie intake and incidence of colorectal cancer (16), there is no correlation between the incidence of the disease and obesity (48), indicating, again, that it is not the direct effect of food on carcinogenesis but some indirect effect. This will be discussed later in the section on metabolic epidemiology.

Histopathology

The histopathology of colorectal cancer is discussed in detail by B. C. Morson (*this volume*). In summary, almost all carcinomas arise in preformed adenomas and there is an adenoma-carcinoma sequence. However, although populations with a high incidence of colorectal adenomas tend to have a high incidence of colorectal cancer and vice versa, there is a very wide range in adenoma prevalence among countries with a low incidence of colorectal cancer. Furthermore, whereas adenomas are evenly distributed along the large intestine, carcinomas are concentrated in the left colon and rectum in high-incidence countries. This indicates that the factors causing the formation of adenomas differ from those causing the progression to malignancy.

Although all adenomas have the potential to become malignant, most remain benign. Whereas the cumulative lifetime risk of colorectal cancer is less than 5% even in the highest

TABLE 10. *Carcinogens detected in the diet*

Carcinogen	Dietary item associated
Polycyclic aromatic hydrocarbons	Smoked foods
N-nitroso compounds	Foods preserved with nitrite
Aflatoxins	Spoiled vegetables
Harman, nor-harman etc.	Grilled meat products
Mycotoxins	Vegetables and vegetable products

incidence countries, the prevalence of adenomas in persons over 75 years old is more than 50% (13). However, the malignant potential is related to adenoma size and large adenomas are likely to contain an area of focal malignancy (Table 11) as are villous adenomas. Large adenomas are much more common in the left colon than in the right colon and have a distribution along the large bowel similar to that of carcinomas. Adenomas are more common in men than in women, but carcinomas have a similar incidence in both sexes (Table 12).

Thus, almost all carcinomas arise in preexisting adenomas; most adenomas are small and are unlikely to become malignant; the risk of malignancy increases with the size of the adenomas are much more common in the left colon than in the right colon and have a distribution along the large bowel similar to that of carcinomas. Adenomas are more common in men than in women, but carcinomas have a similar incidence in both sexes (Table 12). that overall carcinomas are equally likely to develop in men and women.

Genetic Factors

The genetic factors in colorectal cancer have been discussed in detail elsewhere (H. J. R. Bussey, *this volume*). A number of diseases that carry a high risk of colorectal cancer are determined by autosomal dominant genes, including adenomatosis coli (familial polyposis coli), Peutz-Jeghers syndrome, juvenile polyposis, cancer family syndrome, and Turcot's syndrome.

In addition there have been a number of studies showing that relatives of persons with colorectal cancer are more likely than members of the general population to develop the disease (Table 13). Familial studies such as these may show an increased risk because of shared culture or because of shared genes; a recent study by Jensen et al. (28a) showed that spouses of colorectal cancer cases had no excess risk of the disease, indicating that the previous results were due to a genetic predisposition, and Veale (47) has suggested that this is due to an autosomal recessive gene (p) which makes a person "adenoma-prone." Thus persons who are pp will be sensitive to the environmental factors causing adenomas, whereas those who are pn or nn (where n is the "normal" genetic alternative to p) will not develop adenomas however many environmental factors they are exposed to. It is unlikely that this

TABLE 11. *The relationship between histopathological characteristics of an adenoma and its malignant potential*

Type and size of adenoma	Containing a malignant component[a] (%)
Diameter of adenoma	
<5 mm	0
<10 mm	1.3
Between 10 and 20 mm	9.5
>20 mm	46.0
Tubular adenoma	4.8
Villous adenoma	40.7
Intermediate pathology	22.5
Mild dysplasia	Low
Severe dysplasia	High

[a]Data from Morson (38).

TABLE 12. *The sex ratio (M/F) of the prevalence of adenomas and the incidence of carcinomas in various populations*

	Adenomas	Carcinomas
U.S. (New Orleans)		
Black	1.3	0.8
White	1.8	0.9
Sweden (Malmo)	1.6	1.0
U.K. (Liverpool)	1.3	0.9
Japan (Miyagi)	1.1	1.0
Colombia (Cali)	1.0	1.2

Data from Hill (22).

TABLE 13. *Studies of the risk of colorectal cancer in parents and siblings of index cases of the disease[a]*

Ref.	No. of cases of large bowel cancer			
	Parents		Siblings	
	Expected	Found	Expected	Found
Woolf (47a)	1	10	7	16
Macklin (35a)	5.2	17	4.5	14
Burdette (4a)	64	435		
Lovett (34a)	8.3	23	3.4	18

[a]See Hill (22) for details and references.

adenoma-proneness is absolute; it is much more likely that although persons who are *nn* have a risk of developing an adenoma, the risk of persons who are *pp* is very much higher. A measure of the prevalence of persons who are *pp* would then be the prevalence of adenomas in persons less than, for example, 55 years old and in whom there is still plenty of time for the adenoma to progress to malignancy.

Metabolic Epidemiology

There have been no studies on the etiology of colorectal adenomas because, at present, there is a total dearth of hypotheses concerning environmental causes. However, there have been many studies of the metabolic epidemiology of colorectal cancer overall.

Large bowel cancer is correlated with diet and there have been many studies of the carcinogens and mutagens present in food [food is a rich source of carcinogens (Table 10)], and reports of the presence of aflatoxins and other mycotoxins, polycyclic hydrocarbons, N-nitroso compounds, and the pyrolysis products harman, nor-harman, etc. None of these correlates with the risk of colorectal cancer and it was hypothesised (2) that the carcinogen or cocarcinogen responsible is produced *in situ* in the colon by bacterial action on some benign substrate. A range of possible substrates has been investigated (20), including tryptophan, tyrosine, methionine, cholesterol, and bile acids (Table 14); all are related to meat intake, because the strongest data relating diet to colorectal carcinogenesis incriminates meat

TABLE 14. *Some of the possible carcinogens or tumour promoters known to be produced by gut bacteria from dietary substrates*

Food item	Substrate	Product	Action
Meat protein	Tyrosine	Phenol, p-cresol	Promoter
	Tryptophan	Range of metabolites	Promoter
	Basic amino acids	Secondary amines giving N-nitroso compounds	Carcinogen
	Methionine	Ethionine	Carcinogen
Meat fat	Lecithin/choline	Dimethylamine giving N-nitroso compound	Carcinogen
	Cholesterol	Epoxide	Mutagen ?
	Bile acid (secreted in response to fat)	Metabolites	Promoter

or its component animal protein and fat. Of these the data is strongest in support of the bile acids from studies of populations in various parts of the world, racial groups in New York, social classes in Hong Kong, religious subgroups in Southern California, and populations in Scandinavia (Table 15).

There have been three studies in Scandinavia which, when added together, provide a good correlation between faecal bile acid (FBA) concentration and bowel cancer incidence (Fig. 4). Case-control studies have shown less agreement (21) and in this respect are similar to those relating bowel cancer to diet. In addition to these studies in humans there have been many studies of animal models indicating a role as tumour promoters for the bile acids [summarised by Hill (21)]; these have included investigations of dietary changes, bile diversion studies, and experiments on the effect of pure bile acids introduced directly into the rectum. The major problem with the animal models is that the rat and mouse strains used are highly inbred and that in some animal strains the dimethylhydrazine tumours appear to arise *de novo* (36), whereas in others there is an adenoma-carcinoma sequence analogous to that in humans (49). The experiments using strains in which tumours arise *de novo* are clearly irrelevant to human colorectal carcinogenesis; most of the investigators who have

TABLE 15. *Population studies relating large bowel cancer incidence to FBA concentration[a]*

Study	Observed correlation
1. Comparison of 6 populations in various parts of the world	Good correlation
2. Comparison of 5 racial and religious groups in New York	Good correlation
3. Comparison of 2 racial groups in South Africa	Good correlation[b]
4. Comparison of rural Finns and urban Danes	No correlation
6. Comparison of rural Finns and New Yorkers	Good correlation
7. Comparison of urban and rural Finns and urban and rural Danes	Good correlation
8. Comparison of 3 dietary groups of 7th Day Adventists and control Californias	Good correlation

[a]See Hill (22).
[b]Not the original subject of the study but deduced later from the results.

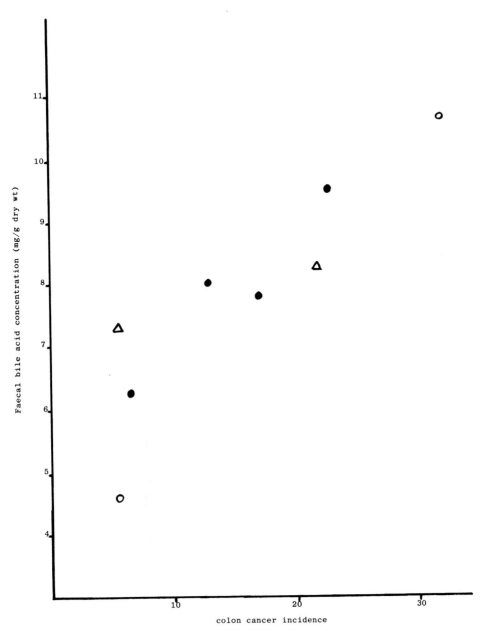

FIG. 4. The relation between faecal bile acid (FBA) concentration and large bowel cancer incidence from three studies in Scandinavia.

looked at the effects of diet change, bile diversion, rectal instillation of bile acids, etc., do not state if in their model there is an adenoma-carcinoma sequence.

The evidence regarding the type of bacterial metabolite implicated in colorectal carcinogenesis is much less clear. The results on rectal installation of pure bile acids show that the primary bile acids are not cocarcinogenic and that of the secondary bile acids tested, only deoxycholic and lithocholic acids are cocarcinogens in this model. There is other evidence indicating that these bile acids are tumour promoters (Table 16) and early studies

TABLE 16. *The evidence indicating that deoxycholic and lithocholic acids may be mutagens, co-mutagens of tumour promoters[a]*

Bile acid	Test system used	Effect observed
Deoxycholic acid	Skin painting on rodents	Tumour promotion
	Rectal instillation	Tumour promotion
	Salmonella mutagenesis	Co-mutagenicity
	Drosophila	Mutagen
Lithocholic acid	Rectal instillation	Tumour promotion
	Salmonella mutagenesis	Co-mutagenicity
	Cell transformation test	Mutagen

[a]See Hill (22).

indicated that the faecal concentrations of deoxycholic acid in various populations correlated well with the incidence of large bowel cancer (24). Deoxycholic and lithocholic acids are produced from the primary bile acids cholic and chenodeoxycholic acids, respectively, by the action of bacterial 7α dehydroxylase; Mastromarino et al. (37) showed that the faecal activity of bacterial 7α dehydroxylase was much higher in colorectal cancer patients than in control persons, a result that has been confirmed by T. Jivraj and M. J. Hill (*unpublished results*). In addition, there is evidence, summarised in Table 17, that clostridia capable of producing unsaturated bile acids (referred to as NDC) may also be implicated in colorectal carcinogenesis. This includes population studies, case-control studies, and studies of high-risk patient groups. In order to combine this evidence, which implicates FBA concentration, 7-dehydroxylase, and the NDC, Hill (19) suggested that the metabolite causing bowel cancer might be 3-oxo-4,6-choladien-24-oic acid (Fig. 5).

Histopathogeneis of Large Bowel Cancer

Studies of the histopathology of large bowel cancer indicate that (a) most colorectal carcinomas arise in preformed adenomas, (b) small adenomas rarely become malignant, but large adenomas have a high malignant potential; small adenomas are evenly distributed along the colorectum, whereas large adenomas are more common in the sigmoid colon and rectum, as are carcinomas; (c) there is good evidence that the factors causing the formation of small adenomas differ from those causing adenomas to grow in size, and that the factors causing the development of increasingly severe dysplasia and malignancy are different again; (d) the factors causing the formation and the growth of adenomas are environmental, but there

TABLE 17. *Evidence indicating a role for NDC in colorectal carcinogenesis*

Type of study	Observation
Comparison of carriage rates of NDC in 8 populations	Good correlation between NDC carriage rate and large bowel cancer incidence
Case-control study in England	Both studies show much higher carriage rate of NDC in cases than in controls
Study of adenomas	Carriage rate of NDC increases with increased adenoma size (as does their malignant potential)

Data from Hill (23).

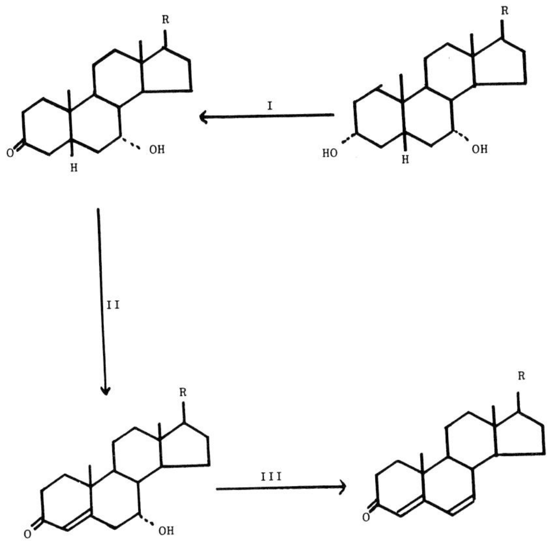

FIG. 5. The production of 3-oxo-4,6-choladien-24-oic acid from chenodeoxycholic acid by gut bacteria.

is no evidence on the origin of the factors causing malignancy; and (e) there is evidence that genetic factors are important in determining which persons are adenoma-prone. On the basis of this analysis, Hill and co-workers (25) postulated a mechanism for the histopathogenesis of colorectal cancer (Fig. 6).

Small adenomas are formed in adenoma-prone persons by the action of an environmental factor E1 but rarely in persons who are not adenoma-prone. However, a further environmental factor E2, which is present in relatively high concentrations in the left colon of western persons but at relatively low concentrations in the colons of Asian and Andean persons, causes small adenomas with a low malignant potential to grow to a large size with a proportionately high malignant potential. A further factor C causes benign adenomas to have increasing epithelial dysplasia and eventually neoplasia.

Migrants from Japan to the United States have a higher prevalence of adenomas than do Japanese who remain in Japan, and similarly for other migrant groups, indicating that E1 is, indeed, an environmental factor. The prevalence of adenomas in Americans, in Japanese living in America, in Sweden and England is similar at all ages, indicating that the proportion of persons who are adenoma-prone is similar in all four populations. Adenomas are evenly distributed along the length of the colorectum in postmortem studies in England, Sweden, the United States, Australia, Colombia, and Japan (Table 18), indicating that all sections of the large bowel are equally exposed to E1. This indicates that E1 is either systemic, reaching the intestinal mucosa from the vascular system, or enters the caecum preformed, or is readily released in the caecum by bacterial action (e.g., by the action of β-glucuronidase on a glucuronide produced as a result of hepatic detoxification of a carcinogen and then secreted in the bile).

It is clear from the variation in adenoma prevalence with age that adenoma-proneness must be relative rather than absolute; normal mucosa must have some sensitivity to E1 but in adenoma-prone persons the sensitivity is greatly enhanced. However, because of the time necessary for adenomas to grow and become malignant, it is likely that only adenomas formed before the age of 55 are likely to have time to become malignant within the normal life-span. Perhaps the concept of adenoma-proneness is best expressed as the likelihood of developing an adenoma in the first 50 years of life; under current environmental conditions this is only likely to occur in persons who have a genetic predisposition to sensitivity to E1.

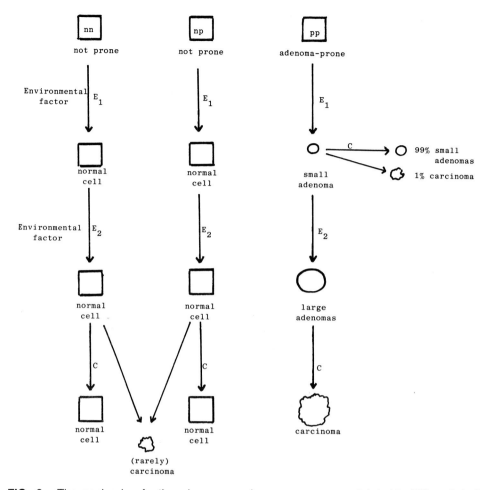

FIG. 6. The mechanism for the adenoma-carcinoma sequence postulated by Hill et al. (25).

TABLE 18. *The distribution of adenomas along the gastrointestinal tract*

	U.S. (%)	Sweden (%)	England (%)
Caecum and ascending colon	31	24	27
Transverse and descending colon	26	31	44
Sigmoid colon	27	29	17
Rectum	16	16	12

We can then envisage a spectrum of sensitivity. In normal persons the mucosa is unlikely to become adenomatous until the person has reached an old age; adenoma-prone persons are likely to develop an adenoma during middle age; and persons with adenomatosis coli develop large numbers of adenomas in early adulthood. In Western countries, most adenoma-prone persons probably develop adenomas, but this is not so in Eastern countries because of the lack of the environmental factor E1. Thus, the amount of E1 determines the prevalence of adenomas in a population, but genetic factors determine which persons in a uniformally exposed population actually develop adenomas.

Adenomas have a higher prevalence in men than in women at all ages (Table 19); this could be because men are more likely to be adenoma-prone, or it could reflect the higher exposure of men to industrial agents. It is of interest that the sex-ratio of colorectal adenomas is similar to that for most carcinomas (e.g., stomach, rectum, kidney, oesophagus, liver, pancreas).

Although large adenomas are relatively rare in Japan, their malignant potential is as high as that of large adenomas in Britain and other Western countries. This indicates that factor C is as common in Eastern as in Western populations; it may be environmental or genetic or may simply be due to "chance" (the malignant potential appears to correlate with adenoma volume or the number of adenomatous cells).

In summary, the incidence of carcinoma of the large bowel in a population is determined by at least two environmental factors, E1 and E2, and by at least one other factor, C. However, genetic factors (adenoma-proneness) determine which persons in a uniformly exposed population actually develop a malignancy.

Since large adenomas are rare in Japanese living in Japan and are much more common in Japanese living in the United States, the prevalence of adenomas in populations around the world is closely correlated with that of colorectal carcinomas, and the distribution of large adenomas along the colorectum correlates with the distribution of carcinomas, it is clear that factor E2, the factor that stimulates or permits adenoma growth, is environmental.

Although large adenomas are relatively rare in Japan, their malignant potential is as high as that of large adenomas in Britain and other Western countries. This indicates that factor C is as common in Eastern as in Western populations; it may be environmental or genetic or may simply be due to "chance" (the malignant potential appears to correlate with adenoma volume or the number of adenomatous cells).

In summary, the incidence of carcinoma of the large bowel in a population is determined by at least two environmental factors, E1 and E2, and by at least one other factor, C. However, genetic factors (adenoma-proneness) determine which persons in a uniformly exposed population actually develop a malignancy.

The Role of Bile Acids and Bacteria in Colorectal Carcinogenesis

It is essential to relate the findings of metabolic epidemiology to those of histopathology. To do this we have studied the faecal analyses of persons with large bowel polyps (21) and have shown that the FBA concentration and the carriage rate of NDC in the group of adenoma

TABLE 19. *Prevalence of adenomas in men and women at various ages (Liverpool, England)*

	Men (70)	Women (70)
<54 years	20	15
55–64 years	34	20
65–74 years	44	35
>75 years	52	33

Data from Day (13).

TABLE 20. *The mean FBA concentration and NDC carriage in adenomas of various sizes*

	No. of specimens	Mean FBA concentration	% Carriage of NDC
All polyps patients	134	8.4	38
Nonadenomatous polyps	20	6.9	38
Adenoma patients	114	8.7	38
Adenomas <5 mm diam.	26	6.8	6
5–10 mm diam.	29	8.2	39
10–20 mm diam.	35	8.8	48
>20 mm diam.	24	11.3	60
Normal persons		8.3	37

patients, the group of patients with nonadenomatous polyps, and control patients were very similar, indicating that the FBA/NDC factor is not related to E1, the factor causing the formation of adenomas. However, when the adenoma patients were subdivided on the basis of adenoma size, the FBA concentration and the carriage rate of NDC increased with increasing adenoma size (Table 20), indicating that the FBA/NDC discriminant might be a measure of factor E2, the factor causing adenoma growth. The faecal analyses of persons with large adenomas did not differ from those of patients with Dukes A carcinoma, indicating that the FBA/NDC discriminant is not related to factor C.

CONCLUSIONS

In this review I have attempted to summarise our knowledge of the causation of gastric and of colorectal cancer. From this we can make deductions concerning ways of preventing carcinogenesis in the gastrointestinal tract. It is important to draw attention to the fact that many dietary items that appear to correlate with cancer at one site are inversely correlated with the other site of carcinogenesis. Gastric cancer has a poor prognosis, but its incidence is decreasing throughout the world. Colorectal cancer is increasing in incidence in much of the world but has a better prognosis. It is essential that we do not attempt to introduce national changes in eating habits that might decrease the risk of colorectal cancer but at the same time increase the risk of gastric cancer.

REFERENCES

1. Aird, I., and Bentall, H. H. (1953): A relationship between cancer of stomach and the ABO blood groups. *Br. Med. J.*, 1:799–801.
2. Aries, V. C., Crowther, J. S., Drasar, B. S., and Hill, M. J. (1969): Degradation of bile salts by human intestinal bacteria. *Gut*, 10:575–577.
3. Armijo, R., and Coulson, A. J. (1975): Epidemiology of stomach cancer in Chile: the role of nitrogen fertilisers. *Int. J. Epidemiol.*, 4:301–310.
4. Blackburn, E. K., Callender, S. T., Dacie, J. V., Doll, R., Girdwood, R. H., Mollin, D. L., Saracci, R., Stafford, J., Thompson, R. B., Varadi, S., and Wetherly-Mein, G. (1968): Possible association between pernicious anemia and leukemia: a prospective study of 1625 patients with a note on the very high incidence of gastric cancer. *Int. J. Cancer*, 3:163–170.
4a. Burdette, W. J. (1965): Carcinoma of the Alimentary Tract. Utah Univ. Press, Salt Lake City.
5. Callender, S., Langman, J. J. S., Macleod, I. N., Mosbech, J., and Rahjkens, N. (1971): ABO blood groups in patients with gastric carcinoma with pernicious anemia. *Gut*, 12:465–467.
6. Carter, C. O. (1969): Genetics of common disorders. *Br. Med. Bull.*, 25:52–57.
7. Chilvers, C., and Adelstein, A. (1980): Cancer mortality: the regional pattern. *Population Trends*, 13:4–9.
8. Correa, P. (1970): Geographic pathology of cancer in Colombia. *Int. Pathol.*, 11:16–22.

9. Correa, P., Cuello, C., Duque, E., Burbano, L., Garcia, F., Bolanos, O., Brown, C., and Haenszel, W. (1976): Gastric cancer in Colombia. III. Natural history of the precurser lesion. *J. Natl. Cancer Inst.*, 57:1027–1035.

10. Correa, P., and Haenszel, W. (1978): The epidemiology of large bowel cancer. *Adv. Cancer Res.*, 26:1–141.

11. Correa, P., Haenszel, W., Cuello, C., Tannenbaum, S., and Archer, M. (1975): A model for gastric cancer epidemiology. *Lancet*, ii:58–60.

12. Correa, P., Sasano, N., Stemmerman, G., and Haenszel, W. (1973): Pathology of gastric carcinoma in Japanese populations: comparisons between Miyagi Prefecture, Japan, and Hawaii. *J. Natl. Cancer Inst.*, 51:1449–1459.

13. Day, D. W. (1981): Epidemiology of colorectal adenomas. In: *Colonic Carcinogenesis*, edited by R. Malt and R. Williamson pp. 135–144. MTP, Lancaster.

14. Doll, R. (1969): The geographical distribution of cancer. *Br. J. Cancer*, 23:1–8.

15. Doll, R., Muir, C. S., and Waterhouse, J. (1970): *J. Cancer in Five Continents, Vol. II*. Springer, Berlin.

16. Heaton, K. W. (1977): Dietary factors. *Top. Gastroenterol.*, 5:29–44.

17. Hermans, P. E., Diax-Buxo, J. A., and Stobo, J. D. (1976): Idiopathic late-onset immunoglobulin deficiency. Clinical observations in 50 patients. *Am. J. Med.*, 61:221–237.

18. Hill, M. J. (1975): The role of colon anaerobes in the metabolism of bile acids and steroids and its relation to colon cancer. *Cancer*, 36:2387–2400.

19. Hill, M. J. (1975): The etiology of colon cancer. *CRC Crit. Rev. Toxicol.*, 4:31–82.

20. Hill, M. J. (1977): Bacterial factors. *Top. Gastroenterol.*, 5:45–64.

21. Hill, M. J. (1980): The aetiology of colorectal cancer. In: *Recent Advances in Gastrointestinal Pathology*, edited by R. Wright, pp. 297–310. Saunders, London.

22. Hill, M. J. (1981): Metabolic epidemiology of large bowel cancer. In: *Gastrointestinal Cancer* edited by J. De Cosse and P. Sherlock, pp. 187–226. Martinus Nijhoff, The Hague.

23. Hill, M. J. (1982): Lipids, intestinal flora and large bowel cancer. In: *Dietary Fats and Health*, edited by E. G. Perkins, W. J. Visek, and J. C. Lyon. A.O.C.A.

24. Hill, M. J., Drasar, B. S., Aries, V. C., Crowther, J. S., Hawksworth, G. M., and Williams, R. E. O. (1971): Bacteria and aetiology of cancer of large bowel. *Lancet*, i:95–100.

25. Hill, M. J., Morson, B. C., and Bussey, H. J. R. (1978): Aetiology of the adenoma-carcinoma sequence in large bowel. *Lancet*, ii:535–538.

26. Hirayama, T. (1981): Changing patterns in the incidence of gastric cancer. In: *Gastric Cancer*, edited by J. Fielding, C. Newman, C. Ford, and B. Jones, pp. 1–16. Pergamon, Oxford.

27. Hoskins, L. C., Loux, H. A., Britten, A., and Samchek, N. (1965): Distribution of ABO blood groups in patients with pernicious anemia, gastric carcinoma and gastric carcinoma associated with pernicious anemia. *N. Engl. J. Med.*, 273:633–637.

28. IARC Working Party (1977): Dietary fibre, transit time, faecal bacteria, steroids and colon cancer in two Scandinavian populations. *Lancet*, ii:207–211.

28a. Jensen, O. M., Bolander, A. M., Sigtryggsson, P., Vercelli, M., Nguyen-Dinh, X., and MacLennan, R. (1980): Large bowel cancer in married couples in Sweden. A follow-up study. *Lancet*, i:1161–1163.

29. Jones, S. M., Davies, P. W., and Savage, A. (1978): Gastric juice nitrate and gastric cancer. *Lancet*, i:1355.

30. Joossens, J. V., and Geboers, J. (1981): Nutrition and gastric cancer. *Nutr. Cancer*, 2:251–261.

31. Kaipainen, W., and Vuorinen, Y. (1960): ABO blood groups in pernicious anemia and pernicious tapeworm anemia. *Ann. Med. Exp. Fenn.*, 38:1–2.

32. Lauren, P. (1965): The two histological main types of gastric carcinoma: diffuse and so-called intestinal type. *Acta Pathol. Microbiol. Scand.*, 64:31–49.

33. Lehtola, J. (1978): Family study of gastric carcinoma; with special reference to histological types. *Scand. J. Gastroenterol. (Suppl.)*, 13(50):1–54.

34. Levin, A. E., and Kuchur, B. A. (1937): An investigation of the relatives of patients with gastric cancer. *Lancet*, i:204–205.

34a. Lovett, E. (1974): Familial factors in the etiology of cancer of the bowel. *Proc. R. Soc. Med.*, 67:751–755.

35. Lynch, H. T., Giurgis, H. A., Harris, R. E., Lynch, P. M., Lynch, J. F., Elston, R. C., Go, R. C. P., and Kaplan, E. (1979): Clinical, genetic and biostatistical progress in the cancer family syndrome. *Front. Gastrointest. Res.*, 4:142–150.

35a. Macklin, M. T. (1969): Inheritance of cancer of the stomach in man. *J. Natl. Cancer Inst.*, 24:551–555.

36. Maskens, A. P. (1976): Histogenesis and growth pattern of 1,2 dimethylhydrazine induced rat colon adenocarcinoma. *Cancer Res.*, 36:1585-1592.

37. Mastromarino, A., Reddy, B. S., and Wynder, E. L. (1976): Metabolic epidemiology of colon cancer: Enzymic activity of the fecal flora. *Am. J. Clin. Nutr.*, 29:1455–1460.

38. Morson, B. C. (1974): The polyp-cancer sequence in the large bowel. *Proc. R. Soc. Med.*, 67:451–457.

39. Mosbech, J. (1961): Genetic considerations in polyps and cancer of the gastrointestinal tract. *Acta Un. Int. Cancer*, 17:302–306.

40. Munoz, N., and Asvall, J. (1971): Time trends of intestinal and diffuse types of gastric cancer in Norway. *Int. J. Cancer*, 8:144–157.

41. Ruddell, W. S. J., Bone, E. S., Hill, M. J., and Walters, C. L. (1978): Pathogenesis of gastric cancer in pernicious anemia. *Lancet*, i:521–523.

42. Schottenfield, D., Berg, J. W., and Vitsky, B. (1969): Incidence of multiple primary cancers. II. Index cancers arising in the stomach and lower digestive system. *J. Natl. Cancer Inst.*, 43:77–86.

43. Segi, M., and Kurihara, M. (1972): *Cancer mortality for selected sites in 24 countries No. 6 (1966-1967)*. Japan Cancer Soc. Tokyo.

44. Stahlsberg, H., and Taksdal, S. (1971): Stomach cancer and gastric operations. Stomach cancer following gastric surgery for benign conditions. *Lancet*, ii:1175.

45. Swedish Cancer Registry (1971): *Cancer incidence in Sweden: 1959-1965*. Stockholm.

46. Thomason, H., Burke, V., and Gracey, M. (1981): Impaired gastric function in experimental malnutrition. *Am. J. Clin. Nutr.*, 34:1278–1280.

47. Veale, A. M. O. (1965): *Intestinal Polyposis. Eugenics Lab. Memoirs, Series 40.* Cambridge University Press, London.

47a. Woolf, C. M. (1958): A genetic study of cancer of the large intestine. *Am. J. Hum. Genet.*, 10:42–47.

48. Wynder, E. L., and Shigematsu, T. (1967): Environmental factors of cancer of the colon and rectum. Colon cancer and overweight, cholesterol. *Cancer*, 20:1520–1561.

49. Zedeck, M. S., Frank, N., and Wiessler, M. (1979): Metabolism of the colon carcinogen methylazoxymethanol acetate. *Front. Gastrointest. Res.*, 4:32–37.

*Precancerous Lesions of the Gastrointestinal
Tract*, edited by P. Sherlock, B.C. Morson,
L. Barbara, and U. Veronesi. Raven Press,
New York © 1983.

Genetics of Precancerous Conditions of the Gastrointestinal Tract

Richard B. McConnell

*Department of Medicine, University of Liverpool, Gastroenterology Unit, Broadgreen Hospital,
Liverpool L14 3LB, England*

In man there are very few cancers caused entirely by genetic factors, and in the gastrointestinal tract there are only four single-gene conditions associated with a 100% cancer risk. With most of the inherited premalignant conditions the risk is much less, and which people develop the cancer is almost certainly influenced by environmental factors. In the present state of knowledge it is probably best to assume that an interaction between genetic and environmental factors underlies the great majority of gastrointestinal cancers.

COMBINED GENETIC AND ENVIRONMENTAL RESEARCH

A combined genetic and environmental approach to cancer research should prove more profitable than separate studies. It is interesting that a genetic influence can be demonstrated in lung cancer in spite of the strength of the smoking factor. It was found (132) that the nonsmoking relatives of lung cancer patients had an increased risk of lung cancer similar to that of smokers without any such family history of the disease. In addition smokers with a family history of lung cancer had a risk that was greater than the sum of both familial and smoking risks.

In a search for genes that might be contributing to this increased susceptibility to the effects of smoking, an enzyme called aryl hydrocarbon hydroxylase was studied (70). The enzyme is inducible, membrane-bound, and involved in the metabolism of chemical carcinogens found in tars. The extent of induction in cultured human leucocytes is under genetic control, there being a polymorphism in United States whites, with about 10% having high inducibility and 45% low inducibility. In lung cancer patients, all of whom were heavy smokers, the inducibility was high in 30% and low in only 4%. These data suggest that susceptibility to lung cancer is associated with high levels of inducible aryl hydrocarbon hydroxylase activity; Kazazian (68) takes the view that this may be one of many inherited risk factors for lung cancer, with gradations of risk being modulated by different genes acting in combination and by different environmental factors.

GENETIC MECHANISMS

The precancerous lesions of the gastrointestinal tract can be divided into those determined by single genes and therefore inherited in a more or less simple Mendelian manner and those in which the genetic influence is more complex and due to genes at several loci influencing susceptibility to environmental carcinogenic factors (Table 1).

TABLE 1. *Precancerous conditions of the gastrointestinal tract*

Conditions with single gene inheritance and 100% cancer risk
Conditions with single gene inheritance and increased cancer risk
Polygenically inherited conditions with increased cancer risk

---

Single Gene Inheritance

Only a few gastrointestinal cancers are determined by a single gene, but in four instances a cancer develops in nearly all the individuals who carry the abnormal gene (Table 2). In two inherited types of colonic polyps, the adenomas themselves are premalignant, but in the Clarke–Howel-Evans Syndrome, those with the high oesophageal cancer risk can be identified by the palmar-plantar keratosis. There is, however, as yet no marker that can be used in an adenocarcinomatosis family to predict which member will develop cancer.

There are other single gene conditions associated with an increased risk of gastrointestinal cancer (Table 3). In some syndromes, the cancer risk is also in organs of other systems, for instance in ataxia-telangiectasia most of the malignancies are reticuloendothelial, but there is also an association with carcinoma of stomach (45).

In dyskeratosis congenita and Bloom's syndrome, the molecular pathology includes defective DNA synthesis, and one might expect to find an increased incidence of malignancy. Indeed an increased incidence of carcinoma of the oesophagus and carcinoma of the rectosigmoid has been reported (48).

Certain single-gene-determined enzyme deficiencies can lead to an increased cancer risk. For instance, alpha-1-antitrypsin deficiency may influence hepatoma development (9) in addition to predisposing to chronic obstructive airway disease in the presence of cigarette smoking.

Polygenic Inheritance

There are several conditions in which inheritance plays a part and which are associated with a cancer risk higher than that expected from general population frequencies. Examples are inflammatory bowel disease and coeliac disease (Table 4). The hereditary mechanism in this group of conditions is probably not the effect of one gene but rather is multifactorial and due to the effect of several genes as well as a considerable environmental influence. The increased cancer risk in these conditions may be due to a nonspecific effect of the disease or may have a genetic basis associated with the genotype of the condition. For instance, abdominal lymphoma associated with coeliac disease may be associated with the same immunological disturbance that underlies the coeliac disease. There are strong genetic influences in several immunological defects (77).

TABLE 2. *Conditions with single gene inheritance
and 100% cancer risk*

Condition	Site of malignancy
Clarke–Howel-Evans syndrome	Oesophagus
Familial polyposis coli	Colon
Cancer family syndrome	Stomach, colon
Discrete colonic polyps	Colon

TABLE 3. *Conditions with single gene inheritance and increased gastrointestinal cancer risk*

Condition	Site of malignancy
Ataxia-telangiectasis	Stomach
Dyskeratosis congenita	Oesophagus
Bloom's syndrome	Recto-sigmoid
Alpha-1-antitrypsin deficiency	Liver
Hereditary pancreatitis	Pancreas
Peutz-Jeghers syndrome	Stomach, intestines
Haemochromatosis	Liver
Wilson's disease	Liver
Multiple endocrine neoplasia I	Pancreatic islets
Severe atrophic fundic gastritis	Stomach

TABLE 4. *Polygenically inherited conditions with increased gastrointestinal cancer risk*

Condition	Site of malignancy
Pernicious anaemia	Stomach
Coeliac disease	Oesophagus, small bowel
Crohn's disease	Intestines
Ulcerative colitis	Colon
Chronic calcifying pancreatitis	Pancreas
Cirrhosis of liver	Liver
Juvenile polyposis	Stomach, intestines

SINGLE GENE OESOPHAGEAL CANCER: CLARKE–HOWEL-EVANS SYNDROME

The weight of evidence is in favour of the view that heredity plays little or no part in the aetiology of sporadic oesophageal cancer. It is, therefore, a surprise to find that there are families in which the disease is inherited in a simple Mendelian dominant manner in association with the late onset type of tylosis (hyperkeratosis palmaris et plantaris). The first report of such families came from Liverpool (19,60) and there has been a follow-up on them (54). In these families at least 24 cases of carcinoma of the oesophagus have occurred during the past 50 years, all of them in members with tylosis, which is determined by a single gene. It has been calculated that members with the abnormal gene have a 95% risk of developing the cancer by the age of 65.

The association of tylosis and oesophageal carcinoma in these families is likely to have only one genetic explanation, and that is the existence of a single mutant gene that causes both tylosis and carcinoma of the oesophagus. This gene may or may not be at the same locus as the usual gene for late onset tylosis. A less likely, though possible, explanation is that there are two separate genes, one for tylosis and the other for carcinoma of oesophagus, so closely linked on a chromosome that no crossing-over has taken place in these large families.

Tylosis and oesophageal cancer have been reported together in other families (31,54,121) and it is therefore worthwhile to examine carefully the palms and soles of the feet of any patients who develop carcinoma of the oesophagus under the age of 50 years. Any sign of hyperkeratosis would be an indication for study of other members of the patient's family. Though prophylactic oesophagectomy is not yet a practical proposition, there is no doubt that one day it will be carried out in tylotic members of these families in the same way that prophylactic colectomy is done in affected members of polyposis coli families. In the meantime all that can be done is to tell the tylotics who are aware of their great cancer risk that they should report immediately even slight dysphagia or chest discomfort. Periodic oesophageal washing for cytology and endoscopy may be of value. The tylotics who are not aware of the risk can be told of it if it is judged that they are sufficiently stable to accept the news without the development of an anxiety state. In the Liverpool families there are few in this category, and, so far, most of the tylotics have been shielded from the knowledge of the fate that awaits them in early middle life.

In these Liverpool families with late-onset tylosis, oral leukoplakia was noted (135). It is therefore interesting that a 25-year-old Los Angeles patient with both oesophageal cancer and oral leukoplakia had tylosis of the early childhood onset type (113).

THE LARGE BOWEL POLYPOSES

The cancer risk in familial polyposis of the large bowel is firmly established (30). Prophylactic colectomy is indicated as soon as polyposis is diagnosed. Figures from St. Mark's Hospital (16) show that 50% of new patients who present because of symptoms already have carcinoma of the large bowel. On the other hand, only 9% of polyposis patients who are traced through family studies already have cancer. The comparable Swedish figures are 64% and 10%, respectively (2).

In a survey of the condition of Sweden no clear-cut genetic distinction was found between families with extracolonic manifestations (Gardner's syndrome) and those without such lesions (2). In 12 of the 32 families with extracolonic signs, only one member had a lesion of the Gardner type.

Conversely, families in which there have been several cases of Gardner's syndrome have been found to contain an individual with polyposis but no extracolonic lesion. The same overlap between classical familial polyposis and Gardner's syndrome has been found in Japan (138). In a Baltimore study (21) several cases of medulloblastoma were noted in child relatives of polyposis patients. These tumours had developed at an age before colonic polyps might have been expected.

There is therefore a good deal of evidence to support the view that Gardner's syndrome, Turcot's syndrome, and other syndromes of colonic polyposis with extracolonic lesions are not distinct entities. A genetic theory that would explain the family data so far collected is that there is one major pleotropic gene underlying the inheritance of all these syndromes, with other genes determining whether or not extracolonic manifestations develop and also their type (95). From the data so far published, it is not clear if these modifying genes at other loci influence the age of development of the polyps (87), though there is evidence of some genetic predisposition to younger colon cancer (137). This genetic theory received some support from skin fibroblast cultures from members of Gardner's kindred 109, in which increased tetraploidy occurred in cultures derived from branches with the full Gardner's syndrome but not in cultures derived from branches showing only extracolorectal lesions (28). Other culture studies indicated genetic heterogeneity, which might be attributed to modifying genes (27).

Not only are the familial polyposes of adenomatous type associated with colonic cancer but so also are the inherited hamartomatous types such as Peutz-Jegher's syndrome (117) and juvenile polyposis (127), though in these latter polyposes, carcinoma of the stomach and duodenum are more frequent than large bowel cancer. To complete the versatility of the polyposes, some patients with familial polyposis of the colon have polyps in the stomach and can develop gastric carcinoma (35), and ampullary carcinoma occurs in both Gardner's syndrome (66) and familial colonic polyposis (100). Another family had members with colonic and gastric polyps, and one member with a medulloblastoma of the cerebellum (13). There were sebaceous cysts but no osseous lesions in this family. Both colonic and gastric cancer had occurred. There seems to be no limit to the permutations of lesions within families and this is in keeping with the genetic theory mentioned above. Theoretically one family could have so many of the modifying genes that the various members could have skin, gastric, osseous, and cerebral lesions (95).

CANCER FAMILY SYNDROME

Families in which many members have been affected by cancer of various organs are often reported in the literature. The name *adenocarcinomatosis* has been applied but, more often, the term *cancer family syndrome* is used.

During the past decade many cancer families have been studied by Lynch and his Omaha group and a good deal of progress has been made in subdividing this heterogeneous group into different types (85). One of the features of the cancer families is that by far the most common tumour has been cancer of the large bowel and, particularly, of the proximal colon (88). In some of the families the only cancer found is in the large bowel; in others there have been, in addition, many members with carcinoma of the endometrium and ovary (74), and in yet other families the additional malignancy has been of the breast (61) or elsewhere in the gastrointestinal tract. Other features of the cancer family syndrome are an early age at onset of malignancy, usually between 30 and 50 years of age, though occasionally earlier (4), and multiple primary cancers (86).

There can be little doubt that in many of these families cancer is being inherited in a dominant manner, presumably owing to the presence of single genes or, possibly, one gene, the expression of which varies from family to family as a result of other modifying genes. There have been far too many of these large families described to be merely due to chance aggregations of cancer. *In vitro* defects of cellular immunity have been demonstrated in cancer family syndrome patients (11).

Although it would be unwise to exclude the involvement of environmental factors in the production of cancer in the members of these families, the evidence suggests that they are not of much importance in deciding which members develop a carcinoma.

It is not known what proportion of sporadic large bowel cancers encountered in clinical practice are due to these major genes, but the finding of a strong family history of the disease when the patient is below 50 years of age or has multiple large bowel cancers (83) suggests that single gene cancers make up as much as 10% of the total. It may be that because people have so few offspring nowadays the familial nature of the disease is often not apparent.

THE GENETIC BASIS OF GASTRIC CANCER

Intense research during the past decade has resulted in several discoveries suggesting not only that there are a number of genes that play a relatively minor role in susceptibility of gastric cancer, such as the gene for blood group A, but also that there may be genes that are able to make a major contribution to cancer susceptibility.

Immunologic Defects

Isolated reports of large families with many affected relatives are not usually very informative because with such a common disease large aggregations are likely to occur by chance alone. One study, however, is worthy of particular note, not because 12 members developed stomach cancer, but because a battery of laboratory studies was applied to 16 family members in an attempt to elucidate mechanisms underlying susceptibility (24). Evidence was found of cell-mediated immunodeficiency and a number of relatives showed antibodies to gastric parietal cells. It was suggested that a genetic defect of T lymphocytes might be involved in the concentration of cases in this family. Because of the parietal cell antibodies and the fact that several members of the family showed macrocytosis, the authors also suggested a subclinical process related to pernicious anaemia, perhaps a genetically mediated autoimmune gastritis predisposing to gastric cancer. The subject of immunological dysfunction, atrophic gastritis, and gastric malignancy has been well reviewed (134).

Pernicious Anaemia

Over the past 30 years it has become established that there is a predisposition to develop gastric cancer in people with pernicious anaemia as well as people with severe atrophic gastritis who have not developed pernicious anaemia. The importance of heredity in these two conditions has also been demonstrated. More recently there have been important advances in the understanding of their genetic bases, which may underlie a large proportion of sporadic, apparently nonfamilial cases of carcinoma of the stomach (see chapter by K. Varis, *this volume*).

Severe Atrophic Fundic Gastritis

Siurala et al. (124) demonstrated that atrophic gastritis was associated with the development of gastric carcinoma. It was found during a 10- to 15-year follow-up that 9 of 10 previously diagnosed gastritis patients had developed carcinoma of the stomach. Subsequently the genetics of chronic gastritis has been extensively investigated by this Helsinki group and it has been shown that severe atrophic gastritis is largely genetically determined (140). The liability to severe atrophic fundic gastritis was shown to be significantly higher in the first-degree relatives of patients with this type of gastritis.

Although family members tended to have similar gastric mucosal changes, patients with severe gastritis had some relatives whose fundic mucosa was normal in all biopsy specimens, even in the oldest age groups. When the liability to fundic gastritis in these subjects was measured as age-adjusted score values, it formed a biomodal curve indicating two populations, one with very high liability to severe fundic gastritis, whereas the other family members did not have this liability (59). There is a strong probability that this liability to fundic gastritis may be due to a single genetic factor rather than to the common family environment.

The term *A-gastritis* has been introduced (129) for the mucosal picture of severe atrophic fundic gastritis accompanied by functional changes in the form of achlorhydria, low vitamin B_{12}, low intrinsic factor levels, and immunological alterations such as a high serum gastrin with parietal cell and intrinsic factor antibodies. The antral mucosa is normal or only slightly altered and A-gastritis is now further defined by having high serum gastrin and low serum pepsinogen I levels (142). It would seem likely that there is a major gene underlying liability to severe fundic gastritis and that the gene is very pleotropic. Alternatively, the nonhistological features of A-gastritis may have separate genetic bases. There is a good deal of evidence of an hereditary basis of gastric acid output (43) and a relationship has been found between low serum pepsinogen activity, achlorhydria, and the subsequent development of gastric cancer (108).

It has been shown that severe atrophic fundic gastritis is significantly more frequent in the relatives of patients with gastric carcinoma than in controls (62,69). It was found particularly when the proband had diffuse gastric carcinoma. This type of carcinoma has been shown to be associated with a greater frequency of affected relatives than is the intestinal type of gastric carcinoma (75).

The diffuse type of carcinoma has been found to be particularly associated with blood group A, and it was suggested that individual, presumably genetic factors are of great importance in its aetiology, whereas the development of the intestinal type of gastric carcinoma is influenced by environmental factors (23). It is not known if the two histological types of carcinoma are associated within families.

Studies of first-degree relatives of patients with severe atrophic gastritis, pernicious anaemia, and carcinoma of the stomach have indicated that the tendency to develop atrophic gastritis is influenced by one gene (141). This genetically determined "A" type of gastritis is connected with a high risk of developing gastric cancer. It is not yet known if this severe atrophic fundic gastritis is a common precursor of sporadic, apparently nonfamilial cases of gastric cancer, but there is much evidence to suggest that it underlies at least some of them.

From the practical point of view, the most satisfactory way to screen people for this premalignant type of chronic gastritis is to test their serum for pepsinogen I and gastrin levels. A low serum pepsinogen I level accompanied by the finding of hypergastrinaemia, in the absence of total gastrectomy for Zollinger-Ellison syndrome, should be diagnostic of this type of gastritis (142). A low serum pepsinogen I level would appear to be the most useful single subclinical marker of increased risk of developing gastric cancer.

ABO Blood Groups

The results of the investigations of families with carcinoma of the stomach suggested that genetic factors are involved in the aetiology of the disease, but they did not conclusively prove it. The demonstration that people of blood group A are more prone to develop the disease than people of blood groups O, B, and AB proved that heredity is concerned, since the ABO blood group is determined solely by what genes the individual inherits from his parents. The ABO genes are therefore involved in determining liability to the disease, and the ABO locus is probably only one of several that play a part.

The relationship between the ABO blood group genes and carcinoma of the stomach was established in 1953 (1) and since then the association has been confirmed all over the world. In 1967, 71 series were summarised (94). Fifty-five showed an excess of group A and 14 showed little difference from the control. In only two series was there a considerable deficiency of group A and one of these was a series of only 112 cases from Jerusalem. Considering the marked heterogeneity of the ABO blood groups over quite small distances and the consequent difficulty in obtaining good controls, these data leave no doubt of the true causal nature of the relationship. The increased risk of group A people is a modest 20% over the general population risk.

Of the more recent reports, one from Amsterdam (144) analysed the data of 874 patients according to the site of the tumour within the stomach and found that group A was especially increased in the series of tumour of the antrum. Previous reports had given conflicting answers to the question of site of tumour and blood groups (94). In a Japanese population, blood group A was associated only with the diffuse-type histology of carcinoma (52). This is the histological type of gastric cancer that has been found to be familial in contrast to the intestinal type in the relatives of whom no increased carcinoma of stomach incidence has been found (75).

There is no evidence that secretor character is concerned in the aetiology of gastric cancer, but a remarkable absence of Lewis negative individuals in 320 stomach cancer patients has been reported (94). Of 1,000 healthy Liverpool controls, 34 were Lewis negative. The significance of this finding awaits the tests of a series of patients in a part of the world, such as Japan, with a much higher incidence of Lewis negative in the population.

In spite of much research the reason for the blood group A association is still unknown. It seems likely that the ABO blood group genes are pleotrophic, with many different effects in various systems in addition to their role in determining the serological specificity of antigens on red cells and water soluble glycoproteins, which are found in most body fluids, including saliva and gastric juice (93). The influence on liability to gastric cancer may be due to one of these effects and may have nothing to do with the blood group antigens or it may be due to the blood group specific substance themselves. An equally high incidence of blood group A is found in series of patients with pernicious anaemia (58), and it has even been suggested that this high incidence of group A in pernicious anaemia may be the reason for the apparent excess of group A in carcinoma of stomach (120).

Work with tumour tissue involving carcinoembryonic antigens that are molecularly similar to blood group antigens has shown that changes in phenotype of blood group antigens in tumour tissue may result from altered glycoprotein synthesis by diseased mucosal cells (33,34). The significance of this work is not obvious. The changes may be due to the cancerous changes within affected cells.

Ataxia-telangiectasia

Carcinoma of the stomach occurs in immunodeficiency diseases such as common variable immunodeficiency and ataxia-telangiectasia (56,125,130). Ataxia-telangiectasia (Louis-Bar syndrome) is inherited as an autosomal recessive condition with neurological, cutaneous, and immunological abnormalities (99). A study of 27 families has been made to see if external factors could explain the increased cancer risk (26). The malignancies are often reticuloendothelial, though carcinomas of the biliary system, ovary, and stomach have been described.

In one reported family (53), two sibs with ataxia-telangiectasia developed mucinous gastric carcinoma before the age of 20. Their mother had also developed gastric cancer. She must have been heterozygous for the gene for ataxia-telangiectasia. This report raised the possibility of an increased cancer risk in those who carry one dose of this gene. This possibility received some support from family studies (26) as an increased susceptibility to malignant tumours was found in heterozygotes.

Ionising radiation of ataxia-telangiectasia lymphocytes produced up to a 10-fold excess of chromatid breaks compared with normal lymphocytes (131). A slower repair of double-strand breaks was suspected. It is interesting that gastric cancer seems to be unduly frequent in heterozygotes for some other recessive defects of DNA repair (56).

Heterozygotes for the ataxia-telangiectasia gene make up about 1% of the general European population. If it is true that they share with homozygotes a high predisposition to cancer (130), their identification becomes a matter of considerable importance in cancer prophylaxis. There has been an encouraging report of laboratory identification of heterozygotes, based on the sensitivity of lymphoblastic cell lines to ionising radiation (18).

INHERITED PRECANCEROUS CONDITIONS OF THE SMALL BOWEL

Heredity is concerned in three conditions predisposing to small bowel malignancy: Peutz-Jeghers syndrome, coeliac disease, and Crohn's disease. Small bowel tumours not associated with these conditions are so uncommon that there is little data available concerning a possible place of heredity in their aetiology. Only isolated reports of familial aggregation have been made and these fall into two categories—carcinoma and lymphoma. Reports of duodenal carcinoma within families without polyposis are very rare (136), but periampullary malignancy has been described in patients with familial polyposis coli with sufficient frequency to justify its being recognised as one of the extracolonic manifestations of the disease and be considered a variant of Gardner's syndrome (66). Reports of abdominal lymphoma in several members of a family are also rare (47) and raise the suspicion of coeliac disease. They have, however, been associated with immunological deficiency (91).

Peutz-Jeghers Syndrome

Compared with the risk of familial polyposis coli in which the development of malignancy is the rule, the cancer risk in Peutz-Jeghers syndrome is slight. There is, however, growing evidence that the syndrome is associated with a frequency of intestinal cancer much higher than one would expect by chance. Because the polyps are hamartomas rather than adenomas, it was at one time thought there might be no increased cancer risk. However, by 1957 one author had found that 13 of the 67 cases reported up to that time had developed small bowel carcinoma (7). Since then there has been a steady flow of reports of carcinoma in the small bowel and elsewhere in the gastrointestinal tract (36,37,109,126,146). The problem has been reviewed (16). In the latest report a 56-year-old woman died of a duodenal carcinoma and her son died at the age of 29 of a gastric carcinoma (20). It was thought that the metastasising tumours developed in hamartomatous polyps.

The genetics of Peutz-Jeghers syndrome has been reviewed (2). There seems little doubt that it is due to a single mutant pleiotropic gene inherited as a Mendelian dominant. Gastrointestinal polyps are not found in all carriers of the gene, nor is mucosal pigmentation invariably present. The cutaneous pigmentation around the mouth and eyes and on the fingers tends to fade gradually after the age of 30 years, so parents of a case may not exhibit this sign. Not only may patients be unaware of any other sufferer in the family, but even examination of the relatives may fail to reveal a few polyps or minute mucous membrane pigmentation.

Fortunately there is no clinical need to diagnose which relatives are affected, as no prophylactic measures are possible to avoid the two common complications of the polyposis—chronic blood loss and attacks of intestinal obstruction due to intussusception. Several operations may be needed for the latter and surgical removal should be as restricted as possible if malabsorption is to be avoided. Even though the exact degree of risk of the development of gastrointestinal malignancy is still not known, it is certainly not high enough to warrant prophylactic resection of large parts of the bowel.

Coeliac Disease

An association between steatorrhoea and malignant lymphoid tumours of the gut was recognised 40 years ago (41) but up to 1962 the steatorrhoea was considered to be secondary to the lymphoma. Then it was suggested (50) that the lymphoma was a complication of adult coeliac disease. This suggestion was supported by further evidence (6) and the relationship of coeliac disease to malignancy is reviewed by Swinson (*this volume*).

Failure of a newly diagnosed patient to respond to gluten withdrawal, or the return of symptoms for no apparent reason in a patient previously well controlled on a gluten-free diet, should raise the possibility that a malignant tumour has arisen. Rising values of serum IgA may be associated with the onset of lymphoma (5). In a survey of the incidence of malignancy in 208 coeliacs (128), 113 had been on a strict gluten-free diet for at least 12 months and 67 had never taken the diet. In these 180 patients there had been 12 cancer deaths and 6 lymphoma deaths. The authors concluded that the gluten-free diet reduces the incidence of carcinomatous complications to approximately that of the normal population, but in a later report (57) the same group reported on a longer follow-up and were unable to confirm the observation.

The magnitude of the association is yet to be uncovered, mainly because it is only in recent years that it has been realised that relatively symptomless coeliac disease is not uncommon in adult life. Perhaps a gluten-free diet will become an important factor in cancer prevention. If so, an understanding of the genetic basis of coeliac disease will be important in detecting symptomless coeliacs who need to be on a gluten-free diet if they are to escape gastrointestinal malignancy.

The Genetics of Coeliac Disease

The genetics of coeliac disease has been intensively studied in recent years. The explanation of one incompletely penetrant autosomal gene (29) is unlikely. Discordant monozygotic twins have been reported (143). The most informative surveys have been those in which jejunal biopsies were carried out in the relatives of coeliacs. Usually these have shown that about 10% to 12% of first-degree relatives have the flat mucosa typical of coeliac disease (98,103,114). However, only 4 of 72 (5.5%) first-degree relatives of 15 child coeliacs were found to have a flat mucosa and all 4 were asymptomatic (115). On the other hand, 35 of 182 (19.2%) first-degree relatives of adult coeliacs were found to have a flat mucosa, and, though many were symptomless, each had at least one abnormality of red cells or other evidence of malabsorption (127).

Identifying Potential Coeliacs

If there is, as seems likely, a considerable cancer risk in coeliacs and if this risk can be lessened by adherence to a gluten-free diet, it becomes a matter of some importance to identify coeliacs as early as possible, perhaps even before they develop symptoms. In Western Europe between 1 in 250 and 1 in 750 people have been estimated to be coeliac. Therefore, the early identification of coeliacs may make up an important part of any large-scale cancer prevention programme (97).

Considerable progress has been made in developing a technique for coeliac identification without carrying out jejunal biopsy, but at present it is possible only in families in which one coeliac has already been identified. HLA typing of the coeliac and the first-degree relatives can point to possible coeliacs, who can thereafter be examined clinically and biopsied. At first the HLA type associated with coeliac disease was HLA-B8, but work on the B-cell antigens has shown that DR3 is much more strongly associated with the disease: about 95% of coeliacs have this antigen (12,110).

It is not known for certain whether the HLA antigen itself is concerned in the aetiology of coeliac disease or whether there is linkage disequilibrium between the HLA locus and a coeliac locus. Such a major locus cannot constitute the whole genetic basis for the disease. Other loci and environmental factors, in addition to wheat gluten, must influence the age of onset of symptoms of the condition. There is a suggestion that the genes determining urinary pepsinogen phenotype, alpha-1-antitrypsin and AB secretor character may be contributing to a coeliac genotype (40). In cancer prevention, however, merely typing for HLA-DR within coeliac families could result in the identification of the majority of the coeliacs or potential coeliacs.

Crohn's Disease

The increased risk of intestinal malignancy in patients with Crohn's disease is not yet firmly established on a statistical basis. There have been rather more reports of small bowel cancer than would be expected by chance alone (8,78). Carcinoma can develop in fistulous tracts (79). Colonic Crohn's disease has been so recently separated from ulcerative colitis that its relationship to colonic cancer may well have to wait some more years before it is clarified, although a relationship has been suggested (42,145). Its genetic basis is bound up with that of ulcerative colitis (96).

INHERITED COLON CANCERS WITHOUT POLYPOSIS

There are inherited types of large bowel cancer not associated with polyposis. The inherited polyposes probably account for 1% or less of all large bowel cancers, whereas the inherited types not associated with polyposis account for at least 10% and perhaps 25% of the total (3). The largest group of colon cancer families are those with cancer family syndrome described above. Families in which only colonic cancer occurs may be a variant of these, as the cancers share the characteristics of a dominant mode of inheritance, an early age of onset, and multiple cancers of the large bowel, particularly in the proximal colon (88). A third type of hereditary colonic cancer is that in which some family members develop stomach cancer. In this hereditary gastrocolonic cancer, there may be double primaries in one individual or a combination of single primaries among relatives (3).

In Muir's or Torre's syndrome (101,133) multiple skin tumours occur in conjunction with large bowel cancer. Some relatives may have duodenal, gastric, or urinary tract malignancy and the syndrome has a dominant mode of inheritance. It may be part of the cancer family syndrome, but it seems likely that it is a distinct clinicogenetic entity (3). An isolated report of colon cancer in a family with the nail-patella syndrome raises the possibility of an association with this condition, which has a Mendelian dominant mode of inheritance (49). A man and two of his daughters died of colonic cancer.

It is difficult not to conclude that a simple major gene for colonic cancer is operating in a family in which 27 cases had developed by 1972 (38). Of 50 deaths in the family, 22 have been due to cancer of the colon and rectum, and no environmental basis was postulated because they lived in a circumscribed area and no special family quirks of dietary habit were discovered. An alternative explanation is that there exists in this type of family (84) a form of polyposis with very few polyps determined by a single gene. Consistent with this possibility is a large family in which solitary polyps were found in nearly 50% of one generation and in which a third of the previous generation had died of gastrointestinal cancer

(112). Such small adenomatous lesions of the rectum and sigmoid might easily be missed, and the cases of cancer would then be considered to be ordinary sporadic carcinoma.

Ulcerative Colitis

The cancer risk in ulcerative colitis may have been exaggerated in the past, but there is certainly some risk of developing colon cancer in people who have had total involvement of the colon by ulcerative colitis for a number of years (51,72,76; E. E. Deschner, *this volume*). With Crohn's disease, the position is much less certain and consensus of opinion is that cancer is very much less liable to develop in Crohn's colitis than in ulcerative colitis.

The most striking result of studying the families of ulcerative colitis patients is the number of relatives affected by Crohn's disease. The converse is also true with many relatives of Crohn's patients having ulcerative colitis. There is no doubt that within families there is a strong association of the two conditions (73,96).

An association between inflammatory bowel disease and the chromosomal abnormality, Turner's syndrome, has been reported (111). Of 135 adults with this syndrome, 2 developed severe ulcerative colitis and 2 Crohn's disease.

There has been a report of identical male twins, one of whom developed ulcerative colitis at the age of 6 and multifocal anaplastic colon cancer at the age of 22 (14). His twin brother was quite healthy. Discordance for inflammatory bowel disease in identical twins is not unusual and there is no evidence of an inherited tendency for colitics to develop colon cancer. Rather, it is likely that the development of malignancy is related to long-standing inflammatory disease, especially if it begins in youth.

A relationship between ulcerative colitis and carcinoma of the proximal bile ducts (110) has been reported.

THE GENETIC BASIS OF SPORADIC LARGE BOWEL CANCER

The incidence of large bowel cancer varies approximately 10-fold from one part of the world to another. It is common in the British Isles, North America, Australia, and Denmark, but it is relatively rare in countries where carcinoma of the stomach is common, such as Poland, Finland, Iceland, and Japan. In Africa it is particularly rare, except in the white population of South Africa. There are no localities with extremely high incidence as is found with carcinoma of the oesophagus.

Incidence in Relatives

Each of the studies that have been made of the incidence of colonic cancer in the relatives of patients with the disease have showed a much higher figure than that in controls. In one survey (147), 26 of 763 relatives had died of large bowel cancer compared with 8 of 763 controls. In another (89), the finding was 31 cases in 392 relatives compared with 9.7 expected. In a painstaking survey of the causes of death in the families of 209 patients who had been admitted to St. Mark's Hospital, London (83), the overall percentage of large bowel cancer in 430 first-degree relatives was 10.9%. The number of large bowel malignancies in the 218 males was 25 (expected 4.5) and in the 212 females it was 22 (expected 6.3). Among the 209 patients investigated, 8 were aged 40 or under when their cancer was diagnosed. Of these 8, 5 had at least 1 affected relative. Of the 15 index cases who had eight or more adenomas in the specimen of bowel removed at operation, 8 had a positive family history. Of the 7 index cases who had two or more carcinomas in the bowel, 3 had a positive family history. Of the 7 index cases who gave a history of previous carcinoma of the large bowel, 5 had a positive family history.

These findings indicate that if a patient with large bowel cancer has a positive family history, the clinician should examine the bowel carefully for neoplasms other than the presenting lesion. After operation he should be followed up because of the increased risk that he may develop a new primary colonic tumour.

There has been an excellent survey of the individuals at high risk for large bowel cancer (81), which includes a review of the genetics of spontaneous colon cancer in rats. This rodent model develops cancer of the ascending colon resembling the human familial aggregates of colon cancer.

Incidence in Spouses

There has been one study that has shown a high incidence of large bowel cancer in the spouses of large bowel cancer patients (83). Of 34 spouses who had died, death certificates were obtained for 27 and 3 had died of large bowel cancer. This 11% incidence in spouses was similar to the 10.9% incidence in the relatives of this study and much higher than the 3% mortality in the general London population.

These London data suggest that the increased incidence in relatives of large bowel cancer patients is due to the environment rather than genetic factors. On the other hand, in a large-scale survey of mortality of married couples in Sweden (63), it was found that 1,716 people had died of colorectal cancer in 1961. The cause of death was determined in 1,094 of their spouses (99.6% of those eligible for the survey), and it was found that the risk of colorectal cancer and other possibly aetiologically related diseases was no higher in the spouses than in a matched population. The authors concluded that if eating a diet identical with that of patients with bowel cancer is not associated with an increased risk, the current view of colon cancer aetiology may need to be revised and dietary patterns before marriage investigated. Studies of the risk in sibships would be an important approach.

Clinical Implications

There are certain clinical conclusions that can be drawn from these data on whether there is a quantitative inherited tendency to develop sporadic large bowel cancer or whether large bowel cancer is mainly environmental in origin, the inherited type being found only in certain families. These clinical conclusions are that, if a patient with large bowel cancer gives a family history that includes a relative who has had bowel cancer, then the whole of his bowel must be thoroughly examined to exclude other lesions, as he may well have two separate cancers at the time of first presentation. If any bowel remains after the initial operation, he must be followed up regularly in case a new primary carcinoma develops.

The occurrence of carcinoma of the large bowel in someone under 40 years of age, someone who has eight or more adenomas in the operative specimen removed for carcinoma of the colon, or someone who has two or more carcinomas at presentation means that the risk in other members of his family is considerable and they should be warned to report immediately any intestinal symptoms. They also ought to undergo periodic surveillance with occult blood testing and colonoscopy.

PRECANCEROUS CONDITIONS AND PANCREATIC CANCER

The only firm evidence of a genetic influence in pancreatic cancer is that there is a high risk in hereditary pancreatitis and malignant islet cell tumours of the endocrine pancreas occur in multiple endocrine neoplasia, type 1.

Hereditary Pancreatitis

Since the first report in 1952 (22), many families have been described in which chronic calcifying pancreatitis is inherited in an autosomal Mendelian dominant manner, even though penetrance is not complete. Nearly 30 large families have been reported, mainly in the United States (90) and the United Kingdom (122). In some families the affected individuals have amino-aciduria, which may be secondary to the disease. In others, pancreatic duct anomolies are found and it is possible that the genetic abnormality is at the sphincter of Oddi rather than in the substance of the gland. Against this is the frequent finding of pancreatic calcification in members of these families who have minimal symptoms.

The disease is similar to sporadic chronic pancreatitis with the development of steatorrhoea and diabetes, but the usual age of onset of abdominal pain ranges from 4 to 14 years. The pathological features are also very similar. Although childhood onset is the rule, families with several adult-onset cases have been reported (105). Among 300 adult cases in France, three families of this type were found (118). Another report is of a 61-year-old man whose first attack of pain was at 17 years of age, and whose daughter and granddaughter became symptomatic at 12 and 9 years, respectively (10). At the present time the position is uncertain, but it seems possible that there is no clear-cut genetic distinction between hereditary pancreatitis and many cases of sporadic adult chronic calcifying pancreatitis.

Attention was first drawn to the cancer risk in hereditary pancreatitis in 1968 (82). It was thought that possibly as many as 30% developed carcinoma of the pancreas and this rate was found in another review (17). On the other hand, in three kindred reported later, only 8 of 54 deaths were found to have been due to pancreatic carcinoma (67) and none was found in 72 patients from seven families (122). Members of hereditary pancreatitis families have developed pancreatic carcinoma without having had clinical pancreatitis (17).

Multiple Endocrine Neoplasia

Islet cell tumours are commonly familial, many of them being the gastrointestinal expression of multiple endocrine neoplasia I (MEN I), characterised by tumours in the pituitary, adrenal cortex, and pancreas. The islet-cell lesion is the most likely to be malignant. MEN I is inherited as an autosomal dominant disorder (119). Penetrance is nearly complete if at-risk individuals below the age of 20 are excluded. Parathyroid or pancreatic tumours are present in over 75% of affected individuals, pituitary involvement occurs in nearly 66%, and the adrenal is affected in about 33%. The various endocrine glands are usually not affected simultaneously, so long-term evaluation is needed to assess the degree of expressivity.

CARCINOMA OF THE LIVER

Malignant hepatoma in Europe and North America usually develops in a cirrhotic liver. Among the genetic causes of cirrhosis is haemochromatosis, which was thought to have a dominant mode of inheritance (15). There have been several studies of HLA antigens in patients with this disease and in their families (39). In one large French investigation (123) it was concluded that the disease is determined by two homologous alleles giving recessive inheritance. The data from various sources are difficult to interpret, but it seems likely that the genetic basis of haemochromatosis is a polygenic system with at least one major gene, which may be HLA-A3 or a gene on chromosome 6 in linkage disequilibrium with it. Some of the genes are probably responsible for increased exchange of iron from plasma to storage and others for increased iron absorption and increased serum iron.

The early detection of affected family members and subsequent regular venesections should prevent the onset of cirrhosis and therefore of malignant hepatoma. Though malignant hepatoma is much less common in Wilson's disease than in haemochromatosis (139), hepatoma also should be preventable by effective treatment of patients with Wilson's disease with D-penicillamine. Wilson's disease has recessive inheritance.

Other inherited conditions that can result in malignant hepatoma are familial cholestatic cirrhosis of childhood (25), familial liver-cell adenoma (44), and alpha-1-antitrypsin deficiency (71). Hepatoblastoma has been reported in infant sisters (46) and infant sister and brother (104). In the Fanconi syndrome, it is uncertain whether hepatoma is a complication of the disease or of oral androgen therapy, but some patients have developed hepatic carcinoma without androgen treatment (102).

In cirrhosis not due to recognisable inborn errors of metabolism, there is a definite though not strong familial tendency (15), which is probably genetic rather than due to the common environment even though reports of familial hepatoma are rare (32,107). In a study of 254 patients who had died with cirrhosis, 24% had developed hepatocellular carcinoma (64). HBsAg-positive chronic active hepatitis was identified as a high-risk group with malignancy in 42%. In the same paper, it was noted that 10 of 16 liver cancer patients who did not have cirrhosis had a family history of various cancers. The father of one of these patients had also died of primary liver cancer. In another family, 2 HBsAg-positive brothers had had hepatocellular carcinoma, but a third brother, also HBsAg-positive, has not yet developed liver cancer (65).

CARCINOMA OF GALL BLADDER AND BILE DUCTS

There is evidence of an association between gallstones and gall bladder neoplasms in Israel (55) and in American Indians (106). The genetic basis of gallstones is not simple (80). Controlled studies have shown that the incidence in sibs of patients is higher than in controls. Parents of patients affected at an early age suffered more often from gallstone disease than did parents of controls. The bile of sisters of young women operated on for gallstones was found to be more lithogenic than that of controls.

It has already been noted that a review of 103 patients with cancer of bile ducts had shown that 8 had ulcerative colitis (116). In 3 the carcinoma of the bile duct developed several years after colectomy, suggesting genetic factors common to the colitis and the malignancy. Seven of the 8 were significantly younger than the median age of the group as a whole, but otherwise there was no other apparent difference. Although this relationship suggests a genetic basis for some cases of bile duct cancer, it should be noted that carcinoma of the bile ducts has been reported in a 45-year-old man (hepatic duct) and his 44-year-old wife (ampulla), both tumours developing in the same year (92). This is a good illustration of the fact that familial occurrences need not be genetic.

REFERENCES

1. Aird, I., Bentall, H. H., and Roberts, J. A. F. (1953): A relationship between cancer of stomach and the ABO blood groups. *Br. Med J.*, 1:799–801.
2. Alm, T., and Licznerski, G. (1973): The intestinal polyposes. *Clin. Gastroenterol.*, 2:577–602.
3. Anderson, D. E. (1980): An inherited form of large bowel cancer: Muir's syndrome. *Cancer*, 45:1103–1107.
4. Arthur, D., Woods, W., Krivit, W., and Nesbit, M. (1978): Hereditary adenocarcinoma of the colon in childhood: Association with the cancer family syndrome. *J. Pediatr.*, 93:318.
5. Asquith, P., Thompson, R. A., and Cooke, W. T. (1969): Serum immunoglobulins in adult coeliac disease. *Lancet*, 2:129–131.
6. Austad, W. I., Cornes, J. C., Gough, K. R., McCarthy, C. F., and Read, A. E. (1967): Steatorrhoea and malignant lymphoma. The relationship of malignant tumours of lymphoid tissue and coeliac disease. *Am. J. Dig. Dis.*, 12:475–490.
7. Bailey, D. (1957): Polyposis of the gastrointestinal tract: the Peutz syndrome. *Br. Med. J.*, 2:433–439.
8. Ben-Asher, H. (1971): Carcinoma in regional enteritis. *Am. J. Gastroenterol.*, 55:391–398.
9. Berg, N. O., and Eriksson, S. (1972): Liver disease in adults with alpha-1-antitrypsin deficiency. *N. Engl. J. Med.*, 287:1264–1267.
10. Bergström, K., Hellström, K., Kallner, M., and Lundh, G. (1973): Familial pancreatitis associated with hyperglycinuria. *Scand. J. Gastroenterol.*, 8:217–223.
11. Berlinger, N. T., and Good, R. A. (1980): Suppressor cells in healthy relatives of patients with hereditary colon cancer. *Cancer*, 45:1112–1116.
12. Betuel, H., Gebuhrer, L., Percebois, H., Descros, L., Minaire, Y., and Bertrand, J. (1979): Association de la maladie coeliaque de l'adulte avec HLA-DRw3 et DRw7. *Gastroenterol. Clin. Biol.*, 3:605.
13. Binder, M. K., Zablen, M. A., Fleischer, D. E., Sue, D. Y., Dwyer, R. M., and Hanelin, L. (1978): Colon polyps, sebaceous cysts, gastric polyps and malignant brain tumour in a family. *Am. J. Dig. Dis.*, 23:460–466.
14. Bisordi, W., and Lightdale, C. J. (1976): Identical twins discordant for ulcerative colitis with colon cancer. *Am. J. Dig. Dis.*, 21:71–73.
15. Brunt, P. W. (1973): Genetics of Liver Disease. *Clin. Gastroenterol.*, 2:615–637.
16. Bussey, H. J., Veale, A. M., and Morson, B. C. (1978): Genetics of gastrointestinal polyposis. *Gastroenterology*, 74:1325–30.
17. Castleman, B., Sculley, R. E., and McNeely, B. U. (1972): Case records of the Massachusetts General Hospital. *New Engl. J. Med.*, 286:1353–1359.
18. Chen, P. C., Lavin, M. F., and Kidson, C. (1978): Identification of ataxia telangiectasia heterozygotes, a cancer prone population. *Nature*, 274:484–486.
19. Clarke, C. A., and McConnell, R. B. (1954): Six cases of carcinoma of oesophagus occurring in one family. *Br. Med. J.*, ii:1137–1138.
20. Cochet, B., Desbaillets, C., Carrel, J. and Widgren, S. (1979): Peutz-Jeghers syndrome associated with gastrointestinal carcinoma. Report of two cases in a family. *Gut*, 20:169–175.
21. Cohen, S. B. (1982): Familial polyposis coli and its extra colonic manifestations. *J. Med. Genet.*, 19:193–203.
22. Comfort, M. W., and Steinberg, A. G. (1952): Pedigree of a family with hereditary chronic relapsing pancreatitis. *Gastroenterology*, 21:54–63.
23. Correa, P., Sasano, N., Stemmerman, G. N., and Haenszel, W. (1973): Pathology of gastric carcinoma in Japanese populations: comparison between Miyagi prefecture, Japan and Hawaii. *J. Natl. Cancer Inst.*, 51:1449–1459.
24. Creagan, E. T., and Fraumeni, Jr., J. F. (1973): Familial gastric cancer and immunologic abnormalities. *Cancer*, 32:1325–1331.
25. Dahms, B. B. (1979): Hepatoma in familial cholestatic cirrhosis of childhood: its occurrence in twin brothers. *Arch. Pathol. Lab. Med.*, 103:30–33.
26. Daly, M. B., and Swift, M. (1978): Epidemiological factors related to the malignant neoplasms in ataxia-telangiectasia families. *J. Chronic Dis.*, 31:625–634.
27. Danes, B. S., and Alm, T. (1979): *In vitro* studies on adenomatosis of the colon and rectum. *J. Med. Genet.*, 16:417–422.
28. Danes, B. S., and Gardner, E. J. (1978): The Gardner syndrome: a cell culture study on kindred 109. *J. Med Genet.*, 15:346–51.
29. David, T. J., and Ajdukiewicz, A. B. (1975): A family study of coeliac disease. *J. Med. Genet.*, 12:79–82.
30. De Cosse, J. J., Adams, M. B., and Condon, R. E. (1977): Familial Polyposis. *Cancer*, 39:267–273.
31. De Dulanto, F., Martinez, F. C., Moreno, M. A., Sintes, R. N., Gonzalez, R. M. R., Dulanto, M. C., Garcia, M. M., and Lloret, S. F. (1977): Sindrome de Clarke–Howel-Evans. *Actas Dermato-sifiliograficas*, 68:127–138.
32. Denison, E. K., Peters, R. L., and Reynolds, T. B. (1971): Familial hepatoma with hepatitis-associated antigen. *Ann. Intern. Med.*, 74:391–394.

33. Denk, H., Tappeiner, G., Davidovits, A., Eckerstorfer, R., and Holzner, J. H. (1974): Carcinoembryonic atigen and blood group substances in carcinoma of the stomach and colon. *J. Natl. Cancer Inst.*, 53:933–942.

34. Denk, H., Tappeiner, G., and Holzner, J. H. (1974): Independent behaviour of blood group A- and B-like activities in gastric carcinoma of blood group AB individuals. *Nature*, 248:428–430.

35. Denzler, T. B., Harned, R. K., and Pergam, C. J. (1979): Gastric polyps in familial polyposis coli. *Radiology*, 130:63–66.

36. Dodds, W. J., Schulte, W. J., Hensley, G. T., and Hogan, W. J. (1972): Peutz-Jeghers syndrome and gastrointestinal malignancy. *Am. J. Roentgenol.*, 115:374–377.

37. Dozois, R. R., Judd, E. S., Dahlin, D. C., and Bartholomew, L. G. (1969): The Peutz-Jeghers syndrome— Is there a predisposition to the development of intestinal malignancy? *Arch. Surg.*, 98:509–516.

38. Dunstone, G. H., and Knaggs, T. W. L. (1972): Familial cancer of the colon and rectum. *J. Med. Genet.*, 9:451–456.

39. Eddleston, A. L. W. F., and Williams, R. (1978): HLA and liver disease. *Br. Med. Bull.*, 34:295–300.

40. Ellis, A., Evans, D. A. P., McConnell, R. B., and Woodrow, J. C. (1980): Liverpool Coeliac Family Study. In: *The Genetics of Coeliac Disease*, edited by R. B. McConnell, pp. 265–286. M.T.P. Press, Lancaster.

41. Fairley, N. H., and Mackie, F. P. (1937): The clinical and biochemical syndrome in lymphoadenoma and allied diseases involving the mesenteric glands. *Br. Med. J.*, 1:375–380.

42. Fielding, J. F., Prior, P., Waterhouse, J. A., and Cooke, W. T. (1972): Malignancy in Crohn's Disease. *Scand. J. Gastroenterol.*, 7:3–7.

43. Fodor, E., Vestea, S., Urcan, S., Popescu, S., Sulica, L., Iencica, R., Goia, A., and Ilea, V. (1968): Hydrochloric acid secretion capacity of the stomach as an inherited factor in the pathogenesis of duodenal ulcer. *Am. J. Dig. Dis.*, 13:260–265.

44. Foster, J. H., Donohue, T. A., and Berman, M. M. (1978): Familial liver-cell andenomas and diabetes mellitus. *N. Engl. J. Med.*, 299:239–241.

45. Frais, M. A. (1979): Gastric adenocarcinoma due to ataxia-telangiectasia (Louis-Bar syndrome). *J. Med. Genet.*, 16:160–161.

46. Fraumeni, J. F., Rosen, P. J., Hull, E. W., Barth, R. F., Shapiro, S. R., and O'Connor, J. F. (1969): Hepatoblastoma in infant sisters. *Cancer*, 24:1086–1090.

47. Freedlander, E., Kissen, L. H., and McVie, J. G. (1978): Gut lymphoma presenting simultaneously in two siblings. *Br. Med. J.*, 1:80–81.

48. German, J., Bloom, D., and Passarge, E. (1979): Bloom's syndrome. VII Progress report for 1978. *Clin. Genet.*, 15:361–367.

49. Gilula, L. A., and Kantor, O. S. (1975): Familial colon carcinoma in nail-patella syndrome. *Am. J. Roentgenol. Radium Ther. Nucl. Med.*, 123:783–790.

50. Gough, K. R., Read, A. E., and Naish, J. M. (1962): Intestinal reticulosis as a complication of idiopathic steatorrhoea. *Gut*, 3:232–239.

51. Greenstein, A. J., Sachar, D. B., Smith, H., Pucillo, A., Papatestas, A. E., Kreel, I., Geller, S. A., Janowitz, H. D., and Aufses, A. H. (1979): Cancer in universal and left sided ulcerative colitis: factors determining risk. *Gastroenterology*, 77:295–297.

52. Haenszel, W., Kurihara, M., Locke, F. B., Shimuzu, K., and Segi, M. (1976): Stomach cancer in Japan. *J. Natl. Cancer Inst.*, 56:265–274.

53. Haerer, A. F., Jackson, J. F., and Evers, C. G. (1969): Ataxia-telangiectasia with gastric adenocarcinoma. *J. Am. Med. Assoc.*, 210:1884–1887.

54. Harper, P. S., Harper, R. M. J., and Howel-Evans, A. W. (1970): Carcinoma of the oesophagus with tlosis. *Q. J. Med.*, 39:317–333.

55. Hart, J., Modan, B., and Shani, M. (1971): Cholelithiasis in the aetiology of gallbladder neoplasms. *Lancet*, i:1151–1153.

56. Hermans, P. E., Diaz-Busco, J. A., and Stubo, J. D. (1976): Idiopathic late-onset immunoglobulin deficiency: clinical observations in 50 patients. *Am. J. Med.*, 61:221–237.

57. Holmes, G. K. T., Stokes, P. L., Sorahan, T. M., Prior, P., Waterhouse, J. A. H., and Cooke, W. T. (1976): Coeliac disease, gluten-free diet and malignancy. *Gut*, 17:612–619.

58. Hoskins, L. C., Loux, H. A., Britten, A., and Zamcheck, N. (1965): Distribution of ABO blood groups in patients with pernicious anaemia, gastric carcinoma and gastric carcinoma associated with pernicious anaemia. *N. Engl. J. Med.*, 273:633–637.

59. Hovinen, E., Kekki, M., and Kuikka, S. (1976): A theory to the Stochastic dynamic model building for chronic progressive disease processes with an application to chronic gastritis. *J. Theor. Biol.*, 57:131–152.

60. Howel-Evans, W., McConnell, R. B., Clarke, C. A., and Sheppard, P. M. (1958): Carcinoma of the oesophagus with keratosis palmaris et plantaris (tylosis)—a study of two families. *Q. J. Med.*, 27:413–429.

61. Howell, M. A. (1976): The association between colorectal cancer and breast cancer. *J. Chronic Dis.*, 29:243–461.

62. Ihamaki, T., Varis, K., and Siurala, M. (1979): Morphological functional and immunological state of the gastric mucosa in gastric carcinoma families: comparison with a computer-matched Family Sample. *Scand. J. Gastroenterol.*, 14:801–812.

63. Jensen, O. M., Bolander, A. M., Sigtryggsson, P., Vercelli, M., Nguyen-Dinh, X., and MacLennan, R. (1980): Large-bowel cancer in married couples in Sweden. A follow-up study. *Lancet*, 1:1161–1163.

64. Johnson, P. J., Krasner, N., Portmann, B., Eddleston, A. L. W. F., and Williams, R. (1978): Hepatocellular carcinoma in Great Britain: influence of age, sex, HBsAg status and aetiology of underlying cirrhosis. *Gut*, 19:1022–1026.

65. Johnson, P. J., Wansbrough-Jones, M. H., Portmann, B., Eddleston, A. L., Williams, R., Maycock, W. D., and Calne, R. Y. (1978): Familial HBsAg-positive hepatoma treatment with orthotopic liver transplantation and specific immunoglobulin. *Br. Med J.*, 1:216.

66. Jones, T. R., and Nance, F. C. (1977): Periampullary malignancy in Gardner's syndrome. *Ann. Surg.*, 185:565–573.

67. Kattwinkel, J., Lapey, A., di Sant'Agnese, P. A., Edwards, W. A., and Hufty, M. P. (1973): Hereditary pancreatitis: three new kindreds and a critical review of the literature. *Pediatrics*, 51:55–69.

68. Kazazian, H. H. (1976): A geneticists' view of lung disease. *Am. Rev. Respir. Dis.*, 113:261–266.

69. Kekki, M., Ihamäki, T., Sipponen, P., and Hovinen, E. (1975): Heterogeneity in susceptibility to chronic gastritis in relatives of gastric cancer patients with different histology of carcinoma. *Scand. J. Gastroenterol.*, 10:737–745.

70. Kellermann, G., Shaw, C. R., and Luyten-Kellermann, M. (1973): Aryl hydrocarbon hydroxylase inducibility and bronchogenic carcinoma. *N. Engl. J. Med.*, 289:934–937.

71. Kelly, J. K., Davies, J. S., and Jones, A. W. (1979): Alpha-1-antitrypsin deficiency and hepatocellular carcinoma. *J. Clin. Pathol.*, 32:373–376.

72. Kewenter, J., Ahlman, H., and Hulten, L. (1978): Cancer risk in extensive ulcerative colitis. *Ann. Surg.*, 188:824–828.

73. Kirsner, J. B. (1973): Genetic aspects of Inflammatory Bowel Disease. *Clin. Gastroenterol.*, 2:557–575.

74. Law, I. P., Herberman, R. B., Oldham, R. K., Bouzoukis, J., Hanson, S. M., and Rhode, M. C. (1977): Familial occurrence of colon and uterine carcinoma and of lymphoproliferative malignancies. Clinic description. *Cancer*, 39:1224–1225.

75. Lehtola, J. (1978): Family studies of gastric carcinoma: with special reference to histological types. *Scand. J. Gastroenterol. (Suppl.)*, 13 (50):11–54.

76. Lennard-Jones, J. E., Morson, B. C., Ritchie, J. K., Shove, D. C., and Williams, C. B. (1977): Cancer in colitis: assessment of the individual risk of clinical and histological criteria. *Gastroenterology*, 73:1280–1289.

77. Lewkonia, R. M. (1973): Inherited immunological abnormality and the gut. *Clin. Gastroenterol.*, 2:645–660.

78. Lightdale, C. J., and Sherlock, P. (1980): Cancer in Crohn's disease: Memorial Hospital experience and review of the literature. In: *Colorectal Cancer: Prevention, Epidemiology and Screening*, edited by S. Winawer, D. Schottenfeld, and P. Sherlock, pp. 341–346. Raven Press, New York.

79. Lightdale, C. J., Sternberg, S. S., Posner, G., and Sherlock, P. (1975): Carcinoma complicating Crohn's disease: Report of seven cases and review of the literature. *Am. J. Med.*, 59:262–268.

80. Linden, W., van der (1973): Genetic factors in gallstone disease. *Clin. Gastroenterol.*, 2:603–614.

81. Lipkin, M. (1977): The identification of individuals at high risk for large bowel cancer: an overview. *Cancer (Suppl.)*, 40:2523–2530.

82. Logan, Jr., A., Schlicke, C. P., and Manning, G. B. (1968): Familial pancreatitis. *Am. J. Surg.*, 115:112–117.

83. Lovett, E. (1976): Family studies in cancer of the colon and rectum. *Br. J. Surg.*, 63:13–18.

84. Lovett, E. (1976): Familial cancer of the gastrointestinal tract. *Br. J. Surg.*, 63:19–22.

85. Lynch, H. T., Guirgis, H. A., Harris, R. E., Lynch, P. M., Lynch, J. F., Elston, R. C., Go, R. C., and Kaplan, E. (1979): Clinical, genetic and biostatistical progress in the cancer family syndrome. *Front. Gastrointest. Res.*, 4:142–150.

86. Lynch, H. T., Harris, R. E., Lynch, P. M., Guirgis, H. A., Lynch, J. F., and Bardavil, W. A. (1977): Role of heredity in multiple primary cancer. *Cancer*, 40:1849–1854.

87. Lynch, H. T., Lynch, P. M., Follett, K. L., and Harris, R. E. (1979): Familial polyposis coli: heterogenous polyp expression in 2 kindreds. *J. Med. Genet.*, 16:1–7.

88. Lynch, P. M., Lynch, H. T., and Harris, R. E. (1977): Hereditary proximal colonic cancer. *Dis. Colon Rectum*, 20:661–668.

89. Machlin, M. T. (1960): Inheritance of cancer of the stomach and large intestine in man. *J. Natl. Cancer Inst.*, 24:551–571.

90. Malik, S. A., Van Kley, H., and Knight, Jr., W. A. (1977): Inherited defect in hereditary pancreatitis. *Am. J. Dig. Dis.*, 22:999–1004.

91. Maurer, H. A., Gotoff, S. P., Allen, L., and Bolan, J. (1976): Malignant lymphoma of the small intestine in multiple family members: association with an immunologic deficiency. *Cancer*, 37:2224–2231.

92. McCarthy, C. F., and Espiner, H. J. (1969): Carcinoma of bile ducts in husband and wife. *Gut*, 10:94–97.

93. McConnell, R. B. (1963): Lewis blood group substances in body fluids. *Proc. 2nd Int. Congr. Human Genetics (Rome)*, 858–861.

94. McConnell, R. B. (1967): The genetics of carcinoma of the stomach. In: *Racial and Geographical Factors in Tumour Incidence*, edited by A. M. Shivas, pp. 107–113. University Press, Edinburgh.

95. McConnell, R. B. (1980): Genetics of Familial Polyposis. In: *Colorectal Cancer: Prevention, Epidemiology and Screening*, edited by S. Winawer, D. Schottenfeld, and P. Sherlock, pp. 69–71. Raven Press, New York.

96. McConnell, R. B. (1980): Inflammatory bowel disease; newer views of genetic influence. In: *Developments in Digestive Diseases*, edited by J. E. Berk, chapt. 7, pp. 129–137. Lea and Febiger, Philadelphia.

97. McConnell, R. B., editor (1981): *The Genetics of Coeliac Disease*. M.T.P. Press, Lancaster.

98. MacDonald, W. C., Dobbins, W. O., and Rubin, C. E. (1965): Studies of the familial nature of coeliac sprue using biopsy of the small intestine. *N. Engl. J. Med.*, 272:448–456.

99. McFarlin, D. E., Strober, W., and Waldman, T. A. (1972): Ataxia-telangiectasia. *Medicine*, 51:280–314.

100. Mir-Madjlessi, S. H., Farmer, R. G., Hawk, W. A., and Turnbull, Jr., R. B. (1973): Adenocarcinoma of the ampulla of Vater associated with familial polyposis coli: report of a case. *Dis. Colon Rectum*, 16:542–546.

101. Muir, E. G., Yates-Bell, A. J., and Barlow, K. A. (1966): Multiple primary carcinoma of the colon, duodenum and larynx associated with keratoacanthomata of the face. *Br. J. Surg.*, 54:191–195.

102. Mulvihill, J. J., Ridolfi, R. L., Schultz, F. R., Borzy, M. S., and Haughton, P. B. T. (1975): Hepatic adenoma in Franconi anaemia treated with oxymetholone. *J. Pediatr.*, 87:122–124.

103. Mylotte, M., Egan-Mitchell, B., Fottrell, P. F., McNicholl, B., and McCarthy, C. F. (1974): Family Studies in Coeliac Disease. *Q. J. Med.*, 43:359–369.

104. Napoli, V. M., and Campbell, Jr., W. G. (1977): Hepatoblastoma in infant sister and brother. *Cancer*, 39:2647–2650.

105. Nash, F. W. (1971): Familial calcific pancreatitis: an acute episode with massive pleural effusion. *Proc. R. Soc. Med.*, 64:17–18.

106. Nelson, B. D., Porvaznik, J., and Benfield, J. R. (1971): Gall bladder diseases in southwestern American Indians. *Arch. Surg.*, 103:41–43.

107. Oon, C. J., Yo, S. L., Chua, L. F., Tan, L., Chang, C. H., and Chan, S. H. (1978): Familial primary hepatocellular carcinoma. *Singapore Med. J.*, 19:218–219.

108. Pastore, J. O., Kato, H., and Belsky, J. F. (1972): Serum pepsin and tubeless gastric analysis as predictors of stomach cancer. *New Surg. J. Med.*, 286:279–284.

109. Payson, B. A., and Moumgis, B. (1967): Metastasizing carcinoma of the stomach in Peutz-Jeghers syndrome. *Ann. Surg.*, 165:145–151.

110. Peña, A. S., Mann, D. L., Hague, N. E., Heck, J. A., van Leeuwen, A., van Rood, J. J., and Strober, W. (1978): Genetic basis of gluten sensitive enteropathy. *Gastroenterology*, 75:230–235.

111. Price, W. H. (1979): A high incidence of chronic inflammatory bowel disease in patients with Turner's syndrome. *J. Med. Genet.*, 16:263–266.

112. Richards, R. C., and Woolf, C. (1956): Solitary polyps of the colon and rectum: a study of inherited tendency. *Am. Surg.*, 22:287–294.

113. Ritter, S. B., and Petersen, G. (1976): Esophageal cancer, hyperkeratosis and oral leukoplakia: follow-up family study. *JAMA*, 236:1844–1845.

114. Robinson, D. C., Watson, A. J., Wyatt, E. H., Marks, J. M., and Roberts, D. F. (1971): Incidence of small-intestinal mucosal abnormalities and of clinical coeliac disease in the relatives of children with coeliac disease. *Gut*, 12:789–793.

115. Rolles, C. J., Myint, T. O. K., Sin, W. K., and Anderson, C. M. (1974): Family study of coeliac disease. *Gut*, 15:827.

116. Ross, A. P., and Braasch, J. W. (1973): Ulcerative colitis and carcinoma of the proximal bile ducts. *Gut*, 14:94–97.

117. Santos, M. J., Krush, A. J., and Cameron, J. L. (1979): Three varieties of hereditary intestinal polyposis. Johns Hopkins *Med. J.*, 145:196–200.

118. Sarles, H. (1973): Constitutional factors in chronic pancreatitis. *Clin. Gastroenterol.*, 2:639–644.

119. Schimke, R. N. (1976): Multiple endocrine adenomatosis syndromes. *Adv. Intern. Med.*, 21:249–265.

120. Shearman, D. J. C., and Finlayson, N. D. C. (1967): Familial aspects of gastric carcinoma. *Am. J. Dig. Dis.*, 12:529–534.

121. Shine, I., and Allison, P. R. (1966): Carcinoma of the oesophagus with tlosis (keratosis palmaris et plantaris). *Lancet*, 1:951–953.

122. Sibert, J. R. (1978): Hereditary pancreatitis in England and Wales. *J. Med. Genet.*, 15:189–201.

123. Simon, M., Fauchet, R., Hespel, J. P., Beaumont, C., Brissot, P., Hery, B., De Nercy, Y. H., Genetet, B., and Bourel, M. (1980): Idiopathic hemochromatosis: a study of biochemical expression in 247 heterozygous members of 63 families: evidence for a single major HLA-linked gene. *Gastroenterology*, 78:703–708.

124. Siurala, M., Varis, K., and Wiljasulo, M. (1966): Studies of patients with atrophic gastritis—a 10–15 year follow-up. *Scand. J. Gastroenterol.*, 1:40–48.

125. Spector, B. D., Perry, III, G. S., and Kersey, J. H. (1978): Genetically determined immunodeficiency diseases (GDID) and malignancy: report from the immunodeficiency-cancer registry. *Clin. Immunol. Immunopathol.*, 11:12–29.

126. Stemper, T. J., Kent, T. H., and Summers, R. W. (1975): Juvenile polyposis and gastrointestinal carcinoma. A study of a kindred. *Ann. Intern. Med.*, 83:639–646.

127. Stokes, P. L., Ferguson, R., Holmes, G. K. T., and Cooke, W. T. (1976): Familial aspects of coeliac disease. *Q. J. Med.*, 45:567–582.

128. Stokes, P. L., and Holmes, G. K. (1974): Malignancy. *Clin. Gastroenterol.*, 3:159–170.

129. Strickland, R. G., and Mackay, I. R. (1973): A reappraisal of the nature and significance of chronic atrophic gastritis. *Am. J. Dig. Dis.*, 18:426–440.

130. Swift, M., Sholman, L., Perry, M., and Chase, C. (1976): Malignant neoplasms in the families of patients with ataxia-telangiectasia. *Cancer Res.*, 36:209–215.

131. Taylor, A. M. (1978): Unrepaired DNA strand breaks in irradiated ataxia telangiectasia lymphocytes suggested from cytogenetic observations. *Mutant. Res.*, 50:407–418.

132. Tokuhata, G. K., and Lilienfeld, A. M. (1963): Familial aggregation of lung cancer in humans. *J. Natl. Cancer Inst.*, 30:289–312.

133. Torre, D. (1968): Multiple sebaceous tumours. *Arch. Dermatol.*, 98:549–551.

134. Twomey, J. J. (1978): Immunological dysfunction with atrophic gastritis and gastric malignancy. In: *Gastrointestinal Tract Malignancy*, edited by M. Lipkin and R. A. Good, pp. 93–117. Plenum Press, New York.

135. Tyldesley, W. R. (1974): Oral leukoplakia associated with tlosis and esophageal carcinoma. *J. Oral Pathol.*, 3:62–70.

136. Ungar, H. (1949): Familial carcinoma of the duodenum in adolescence. *Br. J. Cancer*, 3:321–330.

137. Utsunomiya, J., Murata, M., and Tanimura, M. (1980): An analysis of the age distribution of colon cancer in adenomatosis coli. *Cancer*, 45:198–205.

138. Utsumoniya, J., and Nakamura, T. (1975): The occult osteomatous changes in the mandible in patients with familial polyposis coli: *Br. J. Surg.*, 62:45–51.

139. Vachon, A., Paliard, P., Barthe, J., Grimaud, J. A., Peyrol, M., Gaillard, L., and Reiss, Th. (1973): Les átapes de l'atteinte hépatique de la dégénérescence hépato-lenticulaire: Lésions précoces-hypertension portale et dégénérescence cancereuse. *Lyon Médical*, 230:591–598.

140. Varis, K. (1971): A family study of chronic gastritis: histological immunological and functional aspects. *Scand. J. Gastroenterol. (Suppl.)*, 6 (13):1–50.

141. Varis, K., Ihamaki, T., Lehtola, J., Sipponen, P., Kekki, M., Isokoski, M., Saukkonen, M., and Siurala, M. (1978): Genetic aspects of gastritis-cancer relationship. *Dtsch. Z. Verdau Stoffwechselkr.*, 38:51–54.

142. Varis, K., Samloff, I. M., Ihamäki, T., and Siurala, M. (1979): An appraisal of tests for severe atrophic gastritis in relatives of patients with pernicious anaemia. *Dig. Dis. Sci.*, 24:187–191.

143. Walker-Smith, J. A. (1973): Discordance for childhood coeliac disease in monozygotic twins. *Gut*, 14:374–375.

144. Wayjen, R. G. A. van, and Linschoten, H. (1973): Distribution of ABO and Rhesus blood groups in patients with gastric carcinoma, with reference to its site of origin. *Gastroenterology*, 65:877–883.

145. Weedon, D. D., Shorter, R. G., Ilstrup, D. M., Huizenga, K. A., and Taylor, W. F. (1973): Crohn's Disease and cancer. *New Engl. J. Med.*, 289:1099–1103.

146. Williams, J. P., and Knudsen, A. (1965): Peutz-Jeghers syndrome with metastisizing duodenal carcinoma. *Gut*, 6:179–184.

147. Woolf, C. M. (1958): A genetic study of carcinoma of the large intestine. *Am. J. Hum. Genet.*, 10:42–47.

Precancerous Lesions of the Gastrointestinal Tract, edited by P. Sherlock, B.C. Morson, L. Barbara, and U. Veronesi. Raven Press, New York © 1983.

Polyposis Syndromes of the Gastrointestinal Tract

H. J. R. Bussey

Research Department, St. Mark's Hospital, London EC1V 2PS, England

An important advance in the understanding of precancerous conditions of the gastrointestinal tract was made when the long controversy over what part adenomas play in the aetiology of intestinal cancer was finally resolved. There is now general agreement that they have a major role and that it may, in fact, be an essential one. Evidence indicating that most cancers of the colon and rectum are derived from preexisting adenomas has been accumulated (10,27,29). Although it is not possible to say that this is true for all intestinal cancers, it is probable that, if exceptions do exist, they must be uncommon. If this is so, the factors influencing the development of adenomas become prime objectives in the search for methods of cancer prevention. Much of the evidence supporting the adenoma-carcinoma sequence was derived from observations made on the condition generally known as familial polyposis coli, which is characterised by the presence of large numbers of adenomas and a high, almost inevitable, incidence of colorectal cancer.

GASTROINTESTINAL POLYPOSIS CONDITIONS

Familial polyposis coli is one of a number of conditions that produce multiple polyps in the gastrointestinal tract. Most of them, such as lymphosarcomatous polyposis, benign lymphoid polyposis, and leukaemic polyposis, are rare as are also the lipomatous and neurofibromatous polyp types. The Peutz-Jeghers syndrome and juvenile polyposis are more frequently encountered, although they are less common than familial polyposis coli, the incidence of which is estimated to be at most only 1 in every 7,000 births. In the western world it is probable that the type of polyposis most likely to be met with is that due to the presence of polyps resulting from chronic inflammatory bowel disease, usually chronic ulcerative colitis and, therefore, confined to the large intestine.

Among the polyposis conditions affecting the gastrointestinal tract, there are three that have a tendency to produce adenomas and to be associated with an increased incidence of malignancy. These are the Peutz-Jeghers syndrome, juvenile polyposis, and familial polyposis coli, and it is proposed to study this group to see what factors they have in common and how these may be related to the behaviour of the much more common adenomas of nonpolyposis patients.

Peutz-Jeghers Syndrome

This condition, generally regarded as being inherited as a Mendelian dominant characteristic, is recognised by the appearance of small melanotic spots on the perioral skin, lips, buccal mucosa, and, in some cases, on the hands and feet as well as by the presence of polyps in the gastrointestinal tract. The pigmentation is usually observed in the first year of life and may fade by the fourth decade. The presence of the polyps is usually indicated in the first decade of life by the onset of recurrent episodes of colicky abdominal pain due to small bowel intussusception. The tumours, which are relatively few in number, usually between 50 and 100, are commonly 2 to 3 cm in diameter and may be larger. They may occur in all parts of the gastrointestinal tract, although they are most frequent in the small intestine where increasing size causes the obstructive symptoms.

Histologically the polyps are hamartomas composed of normal gastric or intestinal epithelium covering a stroma containing fine strands of smooth muscle fibres derived from the muscularis mucosae (28). The juxtaposition of epithelium and muscle in the polyps noted in the early descriptions of the condition suggested in many cases that malignant invasion had taken place. The syndrome was considered, therefore, to be associated with a high incidence of gastrointestinal cancer. Follow-up of the patients, however, produced few of the expected deaths from cancer. Subsequent reviews of the histology of the polyps revealed that the epithelium was normal with only occasional evidence of dysplasia being present and that the polyps were in fact hamartomatous in nature rather than neoplastic (9,26). It was then considered that Peutz-Jeghers polyps had no particular malignant potential, but during the last two to three decades, a small number of genuine malignancies of the gastrointestinal tract have been reported (1,7,8,34). These have usually occurred in the stomach or duodenum with the jejunum, the ileum, and colorectum (in that order) being recorded less frequently. The majority of these cancers have developed in patients less than 40 years of age. Occasionally, the carcinoma has been described as developing within a Peutz-Jeghers polyp of the stomach or duodenum (7). At the International Symposium on Precancerous Conditions of the Gastrointestinal Tract held in Bologna 1981, Monga et al. (25) reported two patients with the Peutz-Jeghers syndrome who had a hamartomatous polyp of the colorectum that showed epithelial dysplastic changes similar to those seen in adenomas. Furthermore, multiple small foci of adenocarcinoma were present in one of the two polyps.

To sum up, there appears to be a slightly increased risk of gastrointestinal cancer in the Peutz-Jeghers syndrome, mainly related to the stomach and duodenum but also, to a lesser degree, to the colorectum. This increased risk appears to be associated with a proneness to dysplastic changes of an adenomatous nature in the gastrointestinal epithelium, which, in at least some cases, have their origins in the hamartomatous polyps themselves.

Juvenile Polyposis

This form of gastrointestinal polyposis has been observed for a relatively short period of time, having been first described in 1964 by McColl et al. (24) and more fully 2 years later by the same group (39). Since then, further reports, mostly of isolated cases or of single family groups, have appeared (18,36), but as yet no systematic survey of a large series of this condition has been undertaken.

Juvenile polyposis and the Peutz-Jeghers syndrome have a number of features in common. It is highly probable that juvenile polyposis is also inherited as a Mendelian dominant characteristic. In addition to the gastrointestinal polyps, other congenital defects are present in unusual numbers in juvenile polyposis patients. Approximately one-fourth of such patients recorded in the St. Mark's Hospital Register have associated defects, the commonest being abnormally shaped skulls, heart lesions, and various intestinal lesions such as malrotation, stenosis, and Meckel's diverticulum. Although the condition was originally described as "juvenile polyposis coli," the polyps can occur in all areas of the gastrointestinal tract and the more general term "juvenile polyposis" is less inaccurate. The juvenile polyps do, however, differ from the Peutz-Jeghers type in being much more commonly found in the large intestine and, in fact, may in many instances be confined exclusively to the colorectum. The number of polyps present varies over a wide range. Sometimes less than 10 may be found, but in most cases the tumours number 50 or more, though sometimes hundreds may be present.

The histopathology of juvenile polyps resembles that of Peutz-Jeghers polyps. They are also hamartomas, composed of normal gastrointestinal mucus-secreting epithelium embedded in an excessive amount of lamina propria. Unlike Peutz-Jeghers polyps, no smooth muscle is present. The juvenile polyps are normally covered by a single layer of columnar epithelium containing goblet cells that is easily damaged with resulting superficial ulceration and secondary inflammation of the polyps. Partly because of this and partly because of the tendency of the polyps to undergo auto-amputation, the main symptom associated with juvenile polyposis is intestinal bleeding, which can produce severe anaemia.

When first reported the condition was considered to have little or no malignant potential because of the hamartomatous nature of the polyps. Subsequent observations have included, however, an increasing number of cases with associated colorectal cancer (13,37), the incidence of which is almost certainly greater than that experienced in the general population. This is particularly noticeable among the patients belonging to families in which more than one member has juvenile polyposis. A possible explanation for this increased incidence of malignancy is to be found in the presence of dysplastic changes in the epithelium of the polyps. The records of the Pathology Department of St. Mark's Hospital contain about 60 cases of juvenile polyposis. A review of the histopathology indicated that some degree of epithelial dysplasia was present in at least one or more of the polyps in approximately 20% of the cases. When dysplastic epithelium was present, it was usually to be seen in polyps that also retained hamartomatous elements (3), but occasionally some polyps were indistinguishable from adenomas. Other observers have reported similar findings (2). In such cases it is not possible to say whether the adenoma had arisen from a preexisting juvenile polyp in which all the epithelium had undergone dysplastic changes or had developed directly from the "normal" epithelium situated between the polyps. In either case the result indicates the increased proneness of the mucus-secreting epithelium in patients with juvenile polyposis to undergo dysplastic change. The malignancies, which in some cases are associated with the dysplasia, have so far been described only in the colorectum, where the incidence rate appears on present evidence to be around 10%. This distribution is not unexpected, for, as already mentioned, the great majority of the polyps are situated in this region. Not only are the cases with polyps in the stomach and small intestine much less common but also they are usually accompanied by greater severity of symptoms from the condition and the associated congenital defects that can lead to an early death before malignancy can occur. The average age at which colorectal cancer is diagnosed in the patients with juvenile polyposis is about 40 years, which is considerably lower than that found in the general population but which approximates to that of familial polyposis coli patients.

The tendency for the epithelium of the gastrointestinal mucosa to undergo dysplastic changes in patients with the Peutz-Jeghers syndrome and a similar but more pronounced tendency in regard to the colorectum in juvenile polyposis patients have been noted. It is, however, in the next polyposis condition to be discussed that this feature of proneness to dysplastic change really comes into its own with domination of the whole clinical picture.

Familial Adenomatous Polyposis

This condition has been known by various names—multiple adenomatosis, adenomatosis of the colon and rectum, and recently more generally as familial polyposis coli. Investigations during the last 5 or 6 years have, however, shown that the polyposis is not exclusively colonic and it is better to use a more general term such as familial adenomatous polyposis. Certainly the main feature of the condition is the presence of many adenomatous tumours, so numerous that often they are to be counted in thousands in the colorectum. It is not surprising, therefore, that the condition is associated with a high incidence of colorectal cancer. Adenomatous polyposis has provided a good deal of supportive evidence for the adenoma-carcinoma sequence, which if correct would demand that increased numbers of adenomas should be accompanied by an increased incidence of colorectal cancer. Since colorectal adenomatous polyposis has the highest incidence of adenomas, it is to be expected that it would have the highest incidence of colorectal cancer. It is well known that cancer is the almost certain outcome of untreated adenomatous polyposis (3).

The adenomas may begin to appear in some patients during the first decade of life but more usually they manifest in the second and third decades. On average, another 10 or 12 years may pass before symptoms of rectal bleeding, mucous discharge, and increasing frequency of loose stools appear, slight at first but gradually worsening. By the time symptoms are severe enough to cause alarm, two out of three patients have already developed colorectal cancer (3). The polyps generally measure less than 1 cm in diameter and usually number between 500 and 5,000. Histologically the tumours are adenomas mostly of the tubular type, although a small proportion show tubulo-villous and villous features. In addition to the visible polyps, microscopical examination of most colectomy specimens removed for polyposis will reveal small areas of intramucosal dysplasia which represent early stages in the formation of adenomas. The epithelial dysplastic change may be in some instances confined to a single crypt of Lieberkühn (4). Occasionally a few metaplastic (hyperplastic) polyps may be present and a solitary juvenile polyp was once found.

Until recently the polyps were thought to be confined to the large intestine, but recent investigations now show that the other regions of the gastrointestinal tract are also frequently involved. In particular, adenomas have been reported in the duodenum in a large proportion of polyposis patients. More than half the patients at St. Mark's Hospital who have been investigated by duodenoscopy and biopsy have been found to have duodenal adenomas and studies from other centres have produced even higher incidence rates (40). Adenomas have also been found, although to a lesser degree, in the jejunal and ileal segments of the small intestine (14,16,40). Nor is the stomach entirely immune, although here the adenomas appear to be confined to the antral region, none having as yet been recorded in the fundus or body (30). Multiple small polyps have, however, been observed in the fundus and body in some cases and these, on histological examination, have proved to be of a hamartomatous nature, being composed of normal epithelium, the glands of which frequently show cystic dilatation (cystic polyps) (30,40). This finding is of considerable interest in view of the fact that the other two inherited gastrointestinal polyposis conditions already discussed have hamartomatous polyps.

It will be asked if the adenomas of the stomach and small intestine are precursors of malignancy in the same manner as those of the colorectum. An affirmative answer can certainly be given in respect of the duodenal adenomas and probably, but to a lesser extent, in regard to the small intestine adenomas. Duodenal adenocarcinomas have been increasingly reported in association with polyposis (5,6,23) and in some cases the cancers have developed from preexisting adenomas. The incidence of associated duodenal cancer is not known with any degree of accuracy. Some idea can be obtained from the St. Mark's Hospital records, which includes at least 9 cases of periampullary carcinoma in a series of about 200 patients who have undergone major surgery. Obviously this is a minimal figure, as further cases can still occur and others may have escaped detection, being considered to be recurrences of colonic cancers.

Examples of jejunal and ileal cancers have occurred (31,35). Gastric carcinoma has also been reported in a few instances, usually of Japanese origin (17) and recently the first case of cancer of the stomach in a St. Mark's Hospital patient was recorded. It is probable that the varying incidence of carcinoma in different regions of the gastrointestinal tract relates to the number of adenomas present and to the local affect of environmental factors.

Gardner's Syndrome

Some polyposis patients may exhibit lesions other than the gastrointestinal polyps. These consist of osteomas (mainly of the skull and mandible), epidermoid cysts, dental abnormalities, and an increased fibroblastic reaction, particularly after surgery, which results in fibrous adhesions and the formation of abdominal desmoid tumours (11,12). It has been argued that there is a genetic difference between patients with and without these additional lesions—perhaps involving a further gene mutation—to produce the condition now called Gardner's syndrome. An alternative view, which appears to be more generally accepted, is that both types of polyposis result from a single gene mutation, but whereas the polyps are a constant feature of the mutation, the extragastrointestinal lesions of Gardner's syndrome show variable expressivity.

Inheritance

The incidence of familial adenomatous polyposis in the population has been variously estimated as from 1 in 6,850 to 1 in 23,790 births (32,33,38). Its genetic nature is now firmly established, the numerous polyps being inherited as a Mendelian dominant characteristic. Thus each child of a polyposis parent has a 50/50 chance of inheriting the condition. The children who do not inherit polyposis cannot pass it on to their children. Polyposis is not sex-linked and may, therefore, be passed by either sex to either sex. Sometimes families are observed in which the polyposis appears to be limited to one sex only, but such distributions are purely fortuitous and all children at risk, of whatever sex, should be kept under surveillance.

Cancer Prevention

In one sense, the inheritability of adenomatous polyposis is a fortunate feature. It has the advantage that it pinpoints the whereabouts of other possible sufferers, namely, within the family circle. Construction of a family pedigree is an important part of the investigation of each new polyposis patient. Not only does this indicate those members at risk and, therefore, in need of examination and treatment if the condition should be found to be present, but it also enables those members to be treated at an earlier stage before cancer has developed. It has already been stated that two-thirds of all propositus cases have cancer when first seen. There is limited scope for cancer prevention in this group of patients but more among their siblings who probably have the condition at an earlier stage. The greatest opportunity, however, occurs with the children at risk who are "called-up" for examination. In the St. Mark's Hospital series, the cancer incidence in this call-up group of sibs and children is currently about 5%. Theoretically, with full knowledge of the family pedigree and complete cooperation of all family members, the figure could fall to zero. It is unlikely that this will be achieved in practise, but the degree of cancer prevention actually obtained is probably unsurpassed in any other malignant condition.

COMPARISON OF THE INHERITED POLYPOSIS CONDITIONS

The three gastrointestinal syndromes that have been discussed, Peutz-Jeghers syndrome, juvenile polyposis, and adenomatous polyposis, differ fairly widely in their clinical behaviour but share a number of other features in common. Each is characterised by multiple polyps, which can involve all regions of the gastrointestinal tract, and in each case some of the polyps are of a hamartomatous nature. All three conditions are associated with other physical defects, usually extragastrointestinal in nature. There is a proneness, of variable degree, for the gastrointestinal mucosa to undergo dysplastic changes and this is paralleled by increased incidence rates of gastrointestinal cancer. Familial adenomatous polyposis is inherited as a Mendelian dominant characteristic and it is highly probable that both the Peutz-Jeghers syndrome and juvenile polyposis are of a similar genetic origin. It is difficult to avoid the conclusion that the three conditions are closely related at the chromosomal level.

ADENOMAS IN NONPOLYPOSIS PATIENTS

The three polyposis syndromes discussed are responsible for only a small fraction of the total colorectal cancers in the population, the majority of which occur in another and much larger group of adenoma producers. In these individuals, the number of adenomas is small, usually less than 10, but occasionally as many as 50 may be found. The proportion that this group forms of the total population is not accurately known and estimates vary considerably (from about 10% to 50%) depending on how the particular series had been selected for investigation.

Only a proportion of these patients will develop colorectal cancer, but those who do so and subsequently succumb to it, will constitute about 3% of the population. Set against that figure, the success in cancer prevention in adenomatous polyposis is negligible. The importance of familial polyposis, however, probably lies more in the extent to which the lessons derived from its study can be applied to the much greater problem of adenomas and carcinomas in the nonpolyposis patients. Two common features of the three polyposis conditions have been a proneness to gastrointestinal epithelial dysplasia, howbeit of widely varying degree, and a genetic origin. In the nonpolyposis adenoma group the first feature is obviously present and it is natural to ask if a genetic factor is also involved. When constructing a family pedigree it is much harder to obtain evidence of intestinal adenomas than it is of cancers. It is not surprising, therefore, that most reports are concerned with families with a high incidence of colorectal cancer (22,41). Investigations were carried out on a broader base by Machlin (21), who investigated the family histories of 145 patients with colorectal cancer and noted an increased incidence of the same condition among relatives over that expected in the general population. Lovett (19), in a larger series, found the observed incidence of colorectal cancer (on the basis of death certificates) in sibs and parents to be approximately five and three times, respectively, greater than that expected. More than a quarter of her index cases had one or more relatives who had suffered from intestinal cancer. A familial incidence of polyps was recorded by Woolf et al. (41) in a family in which there was a high incidence of intestinal cancer in one generation and of polyps in the children of that generation. The polyps, probably adenomas, although this was not specifically stated, were thought to be inherited. The cumulative evidence points to a familial factor in bowel cancer, which could be either genetic or environmental in origin.

Veale's Hypothesis

During his investigation into familial adenomatous polyposis, Veale came to the conclusion that all adenomas were of genetic origin. He considered that three allelic genes could exist at the same locus; x, the normal "wild" type and P and p, two mutated genes. Each of the mutations could be responsible for the presence of colorectal adenomas, P for adenomatous polyposis as a Mendelian dominant characteristic and p for a few isolated adenomas as a recessive characteristic when the homozygous genotype, pp, is present (38). Individuals having the other two possible genotypes, xx and px, do not produce adenomas. Thus, the nonpolyposis patients with adenomas or cancer of the large intestine are all homozygous for the p gene. The hypothesis has the virtue of simplicity while agreeing with much that is known about intestinal tumours. For instance, the possible permutations of the three genotypes in matings could account for the spectrum of family histories encountered. A union involving xx and px would produce no further adenomas in the children. On the other hand, if both parents have the homozygous pp genotype, their children would all develop adenomas and possibly cancer. If the children were numerous, the family could well become one with an incidence of colorectal cancer so high as to suggest a Mendelian dominant, rather than a recessive, mode of inheritance as is claimed by some workers (20).

Again, the idea that the nonpolyposis adenomas have a different mode of inheritance may also explain the fact that they are not similarly associated with hamartomatous polyps and an increased incidence of congenital defects, as are the adenomas of the polyposis syndromes.

An alternative to Veale's hypothesis still involves a genetic factor but of a polygenic nature, although so far little supportive evidence has been produced. The collection of information about a possible genetic origin for nonpolyposis adenomas is likely to be a long process. Several decades were required to establish the inheritance pattern of familial polyposis and polyposis is usually diagnosed by the third decade, using the simple method of sigmoidoscopic examination. Nonpolyposis adenomas are rare below the age of 30 years but show an increasing incidence throughout life. Moreover, to be effective, any examination must include all the colorectum and, therefore, the more expensive and time-consuming techniques of barium enema and colonoscopic examinations are necessary. Unlike polyposis which does not skip generations, the recessive mode of inheritance can do so and time is required to see if the condition will return in a subsequent generation.

While these investigations are being pursued, another method that could possibly give information about the mode of inheritance of the nonpolyposis adenomas and at the same time initiate a degree of cancer prevention could be employed. This is to assume that Veale's hypothesis is correct. The success of cancer prevention in polyposis depends on its mode of inheritance and clinical course being known, thus enabling those at risk to be identified and the adenoma-carcinoma sequence to be broken at the right moment. The same policy can be used in the case of the nonpolyposis patient with adenomas. A family history is taken, and on the basis that the inheritance is recessive, the degree of risk can be assessed for individual family members. Figure 1a shows the pedigree of a small family in which nothing is known of the presence or absence of neoplastic tumours of the colorectum in any of the members. If it is assumed that the incidence of adenomas in the general population is 10%, that is the risk that each member has of developing adenomas. The propositus (marked by the arrow) is examined and found to have an adenoma or cancer. The situation is now changed to that in Fig. 1b. The propositus's risk has risen to 100% because he actually has an adenoma. His brother and sister have a 40% risk and his children a 30% risk (these figures have been rounded off for the sake of simplicity). Should the propositus then say that one of his parents had died of bowel cancer, the risk of adenomas in his

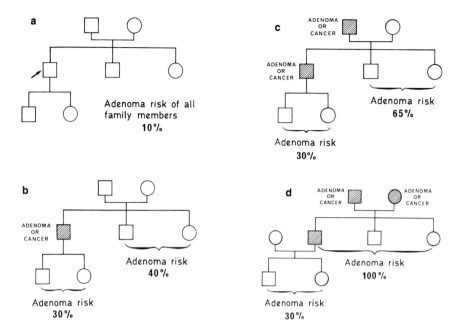

FIG. 1. Variable risk of family members developing adenomas which are inherited as a recessive characteristic with a 10% incidence in the population. **a**: No knowledge of adenomas (or cancer) in family. Propositus case arrowed. **b**: Adenomas diagnosed in propositus. **c**: Propositus and one parent known to have adenomas (or cancer). **d**: Both parents have adenomas (or cancer).

brethren rises to 65% (Fig. 1c). If both parents are known to have had neoplasia of the colon, all their children have a 100% risk of similar tumours (Fig. 1d). It will be noted that the risk in respect of the children of the propositus has remained steady throughout at 30%. They have each received one p gene from the father and no matter how many of their paternal relatives develop adenomas or cancer of the large intestine, their own risk is not increased further on this account. On the other hand, any evidence of colonic tumours in the mother or her family immediately increases the children's risk. It is possible to grade the family members into groups according to the estimated degree of risk. Those at greatest risk could be invited to be examined, the level of risk for investigation being determined by the available facilities. Adenomas might be found in, at least, some of the patients and destroyed. Examinations could be repeated at intervals of perhaps 3 or 4 years. Removal of the adenomas in familial polyposis resulted in a significant decrease in the incidence of colorectal cancer and a comparable decrease is to be expected by the application of the same policy in this group of patients. Moreover, an opportunity of testing Veale's hypothesis would have been created. The expected incidence of colorectal tumours in each group is not likely to be fully realised even after a long period of time. If, however, the ratio of observed tumours and expected tumours in each of the groups with variable risk proved to be reasonably constant, this would be strong support for Veale's hypothesis.

AETIOLOGY OF COLORECTAL ADENOMAS AND CARCINOMAS

In this review, the emphasis has been on the probable part played by genetic factors in the appearance of intestinal adenomas. This is not intended to suggest that environmental factors have little or no role in the process. On the contrary, they are of great importance. Even with a condition like familial polyposis, where at first sight the genetic aspect dominates the picture, there can be wide variations from one case to another, which are most satisfactorily explained as modification of the effects of the genetic factors by environmental factors. In some patients, polyposis is not diagnosed until middle age and then relatively few adenomas, and these only small in size, are found. On the other hand, children not yet of teen age may have enormous numbers of tumours of more than average size. Normally cancer appears in polyposis patients around the fourth decade but it may sometimes be found in teenagers or patients over 60 years of age.

A scheme of the possible mode of interaction between genetic and environmental factors has been suggested by Hill et al. (15). This has been based on a study of epidemiological data from various sources, leading to the conclusion that in addition to the initial genetic factor, at least three environmental factors are required. The genetic factor plays an initial essential role in making the patient adenoma-prone. The first environmental factor (A) causes the formation of small adenomas which rarely become malignant. Since the ratio of small adenomas to large adenomas varies in different regions, a second factor (B) is probably necessary to promote growth. Finally, a third agent (C) is responsible for inducing malignancy in the adenomas, particularly when these are large.

Until a marker for the genetic factor is known, its presence can only be detected for certain by the diagnosis of adenomas or carcinomas in the colorectum. The taking of a family history may indicate the distribution of the factor within the family, at the same time revealing those at most risk and in need of examination, when perhaps adenomas may be found. At this stage, cancer prevention can be achieved by removal of the adenomas before the third factor (C) can become effective. This policy is the basis for the success obtained in reducing the incidence of intestinal cancer in polyposis. A further possibility of attaining the same objective is to identify and eliminate one or more of the three factors involved, thereby interrupting the adenoma-carcinoma sequence in the earlier stages. Perhaps in the future it may be possible to correct the genetic defect. In the meantime the policy of seeking out those most prone to develop adenomas and destroying any tumours found should produce a reduction in the incidence of colorectal cancer.

REFERENCES

1. Achord, J. L., and Proctor, H. D. (1963): Malignant degeneration and metastasis in Peutz-Jeghers syndrome. *Arch. Inter. Med.*, 111:498–502.
2. Beacham, C. H., Shields, H. M., Raffensperger, E. C., and Enterline, H. T. (1978): Juvenile and adenomatous gastrointestinal polyposis. *Am. J. Dig. Dis.*, 23:1137–1143.
3. Bussey, H. J. R. (1975): *Familial Polyposis Coli*. Johns Hopkins University Press, Baltimore, London.
4. Bussey, H. J. R. (1979): Familial polyposis coli. In: *Pathology Annual, Part 1, 1979*, edited by S. C. Sommers and P. P. Rosen, pp. 61–81. Appleton-Century-Crofts, New York.
5. Cabot, R. C. (1935): Case Records of the Massachusetts General Hospital, Case No. 21061. *N. Engl. J. Med.*, 212:263–267.
6. Capps, Jr., W. F., Lewis, M. I., and Gazzaniga, D. A. (1968): Carcinoma of the colon, ampulla of Vater and urinary bladder associated with familial multiple polyposis. *Diseases of the Colon and Rectum*, 11:298–305.
7. Cochet, B., Carrel, J., Desbaillets, L., and Widgren, S. (1979): Peutz-Jeghers syndrome associated with gastrointestinal carcinoma. *Gut*, 20:169–175.
8. Dodds, W. J., Schulte, W. J., Hensley, G. T., and Hogan, W. J. (1972): Peutz-Jeghers syndrome and gastrointestinal malignancy. *Am. J. Roentgenol.*, 115:374–377.
9. Dormandy, T. L. (1957): Gastrointestinal polyposis with mucocutaneous pigmentation (Peutz-Jeghers syndrome). *N. Engl. J. Med.*, 256:1093–1141, 1186.
10. Enterline, H. T., Evans, G. W., Mercado-Lugo, R., Miller, L., and Fitts, W. T. (1962): Malignant potential of adenomas of the colon and rectum. *JAMA*, 179:322–330.

11. Gardner, E. J. (1969): Gardner's syndrome re-evaluated after twenty years. *Proc. Utah Acad.*, 46:1–11.
12. Gardner, E. J., and Richards, R. C. (1953): Multiple cutaneous and subcutaneous lesions occurring simultaneously with hereditary polyposis and osteomatosis. *Am. J. Hum. Genet.*, 5:139–147.
13. Goodman, Z. D., Yardley, J. H., and Milligan, F. D. (1979): Pathogenesis of colonic polyps in multiple juvenile polyposis. Report of a case associated with gastric polyps and carcinoma of the rectum. *Cancer*, 43:1906–1913.
14. Hamilton, S. R., Bussey, H. J. R., Mendelsohn, G., Diamond, M. P., Pavlides, G., Hutcheon, D., Harbison, M., Shermata, D., Morson, B. C., and Yardley, J. H. (1979): Ileal adenomas after colectomy in nine patients with adenomatous polyposis coli/Gardner's syndrome. *Gastroenterology*, 77:1252–1257.
15. Hill, M. J., Morson, B. C., and Bussey, H. J. R. (1978): Aetiology of adenoma-carcinoma sequence in large bowel. *Lancet*, i:245–247.
16. Iida, M., Yao, T., Ohsato, K., Itoh, H., and Watanabe, H. (1980): Diagnostic value of intra-operative fiberoscopy for small intestinal polyps in familial adenomatous coli. *Endoscopy*, 12:161–165.
17. Iowa, T., and Watanabe, H. (1978): Report of case of familial adenomatous coli associated with gastric cancer. *Stomach and Intestine*, 13:1105–1111.
18. Johnson, G. W., Eakins, D., and Gough, A. D. (1968): Juvenile polyposis coli. *Ulster Med. J.*, 37:170–174.
19. Lovett, E. (1976): Family studies in cancer of the colon and rectum. *Br. J. Surg.*, 63:13–18.
20. Lynch, H. T., Guirgis, H. A., Lynch, P. M., Lynch, J. F., and Harris, R. E. (1977): Familial cancer syndrome: a survey. *Cancer*, 39:1867–1881.
21. Macklin, M. T. (1960): Inheritance of cancer of the stomach and large intestine in man. *J. Natl. Cancer Inst.*, 24:551–571.
22. Mathis, M. (1962): Familial carcinoma of the colon. A family tree from the Canton of Argau. *Schweiz Med. Wochenschr.*, 92:1673–1678.
23. MacDonald, J. M., David, W. C., Crago, H. R., and Berk, A. D. (1967): Gardner's syndrome and periampullary malignancy. *Am. J. Surg.*, 113:425–430.
24. McColl, I., Bussey, H. J. R., Veale, A. M. O., and Morson, B. C. (1964): Juvenile polyposis coli. *Proc. R. Soc. Med.*, 57:896–897.
25. Monga, G., Mazzucco, G., and Mollo F. (1981): Adenomatous and carcinomatous transformation in hamartomatous polyps (Peutz-Jeghers type) of the large bowel. *International Symposium on Precancerous Conditions of the gastrointestinal tract*. Fondazione Internazional Menarini, p. 100, Bologna, Italy.
26. Morson, B. C. (1962): Some peculiarities in the histology of intestinal polyps. *Dis. Colon Rectum*, 5:337–344.
27. Morson, B. C. (1974): The polyp-cancer sequence in the large bowel. *Proc. R. Soc. Med.*, 67:451–457.
28. Morson, B. C., and Dawson, I. M. P. (1979): *Gastrointestinal Pathology*, 2nd edition. Blackwell Scientific Publications, Oxford, London, Edinburgh, Melbourne.
29. Muto, T., Bussey, H. J. R., and Morson, B. C. (1975): The evolution of cancer of the colon and rectum. *Cancer*, 36:2251–2270.
30. Ohsato, K., Yao, T., Watanabe, H., Iida, M., and Itoh, H. (1977): Small-intestinal involvement in familial polyposis diagnosed by operative intestinal fiberoscopy: report of 4 cases. *Dis. Colon Rectum*, 20:414–420.
31. Phillips, L. G. (1981): Polyposis and carcinoma of the small bowel and familial colonic polyposis. *Dis. Colon Rectum*, 24:478–481.
32. Pierce, E. R. (1968): Some genetic aspects of familial multiple polyposis of the colon in a kindred of 1,422 members. *Dis. Colon Rectum*, 11:321–329.
33. Reed, T. E., and Neel, J. V. (1955): A genetic study of multiple polyposis of the colon (with an appendix deriving a method of estimating relative fitness). *Am. J. Hum. Genet.*, 7:236–263.
34. Reid, J. D. (1965): Duodenal carcinoma in the Peutz-Jeghers syndrome. *Cancer*, 18:970–977.
35. Ross, J. E., and Mara, J. E. (1974): Small bowel polyps and carcinoma in multiple intestinal polyposis. *Arch. Surg.*, 108:736–738.
36. Smilow, P. C., Pryor, C. A., and Swinton, N. W. (1966): Juvenile polyposis coli: a report of three patients in three generations of one family. *Dis. Colon Rectum*, 9:248–254.
37. Stemper, T. J., Kent, T. H., and Summers, R. W. (1975): Juvenile polyposis and gastrointestinal carcinoma: A study of a kindred. *Ann. Inter. Med.*, 83:639–646.
38. Veale, A. M. O. (1965): *Intestinal Polyposis*, Eugenics Laboratory Memoirs Series 40, Cambridge University Press, London.
39. Veale, A. M. O., McColl, I., Bussey, H. J. R., and Morson, B. C. (1966): Juvenile polyposis coli. *J. Med. Genet.*, 3:5–16.
40. Watanabe, H., Enjoji, M., Yao, I., Iida, M., and Ohsato, K. (1977): Accompanying gastro-enteric lesions in familial adenomatosis coli. *Acta Pathol. Jpn.*, 27:823–839.
41. Woolf, C. M., Richards, R. C., and Gardner, E. J. (1955): Occasional discrete polyps of the colon and rectum showing an inherited tendency in a kindred. *Cancer*, 8:403–408.

Precancerous Lesions of the Gastrointestinal Tract, edited by P. Sherlock, B.C. Morson, L. Barbara, and U. Veronesi. Raven Press, New York © 1983.

High-Risk Conditions and Precancerous Lesions of the Oesophagus

Nubia Muñoz and *Massimo Crespi

*Division of Epidemiology and Biostatistics, International Agency for Research on Cancer, 69372 Lyon Cédex 08, France; and *The Service of Environmental Carcinogenesis, Epidemiology and Prevention, Istituto Regina Elena, 00121 Rome, Italy.*

HIGH-RISK CONDITIONS

Conditions associated with an increased risk for oesophageal cancer can be grouped into four categories: genetic, environmental, a combination of both, and others.

Genetic Susceptibility

The classical example is provided by the joint segregation of oesophageal cancer and "keratosis palmaris et plantaris" (tylosis) observed in some families. The two conditions appear to be due to a single autosomal gene with dominant effect. This association was originally described in 18 patients with oesophageal cancer belonging to two Liverpool families (20). The tylosis in these cases was of the late-onset form, appearing after 1 year of age. The oesophageal malignancies have been diagnosed as squamous cell carcinomas arising mostly in the middle and lower thirds of the oesophagus. The mean age at onset of cancer was 45 years and the youngest patient was 29 years old. Six new cases of oesophageal cancer have been reported in one of these two families (16). In one of them an association between oral leukoplakia and oesophageal cancer was also reported (55), which has also been described in a 25-year-old patient with oesophageal cancer, oral leukoplakia, and hyperkeratosis (49). Two additional families with tylosis, in each of which one member has developed oesophageal carcinoma, have been reported from Liverpool (16). Another family in which tylosis has been associated with a congenital oesophageal stricture and subsequent development of oesophageal carcinoma has been described (51).

A recent report describes tylosis at birth, early-onset form, in 22 out of 45 members of an Indian family spanning five generations. Squamous cell carcinoma of the tylotic skin developed in 3 of the subjects with tylosis. In all of them the skin cancer appeared in the second decade of life and one of them died of squamous cell carcinoma of the oesophagus in the fourth decade (66).

That this genetic susceptibility accounts for only a minimal proportion of oesophageal cancers is suggested by the small number of cases of this cancer associated with tylosis so far reported, and by the negative results obtained in family studies. One of these studies, involving 877 relatives of 101 oesophageal cancer patients and 2,572 relatives of control patients, failed to show any influence by hereditary factors, but showed a clear association of this cancer with alcohol abuse (39). Another study showed an increased risk for oeso-phageal cancer among spouses of patients with this cancer, suggesting exposure to common environmental factors rather than a hereditary component (43). In the high-incidence pop-ulation of Northern Iran, the aggregation of oesophageal cancer in descendants of one family has been described; the occurrence of 13 cases of oesophageal cancer among 19 relatives from three generations is striking (47). However, subsequent studies in the same population, using various genetic markers, such as red blood cell enzymes (28) and human leukocyte antigens (HLA) (17), have yielded negative results. Furthermore, in a recent clinical-en-doscopic survey carried out in three villages of the same area, no clear tylosis was detected in 430 individuals examined, although it would be difficult to differentiate it from plantar or palmar hyperkeratosis due to walking barefoot or manual labour (9).

In high-risk areas for oesophageal cancer in North China, a family history for this cancer has been reported in 25% to 60% of the patients, but no association with tylosis has been noted (32). The analysis of the genealogical history of oesophageal cancer in seven Linxian families shows that most of the cases of oesophageal cancer occurring in these families were distantly related or not related at all (32). It is therefore possible that the high prevalence of a positive family history in North China reflects a common exposure to carcinogens rather than a genetic susceptibility.

Environmental Susceptibility

This type of susceptibility is illustrated by the increased frequency of cancer of the upper oesophagus and hypopharynx in patients with sideropenic dysphagia (3,6,25,52,60). This syndrome was first described by Plummer and Vinson in the United States (56) and by Paterson and Kelly in the United Kingdom (26,45). There is some disagreement in the definition of this syndrome. Plummer-Vinson, or Paterson-Kelly, syndrome is sometimes used to group all epithelial lesions (atrophic changes of nails, mouth, tongue, hypopharynx, oesophagus, and stomach) that may accompany hypochromic anaemia, but in a more re-stricted sense it is reserved for cases with postcricoid dysphagia and the typical radiological changes observed in the hypopharynx and upper oesophagus. Although hypochromic anaemia has been reported to occur frequently in patients with this syndrome (6,35,57,59), dysphagia has been reported to be uncommon in populations with a high prevalence of severe iron deficiency (24). In an attempt to clarify the association between dysphagia and anaemia, subjects with dysphagia were identified in an unselected population and their haematological changes were compared with those of a control group matched for sex and age and chosen at random from the same population (10). No differences were observed between the two groups and it was therefore concluded that there was no association between dysphagia and anaemia in this unselected population and that dysphagia should be regarded as a single symptom (10). This apparent discrepancy may be reconciled if dysphagia and the epithelial lesions are considered as sequelae of sideropenic anaemia and other deficiencies that occurred many years before and that have been treated and have therefore disappeared (30).

Although this condition used to be very common in the northern parts of the world and especially in some rural areas of northern Sweden (58), it is today rare. However, relatively high rates for oesophageal cancer in females are still seen in northern areas of Norway and rural Wales (U.K.) (44). These high rates may be the remnants of a high prevalence of Plummer-Vinson syndrome 40 to 50 years ago. The prevalence of dysphagia in the 40- to 75-year age group of an unselected population of the United Kingdom was found to be between 0.7 and 1.5% in males and between 4 and 6% in females (10).

The pathogenesis of this syndrome is not clear. Although iron deficiency has been considered of prime importance, other nutritional deficiencies, and specifically riboflavin, thiamin, and pyridoxine deficiencies, may be involved (23,24,38,63).

Iron deficiency in tropical regions does not cause dysphagia and the accompanying epithelial lesions, and it has not been possible to induce similar lesions in animals using an iron-deficient diet (2). On the other hand, riboflavin deficiency causes very similar epithelial lesions in humans and animals (38). This vitamin is an essential factor in maintaining the integrity of the skin, and particularly of the squamous epithelium of the oesophagus.

A role of nutritional deficiencies in cancers of the upper alimentary tract has long been suspected, but it has been documented in only a few reports. This suspicion is consistent with the persistent association found with low socioeconomic status. A high frequency of cancer of the oesophagus and hypopharynx in Swedish women, especially in the most northern areas of the country, and a possible association with Plummer-Vinson syndrome, was suspected as early as 1936 (3). This association was confirmed in a large Swedish study, which also linked the occurrence of the Plummer-Vinson syndrome to a restricted diet particularly deficient in iron, vitamin C, and riboflavin (63). In the populations where oesophageal cancer has been associated with alcohol and tobacco, dietary deficiencies, particularly in so far as milk, fruits, and vegetables (sources of riboflavin) are concerned, have also been described, but it is not clear whether such deficiencies or the heavy alcohol intake by itself is the responsible factor for an increased risk of oesophageal cancer (37,61). However, in the high-risk populations of Iran, where alcohol and tobacco have been excluded as risk factors, a low intake of vegetables, fruits, and foods of animal origin, resulting in a low intake of vitamins A, C, and riboflavin, has been associated with this cancer (21).

Clinical and biochemical studies in Iran have revealed widespread riboflavin deficiency in northern Iran, but this is equally prevalent in the high- and low-incidence areas for oesophageal cancer (29). If riboflavin deficiency is involved in the aetiology of this cancer in Iran, it could be facilitating the action of unknown carcinogen(s). Several features of riboflavin deficiency are compatible with this action: the earliest instances of angular stomatitis were seen in children 2 to 3 years old and the highest incidence and most severe lesions were in school children and young adults. Riboflavin deficiency appears to affect both sexes equally and it is probable that almost all members of the low socioeconomic groups of these communities suffer from it at some time, and for considerable periods during their earlier years (29). The finding of a strikingly high prevalence (80%) of chronic oesophagitis in subjects 15 to 70 years of age from the high-incidence areas of Iran suggests that riboflavin deficiency may be involved in this lesion (9).

The experimental evidence linking riboflavin to cancer is complex. Riboflavin deficiency decreases the rates of growth of spontaneous tumours in experimental animals, specifically mammary tumours and lymphosarcoma in mice and Walker carcinoma in rats (50), but it also causes atrophic changes in the epithelium of the oesophagus and forestomach of mice. The earliest atrophic changes in the oesophagus were observed during the third to fifth week of deficiency and later an epithelial hyperplasia and hyperkeratosis were also noted (64). When mice on a riboflavin-deficient diet for 3 to 4 weeks were treated with dimethylbenzanthracene (DMBA) and croton oil, a remarkable increase in the frequency of skin tumours was observed compared with the two control groups, one on a normal diet and the other on a high riboflavin diet. Tumours also appeared more rapidly after application of the carcinogen to the skin of animals on a deficient diet than on the control diets (62). Complete riboflavin in the baboon causes atrophy, ulcers, and some hyperplastic oesophageal lesions interpreted as precancerous (13,14). Although it may be unlikely that a riboflavin deficiency severe enough to produce the lesions described in animals can exist in man, less extreme deficiencies may contribute to create a fertile soil for specific carcinogens.

In relation to other nutritional deficiencies of possible relevance to the development of oesophageal cancer, zinc deficiency deserves special attention. Lower concentrations of zinc in blood, hair, and oesophageal tumour tissue have been reported in patients with oesophageal cancer more than in matched controls (33), and experimental studies suggest that zinc deficiency enhances the induction of oesophageal cancer in rats treated with nitrosobenzyl-methylamine (12). On the other hand, it has been demonstrated that high intake of bread high in fibre causes increased faecal excretion of zinc and other minerals, which could lead to zinc deficiencies (48). This observation is of special relevance to the high-incidence populations for oesophageal cancer in Iran, whose staple diet is bread. All rural and most urban breads in these regions contain substantial amounts of fibre and phytate. A nutritional survey has revealed that up to 70% of households in these areas receive more than 90% of their protein from bread (21).

Genetic and Environmental Susceptibility

A further example of the role of individual susceptibility is provided by the association between oesophageal cancer and idiopathic steatorrhoea and coeliac disease (15,19). This association may be either a genetic or an environmental susceptibility. Coeliac disease is a malabsorptive disorder of the small intestine, characterized by a flat jejunal mucosa whose histological abnormalities and clinical features can be reversed by gluten withdrawal. The main symptoms are diarrhoea, anaemia, weight loss, lassitude and skeletal disorders (8). Since the upper small intestine is the most seriously involved portion of the intestine, iron, folic acid, B12, and pyridoxine deficiency have been reported (18). Deficiency of vitamins A, C, and K has also been observed as well as disturbances of carbohydrate, protein, and calcium metabolisms (18). It is of interest to note that severe zinc deficiency has been observed in patients with coeliac disease who do not respond to gluten-free diets (34). Coeliac disease is a familial condition with approximately 10% of first-degree relatives affected (53). The mode of inheritance remains to be established, but studies of histocom-patibility (HLA) antigens suggest that HLA-B8 and HLA-Dw3 are important factors in the inheritance of this disease (11,27). Malignant lymphoma of the jejunum has been the most common complication of coeliac disease (15–19), but oesophageal cancer has been observed to be almost as common. The patients who developed oesophageal cancer have a long history of coeliac disease (mean age 50 years), and the most frequent location of the tumour was middle or lower thirds (15). An increased incidence of oesophageal cancer has also been reported in male relatives of patients with coeliac disease, but no excess of cancer deaths due to lymphoma was observed in either sex (54).

The increased susceptibility to oesophageal cancer in these patients may be the result of both genetic factors and nutritional deficiencies. The long latent period between the onset of coeliac disease and the development of oesophageal cancer may favour the nutritional hypothesis.

Other High-Risk Conditions

Achalasia

Achalasia is a motor disorder of the oesophagus characterized by aperistalsis, partial or incomplete lower-oesophageal sphincter relaxation, and increased lower-oesophageal sphincter pressure. Neural lesions have been described in the dorsal vagal nucleus in the brainstem, in the vagal trunks, and in myenteric ganglions in the oesophagus. They may be caused by a neurotropic virus, such as herpes zoster (7). Squamous cell carcinoma of the oesophagus has been described in 5% to 10% of patients with achalasia (7).

Oesophageal Lye Corrosion

Cicatricial strictures of the oesophagus due to the ingestion of corrosive substances occasionally give rise to malignant tumours. Most of the strictures resulting in oesophageal cancer are caused by lye burns. A history of lye burns has been reported in 1% to 4% of patients with oesophageal cancer (5,31). Approximately 70 cases of oesophageal cancer associated with lye corrosion have been reported in the literature. A recent review describes the features of 63 of these cases (4). In 52 out of 63 cases the lye burn occurred before 10 years of age and the mean age of the patients at lye ingestion was 6.2 years. The mean interval between the lye burns and the diagnosis of oesophageal cancer was 41 years and all cancers were diagnosed histologically as squamous cell cancers (4).

PRECURSOR LESIONS OF OESOPHAGEAL CANCER

Little is known about the precancerous lesions of oesophageal cancer in man. The available information is derived from a limited number of studies analysing postmortem and surgical specimens in the presence of cancer or in subjects dying from diseases other than oesophageal cancer. In this way dysplasia has been proposed as a precancerous lesion, but up to now no information was available on the lesions preceding this dysplasia (36,40,46,65). To gather information on these lesions that will enable us to construct the natural history of this disease, endoscopic surveys have been carried out in two high-risk populations for oesophageal cancer in Northern Iran and Northern China.

In Northern Iran a total of 430 subjects (218 males and 212 females) from the villages of Khoran, Hottan, and Ghappan were included in this study. Initially, persons with gastrointestinal symptoms and those with close relatives who had had cancer of the oesophagus were encouraged to attend. Later in the study symptom-free individuals and individuals with no family history of oesophageal cancer were also included. Results of this survey have been published elsewhere (9).

In Northern China 527 individuals (292 males and 235 females) from the Chen Guam commune of Linxian were included in the study. Two hundred and fifty of these individuals had been examined in 1975 by cytological screening by the Chinese balloon technique and 277 were not included in the 1975 survey. Detailed results of this survey are being published in a separate report (41).

The following procedure was followed with each of the subjects examined:

1. A questionnaire containing information on basic demographic data and information on smoking and drinking habits and cancer family history was completed together with a clinical form recording personal medical history and symptoms of upper gastrointestinal disease. In addition, in the Iranian village of Ghappan questions on opium smoking or eating of opium pyrolysates were asked and in Northern China information on dietary habits before 1950 and in 1979 was also obtained.
2. A physical examination including evaluation of general health and signs of specific vitamin deficiencies was performed.
3. Specimens of blood and hair were collected in a sample of the subjects included in the China survey for analysis of vitamin A, riboflavin, and zinc.

4. An endoscopic examination was performed and guided cytology and at least two biopsies were taken from each individual.
5. The histological slides were read without knowledge of any clinical data.

The oesophagitis detected endoscopically and histologically in these two populations was classified according to criteria described in a previous report (11) in mild, moderate, and severe. The results of the endoscopical findings are summarized in Table 1.

Oesophagitis was found in 85.3% and 88.4% of the males in Iran and China, respectively and in 87.7% and 70.2% of the females in Iran and China, respectively. Most of the oesophagitis was classified as mild or moderate and the severe type was found more frequently among the males than among the females in both populations. Oesophageal varices, single or multiple, were observed in 13.2% and 7.2% among the males and in 18.4% and 9.4% among the females in Iran and China, respectively. Incompetent cardia was found in 7.3% and 9.2% of the males and in 8.5% and 9.8% of the females in Iran and China, respectively. Hiatus hernia was observed in approximately 1% of the populations examined except among the Chinese females. Oesophageal cancer was diagnosed endoscopically in 7 patients from Iran and in 5 patients from China, and cancer of the cardia was found in 5 patients from China.

Table 2 summarizes the results of the histological evaluation. It shows that most of the oesophagitis diagnosed endoscopically was confirmed histologically. The great majority of the cases were classified as mild oesophagitis followed by the moderate type. The severe type was diagnosed only in 1% to 3% of the individuals and it was more common among males than among females. The oesophagitis was characterized by papillomatosis, lympho-plasmocytic infiltration and proliferation, and dilatation of blood vessels in the submucosa and in the epithelium. The second most common lesion was clear cell acanthosis, corresponding both to a thickened epithelium by swollen clear cells, which in most cases were Periodic Acid Schiff (PAS) negative, and endoscopically to white patches or whitish mucosa. This clear cell acanthosis accompanied the oesophagitis in most cases. In 12.7% and 11.6% of the males and 9.8% of the females in Iran and China, respectively, the chronic

TABLE 1. *Endoscopical findings in high-risk populations for oesophageal cancer in Iran and China*

	% Males		% Females	
	Iran (218)	China (292)	Iran (212)	China (235)
Oesophagitis				
Mild	37.6	41.1	59.9	53.6
Moderate	36.7	38.4	23.1	14.9
Severe	11.0	8.9	4.7	1.7
Total	85.3	88.4	87.7	70.2
Varices				
Single	5.9	5.1	6.1	5.1
Multiples	7.3	2.1	12.3	4.3
Total	13.2	7.2	18.4	9.4
Incompetent cardia	7.3	9.2	8.5	9.8
Hiatus hernia	0.9	0.7	0.9	0
Cancer	2.8	2.1	1.3	1.3

Number of subjects examined is shown in parentheses.

TABLE 2. *Histological findings in high-risk populations for oesophageal cancer in Iran and China*

	% Males		% Females	
	Iran (213)	China (292)	Iran (205)	China (235)
Oesophagitis				
Mild	58.7	55.8	57.6	56.2
Moderate	21.6	7.5	17.6	6.4
Severe	2.8	1.7	1.0	0.9
Total	83.1	65.0	76.2	63.5
Clear cell acanthosis	66.2	80.8	64.9	72.4
Atrophy	12.7	11.6	8.3	9.8
Dysplasia	4.7	7.9	2.9	8.1
Cancer				
Oesophagus	2.8	1.4	2.0	0.4
Cardia	0	0.7	0	1.3

oesophagitis was accompanied by atrophic changes in the epithelium. Dysplasia was diagnosed among males in 4.7% and 7.9% and among females in 2.9% and 8.1% in Iran and China, respectively. The frequency of dysplasia was therefore more common in China than in Iran. In the Iran group carcinoma was diagnosed in 11 subjects and in 4 of these cases the diagnosis was made only after histological examination. In China squamous cell carcinoma of the oesophagus was diagnosed in 5 individuals, adenocarcinoma of the cardias also in 5, and adenocarcinoma of the stomach in 4. Two of the squamous cell cancers of the oesophagus were diagnosed only after histological examination and only one at cytology. A similar prevalence of oesophagitis was observed in all the age groups in Iran as well as China, as shown in Table 3. It is remarkable that a high prevalence of oesophagitis is present even in the younger age groups.

Twenty of the subjects examined in Linxian were reexamined endoscopically 1 year later. In 12 of them the oesophagitis with or without atrophy had not changed and in 8 a progression was observed. In 4 subjects a progression from mild oesophagitis to oesophagitis with atrophy and dysplasia was observed, and the remaining 4 with oesophagitis with atrophy or dysplasia

TABLE 3. *Age distribution of histologically confirmed oesophagitis in Iran and China—males*

			% Oesophagitis							
	No. of subj.		Mild		Moderate		Severe		Total	
Age	Iran	China	Iran	China	Iran	China	Iran	China	Iran	China
15–24	5		80.0		0.0		0.0		80.0	
25–34	17	21	88.2	61.9	11.8	9.5	0.0	0.0	90.0	71.4
35–44	77	77	58.9	49.4	20.8	10.4	2.6	1.3	82.3	61.1
45–54	54	84	51.8	61.9	29.6	2.4	3.7	2.4	85.1	66.7
≥55	60	110	58.3	54.5	20.0	9.1	3.3	1.8	81.6	65.4
Total	213	292	58.7	55.8	21.6	7.5	2.8	1.7	83.1	65.0

had progressed to cancer. This evolution of the lesions suggests that in fact they are pre-cancerous.

The similarity of the observations in two high-risk populations for oesophageal cancer living in widely separated geographical regions is striking. In both northeast Iran and central China an unusually high prevalence of chronic oesophagitis was found, which contrasts with the lower prevalence of this lesion reported among patients attending gastrointestinal clinics in Europe, where oesophageal cancer is known to be rare. In addition to this fact, the similar location of the oesophagitis and the cancer in the oesophagus suggests that these two lesions are associated.

The oesophagitis described by us in these two high-risk populations differs from that reported from low-risk populations. In Iran and China the oesophagitis is characterized by an irregular friable mucosa with varying degrees of aedema, hyperaemia, and leukoplakia but without ulceration and which usually involves the middle and lower thirds of the oesophagus, leaving the precardial region free. On the other hand, in the low-risk populations in Europe, the oesophagitis is characterized by erosions and ulcerations, which usually involve the precardial region, as it is in general due to reflux.

Based on these observations, we propose the following sequence in the natural history of oesophageal cancer:

$$\text{Chronic oesophagitis} \rightarrow \text{atrophy} \rightarrow \text{dysplasia} \rightarrow \text{cancer}$$

This suggestion is supported by observations in experimental animals. Similar morphological changes have been described in the oesophagus of rats treated with N-methyl-N-nitrosoaniline (42). The oesophagus of rats killed after 3 months of treatment showed inflammatory infiltrate, acanthosis, and slight dystrophic changes. No clear atrophic changes were described after 6 months of treatment but proliferation of the epithelium resulting in the formation of long epithelial downgrowths, progressing later on to the formation of papillomas, then to dysplasia, and finally to cancer. Oesophageal lesions very similar to the ones we have described in human populations from Iran and China have been noted in nonhuman primates after treatment with 1-methyl-1-nitrosourea (MNU) (1). In the monkeys receiving low doses of MNU oesophagitis and diskeratosis of the oesophageal mucosa were observed. In some monkeys the oesophagitis was accompanied by atrophy and hyperkeratosis. Squamous cell carcinoma developed in 71% of the monkeys receiving MNU for more than 57 months.

Concerning the aetiology of the precursor lesions and of the cancer of the oesophagus in Iran and China, there are at least three possibilities:

1. As in the experimental models, the precursor lesions and the cancer may be the result of a given carcinogen(s), the precursor lesions being the manifestations of low doses of the carcinogen and the cancer the result of an exposure to higher doses. In Iran, there is indirect evidence suggesting that one of such carcinogens may be opium tar, but in China the responsible carcinogens remain to be identified.

2. The precursor lesions could be the manifestation of chronic injury resulting from drinking very hot beverages, from eating very coarse food, and from deficiencies of riboflavin and vitamin A. The cancer would be the result of the carcinogen(s) acting on the precursor lesions.

3. The precursor lesions and the cancer may both be the result of a given carcinogen(s) (no. 1) and the effect of the carcinogen(s) could be facilitated or potentiated by the

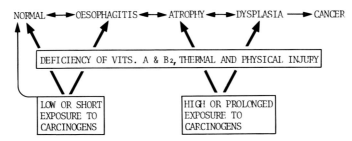

FIG. 1. Natural history of oesophageal cancer.

cofactors responsible for the chronic injury (no. 2). This possibility, which we believe is closest to reality, is illustrated in Fig. 1.

Our understanding of the mechanisms of carcinogenesis will be decisive in determining whether prevention should be aimed primarily at the suspect carcinogen or at eliminating the cofactors responsible for the chronic injury.

REFERENCES

1. Adamson, R. H., Krolikowski, F. J., Correa, P., Sieber, S. M., and Dalgard, D. W. (1977): Carcinogenicity of 1-methyl-1-nitrosourea in non-human primates. *J. Natl. Cancer Inst.*, 59:415–422.
2. Adlington, P., Leedham, P., and Smith, P. (1973): The place of iron deficiency in the Peterson-Brown Kelly syndrome. *J. Laryngol. Otol.*, 87:845–857.
3. Ahlbom, H. E. (1936): Simple achlorhydric anaemic, Plummer-Vinson syndrome and carcinoma of the mouth, pharynx and oesophagus in women. *Br. Med. J.*, 2:331–333.
4. Appelqvist, P., and Salmo, M. (1980): Lye corrosion carcinoma of the esophagus. *Cancer*, 45:2655–2658.
5. Benedict, E. B. (1941): Carcinoma of the esophagus developing in benign stricture. *N. Engl. J. Med.*, 224:408–412.
6. Beveridge, B. R., Bannerman, R. M., Evanson, J. M., and Witts, L. J. (1965): Hypochromic Anaemia. A retrospective study and follow-up of 378 in-patients. *Q.J. Med.*, 34:145–161.
7. Cohen, S. (1979): Motor disorders of the esophagus. *N. Engl. J. Med.*, 301:184–192.
8. Cooke, W. T., and Asquith, P. (1974): Introduction and definition. *Coeliac Disease—Clinics in Gastroenterology*, 3(1):3–11.
9. Crespi, M., Muñoz, N., Grassi, A., Aramesh, B., Amiri, G., Mojtabai, A., and Casale, V. (1979): Oesophageal lesions in northern Iran: a premalignant condition? *Lancet*, ii:217–221.
10. Elwood, P. C., Pitman, R. G., Jacobs, A., and Entwistle, C. C. (1964): Epidemiology of the Paterson-Kelly syndrome. *Lancet*, ii:716–720.
11. Falchuk, Z. M., Rogentine, G. N., and Strober, W. (1972): Predominance of histocompatibility antigen HL-A8 in patients with gluten sensitive enteropathy. *J. Clin. Invest.*, 51:1602–1605.
12. Fong, L. Y. Y., and Newberne, P. M. (1978): Nitrosobenzylmethylamine zinc deficiency and oesophageal cancer. In: *Environmental Aspects of N-nitroso Compounds*, edited by E. A. Walker, M. Castegnaro, L. Griciute, and R. E. Lyle, pp. 503–516. IARC Scientific Publication No. 19, Lyon.
13. Foy, H., Gillman, T., and Kondi, A. (1972): Histological changes in the skin of baboons deprived of riboflavin. In: *Medical Primatology 1972. Proceedings of the Conference on Experimental Medicine and Surgery in Primates*, edited by E. I. Goldsmith and J. Moor-Jankowski, pp. 159–168. Karger, Basel.
14. Foy, H., and Mbaya, V. (1977): Riboflavin. *Prog. Food Nutr. Sci.*, 2:357–394.
15. Harris, O. D., Cooke, W. T., Thompson, H., and Waterhouse, J. A. (1967): Malignancy in adult coeliac disease and idiopathic steatorrhoea. *Am. J. Med.*, 42:899–912.
16. Harper, P. S., Harper, R. M. J., and Howel-Evans, A. W. (1970): Carcinoma of the oesophagus with tylosis. *Q.J. Med.*, 155:317–333.
17. Hashemi, S., Dowlatshahi, K., Day, N., Kmet, J., Takasugi, M., and Modabberg, F. Z. (1979): Esophageal cancer studies in the Caspian littoral of Iran: introductive assessment of the HLA profile in patients and controls. *Tissue Antigens*, 14:422–425.
18. Hoffbrand, A. V. (1974): Anaemia in adult coeliac disease. In: *Coeliac Disease—Clinics in Gastroenterology*, 3(1),71–90.
19. Holmes, G. K. T., Stokes, P. L., Sorahan, T. M., Prior, P., Waterhouse, J. A. H., and Cooke, W. T. (1976): Coeliac disease, gluten-free diet, and malignancy. *Gut*, 17:612–619.

20. Howel-Evans, A. W., McConnell, R. B., Clarke, C. A., and Sheppard, P. M. (1958): Carcinoma of the oesophagus with keratosis palmaris et plantaris (tylosis): A study of two families. *Q. J. Med.*, 27:413–429.
21. Iran-IARC Study Group, (1977): Esophageal cancer studies in the Caspian littoral of Iran: Results of population studies. A prodrome. *J. Natl. Cancer Inst.*, 59:1127–1138.
22. Jacobs, A. (1963): Epithelial changes in anaemic East Africans. *Br. Med. J.*, 454:1711–1712.
23. Jacobs, A., and Cavill, I. A. J. (1968): Pyridoxine and riboflavin status in the Paterson-Kelly syndrome. *Br. J. Haematol.*, 14:153–160.
24. Jacobs, A., and Cavill, I. A. J. (1968): The oral lesions of iron deficiency anaemia: pyridoxine and riboflavin status. *Br. J. Haematol.*, 14:291–295.
25. Jacobsson, F. (1948): Carcinoma of the tongue. A clinical study of 277 cases treated at Radiumhemmet, 1931–1942. *Acta Radiol. (Suppl.)*, 68:1–184.
26. Kelly, A. B. (1919): Spasm at the entrance of the oesophagus. *J. Laryngol. Otol.*, 34:285–289.
27. Kenning, J. J., Peña, A. S., van Leeuwen, A., van Hooff, J. P., and van Rood, J. J. (1976): HLA-DW3 associated with coeliac disease. *Lancet*, i:606–608.
28. Kirk, R. L., Keats, B., and Blake, N. M. (1977): Genes and people in the Caspian littoral. *Am. J. Phys. Anthropol.*, 46:377–390.
29. Kmet, J., McLaren, D. S., and Siassi, F. (1980): Epidemiology of oesophageal cancer with special reference to nutritional studies among the Turkoman of Iran. *Adv. Mod. Hum. Nutr.*, 343–365.
30. Larsson, L. G., Sandstrom, A., and Westling, P. (1975): Relationship of Plummer-Vinson disease to cancer of the upper alimentary tract in Sweden. *Cancer Res.*, 35:3308–3316.
31. Lawler, M. R., Gobbel, W. G., Killen, D. A., and Daniel, R. A. (1969): Carcinoma of the esophagus. *J. Thorac. Cardiovasc. Surg.*, 58:609–613.
32. Li Mingxin, Li Ping, and Li Baorong (1980): Recent progress in research on esophageal cancer in China. *Adv. Cancer Res.*, 33:173–249.
33. Lin, H. J., Chan, W. C., Fong, J. J., and Newberne, P. M. (1977): Zinc levels in serum, hair and tumours from patients with oesophageal cancer. *Nutr. Report Int.*, 15:625–643.
34. Love, A. H. G., Elmes, M., Golden, N. K., and McMaster, D. (1978): Zinc deficiency and coeliac disease. In: *Perspectives in Coeliac Disease*, edited by B. McNicholl, C. F. McCarthy, and P. F. Fottrell, pp. 335–342. MTP Press Ltd.
35. Lundholm, L. (1939): Hereditary hypochromic anaemia. A clinical-statistical study. *Acta. Med. Scand. (Suppl.)*, 102:1–237.
36. Mandard, A. M., Chasle, J., Marnay, J., Villedieu, B., Bianco, C., Roussel, A., Elie, H., and Vernhes, J. C. (1981): Autopsy findings in 111 cases of esophageal cancer. *Cancer*, 48:329–335.
37. Martinez, I. (1969): Factors associated with cancer of the esophagus, mouth and pharynx in Puerto Rico. *J. Natl. Cancer Inst.*, 42:1069–1094.
38. Meulengracht, E., and Bichel, J. (1941): Riboflavin-avitaminose und das Plummer-Vinson-Syndrom. *Klin. Wochschr.*, 20:831–834.
39. Mosbech, J., and Videback, A. (1955): On the etiology of oesophageal carcinoma. *J. Natl. Cancer Inst.*, 15:1665–1673.
40. Mukada, T., Sato, E., and Sasano, N. (1976): Comparative studies on dysplasia of esophageal epithelium in four prefectures of Japan (Miyagi, Nara, Wakayama and Aomori) with reference to risk of carcinoma. *Tohoku J. Exp. Med.*, 119:51–63.
41. Muñoz, N., Crespi, M., Grassi, A., Wang, G. Q., Shen, Q., and Li, Z. C. (1982): Precursor lesions of oesophageal cancer in high-risk populations in Iran and China. *Lancet*, 1:876–879.
42. Napalkov, N. P., and Pozharisski, K. (1969): Morphogenesis of experimental tumors of the esophagus. *J. Natl. Cancer Inst.*, 42:922–940.
43. Nasipov, S. N. (1977): Esophageal cancer morbidity as evidenced by the genealogy of patients registered in the Guryev province. *Vop. Onkol.*, 23(8):81–85.
44. Norwegian Cancer Society (1978): *Geographical variations in Cancer Incidence in Norway, 1966–1975*. The Cancer Registry of Norway, Oslo.
45. Paterson, D. R. (1919): Spasm at the entrance of the oesophagus. *J. Laryngol. Otol.*, 34:289–291.
46. Postlethwait, R. W., and Wendell Musser, A. (1974): Changes in the esophagus in 1,000 autopsy specimens. *J. Thorac. Cardiovasc. Surg.*, 68:953–956.
47. Pour, P., and Ghadirian, P. (1974): Familial cancer of the oesophagus in Iran. *Cancer*, 33:1649–1652.
48. Reinbold, J. G., Faradje, B., Abadi, P., and Isamail-Beigi, F. (1976): Decreased absorption of calcium, magnesium, zinc and phosphorous by humans due to increased fiber and phosphorous consumption as wheat bread. *J. Nutr.*, 106(4):493–503.
49. Ritter, S. B., and Petersen, G. (1976): Esophageal cancer, hyperkeratosis and oral leukoplakia: occurrence in a 25 year old woman. *JAMA*, 235:1723.
50. Rivlin, B. (1973): Riboflavin and cancer: a review. *Cancer Res.*, 37:1977–1986.
51. Shine, I., and Allison, P. R. (1966): Carcinoma of the oesophagus with tylosis (keratosis palmaris et plantaris). *Lancet*, i:951–953.
52. Simpson, R. R. (1939): Anaemia with dysphagia: A precancerous condition? *Proc. R. Soc. Med.*, 32:1447–1454.

53. Stokes, P. L., Asquith, P., and Cooke, W. T. (1973): Genetics of coeliac disease. In: *Clinics of Gastroenterology*, p. 547. Saunders, London.
54. Stokes, P. L., Prior, P., Sorahan, T. M., McWalter, R. J., Waterhouse, J. A. H., and Cooke, W. T. (1976): Malignancy in relatives of patients with coeliac disease. *Br. J. Prevent. Soc. Med.*, 30:17–21.
55. Tyldesdley, W. R. (1974): Oral leukoplakia associated with tylosis and oesophageal carcinoma. *J. Oral. Pathol.*, 3:62–70.
56. Vinson, P. P. (1922): Hysterical dysphagia. *Minn. Med.*, 5:107–108.
57. Waldenstrom, J. (1938): Iron and epithelium. Some clinical observations. Part I. Regeneration of the epithelium. *Acta Med. Scand. (Suppl.)*, 90:380–397.
58. Waldenstrom, J. (1946): Incidence of "iron deficiency" (sideropenia) in some rural and urban populations. *Acta Med. Scand. (Suppl.)*, 170:252–279.
59. Waldenstrom, J., and Kjellberg, S. R. (1939): The roentgenological diagnosis of sideropenic dysphagia (Plummer-Vinson's Syndrome). *Acta Radiol.*, 20:618–638.
60. Wynder, E. L. (1971): Etiological aspects of squamous cancers of the head and neck. *JAMA*, 215:452–453.
61. Wynder, E. L., and Bross, I. J. (1961): A study of etiological factors in cancers of the oesophagus. *Cancer*, 14:389–413.
62. Wynder, E. L., and Chan, P. C. (1970): The possible role of riboflavin deficiency in epithelial neoplasia. II. Effect on skin tumor development. *Cancer*, 26:1221–1224.
63. Wynder, E. L., Huttberg, S., Jacobsson, F., and Bross, I. J. (1957): Environmental factors in cancer of the upper alimentary tract. A Swedish study with special reference to Plummer-Vinson (Paterson-Kelly) syndrome. *Cancer*, 10(3):470–487.
64. Wynder, E. L., and Klein, U. E. (1965): The possible role of riboflavin deficiency in epithelial neoplasia. I. Epithelial changes in mice in simple deficiency. *Cancer*, 18(2):167–180.
65. Ushigome, S., Spjut, H. J., and Noon, G. P. (1967): Extensive dysplasia and carcinoma in situ of esophageal epithelium. *Cancer*, 20:1023–1034.
66. Yesudian, P., Premalatha, S., and Thambiah, A. S. (1980): Genetic tylosis with malignancy: a study of a South Indian pedigree. *Br. J. Dermatol.*, 102:597–600.

Precancerous Lesions of the Gastrointestinal Tract, edited by P. Sherlock, B. C. Morson, L. Barbara, and U. Veronesi. Raven Press, New York © 1983.

Endoscopic Vital Staining of the Oesophagus in High-Risk Patients: Detection of Dysplasia and Early Carcinoma

*K. Jessen, **P. Paolucci, and *M. Classen

*Department of Gastroenterology and **Department of Surgery, Johann-Wolfgang-Goethe-Universität, Frankfurt am Main, Federal Republic of Germany

In western countries the prognosis for carcinoma of the oesophagus is very poor. When the diagnosis is confirmed, only a few patients are considered operable. Metastasis has already occurred in 50% to 80% of the cases (14). The advanced stage of oesophageal carcinoma has a poor chance of curable resectability. To improve therapeutic results, that is, to increase the survival rate to 90% after surgical treatment, earlier diagnosis of the tumour is required (6).

Mass cytology surveys from high-incidence areas in North China and reports from Japan verified this assumption (5–7,9). In West Germany extensive mass screening is unsuitable and uneconomical for low incidence of oesophageal carcinoma. In 1978, 2,128 persons (1,577 men and 591 women) died from this cancer (19).

We looked for a simple and practicable method of detecting early oesophageal carcinomas in high-risk patients. The preliminary data of a current study are presented in this chapter.

MATERIALS AND METHODS

Routine upper GI-endoscopy was performed with Olympus forward-viewing endoscopes, type GIF-D 3 or GIF-HM. The oropharynx was sprayed with a contact anaesthetic before introduction of the endoscope. In general the patient had an i.v. injection of 10 mg diazepam. The oesophagus and cardia were examined carefully for every suspicious lesion (mucosal discoloration, surface irregularity, and motor disorders). Then Toluidine blue *in vivo* staining of the oesophageal mucosa was carried out under direct vision of the endoscope (12,17). The oesophagus was cleaned with a solution of 1% acetic acid and then the epithelium was stained with a solution of 2% Toluidine blue for 2 min. A thorough rinsing using 1% acetic acid again allowed an optimal examination of epithelium lesions that had been staining intensively violet. Multiple forceps biopsies and brush cytology were taken from these areas. The specimens were fixed in formalin and transferred to the pathologist for morphological analysis.

PATIENTS

Ten patients were examined to test the *in vivo* staining technique. These patients were suffering from dyspepsia or had a duodenal ulcer but had no eosophageal disease. Thirty-

TABLE 1. *Precancerous conditions of oesophageal cancer*

Barrett's oesophagus (2)
Achalasia (18)
Lye-strictures (1)
Tylosis palmaris et plantaris (15)
Plummer-Vinson syndrome (10)
Cancer of the stomach and bronchi (16)
Squamous carcinomas of the mouth and laryngo-pharynx (16)
(Celiac sprue disease)
(Scleroderma) (unproven)

Patients suffering from above-mentioned diseases are at high risk for developing carcinoma of the oesophagus. Numbers within parentheses indicate references.

two patients from a high-risk group for developing oesophageal carcinoma (Table 1) underwent our systematic screening program consisting of upper GI-endoscopy, Toluidine blue staining, multiple forceps biopsies, and brush cytology. We expected to find relevant discrepancies between normal mucosa and suspicious lesions.

RESULTS

Control Group

The control group (Table 2) consisted of 10 patients (7 men and 3 women), 28 to 72 years old. Mucosal abnormalities were not noticeable in the oesophagus. After *in vivo* staining with Toluidine blue, no stained areas could be found. Forceps biopsies and brush cytology were taken from the gastro-oesophageal junction and the lower third of the oesophagus showing normal squamous epithelium without inflammation or tumour signs.

High-Risk Patients

In 33 patients (26 men and 7 women), 28 to 87 years old ($\bar{x}$ 63 years); suffering from pyrosis, regurgitation, dysphagia, or already known oesophageal diseases (Table 3), upper

TABLE 2. *Results of endoscopic examination of control group*

Normal oesophagus
No stained areas (Toluidine blue)
Forceps biopsy: normal epithelium
Brush cytology: no tumour cells

Control group data: $n = 10$, 7 males and 3 females; 28–72 years old, $\bar{x} = 45$ years.

TABLE 3. *Data of the patients at high risk for oesophageal cancer*

n: 33, 26 males and 7 females
Age: 28–27 years, $\bar{x} = 63$ years
Symptoms: pyrosis, regurgitation, dysphagia, or known oesophageal disease

TABLE 4. *Results of endoscopy, vital staining, and histology in high-risk patients (n = 33)*

No.	Diagnosis	Endoscopy: suspicious lesions	*In vivo* staining positive[a]	Oesophageal early	Carcinoma advanced
9	Barrett's syndrome	1	6	1	1
6	Achalasia	0	1	1	0
2	Lye-stricture	0	1	0	0
5	Laryngo-pharynx Ca	0	0	0	0
8	Post-operative follow-up	3	3	0	3
1	Dysplasia	?	1	?	?
1	Oesophageal ulcer	1	1	0	1
1	Scleroderma	0	0	0	0

[a]Positive = circumscript stained areas.

GI-endoscopy and *in vivo* staining of the oesophageal mucosa were performed. The results are listed in Table 4.

In a 67-year-old man, a region of prominent epithelial nodules with a central ulcer was found at a distance of 30 cm from the incisor teeth. This lesion was already endoscopically suspected to be malignant. Toluidine blue staining discovered an intensively violet colour area. Biopsies obtained from this region verified a squamous carcinoma.

Two men with lye strictures of the oesophagus and 5 men with histologically proven squamous carcinoma of the laryngo-pharynx showed endoscopically no suspicious lesions or dyed areas. Forceps biopsy analysis from different sites of the oesophagus demonstrated mild dysplasia in one case of lye-stricture.

In the postoperative follow-up group, 3 patients had known recurrent oesophageal cancers proven by endoscopy and X-ray examination. Vital staining was performed to test the validity of Toluidine blue. In all cases the macroscopically visible tumour could be stained and in 2 patients multicentric lesions separated from the tumour could be detected. Biopsies taken from stained violet areas confirmed the diagnosis of carcinoma. The other 5 follow-ups failed to produce stained areas. A 77-year-old woman suffering from Barrett's syndrome for several years revealed on endoscopy oesophageal tumour signs proved by histology. Because of her very poor condition, oesophageal resection was impossible. Up to now one case is unresolved: a 62-year-old man who had histologically determined severe dysplasia in the middle part of the oesophagus. Control endoscopy is intended, since severe dysplasia should be followed by oesophageal resection.

Two interesting cases reflecting the efficiency of our *in vivo* staining method should be mentioned as brief case reports. A young man, age 40, had been suffering from postprandial substernal pain and regurgitation over a period of 3 months. Endoscopy and X-ray examination revealed a beginning achalasia. Some months later at control endoscopy the oesophagus was found dilated and contained some food and fluids. No epithelial abnormality could be demonstrated. Upon retroflexing the endoscope the cardia was normal as well. After Toluidine blue *in vivo* staining was performed, two intensively violet-dyed areas were found at the gastro-oesophageal junction. Forceps biopsies taken from these regions verified an adenocarcinoma. Although aware of the diagnosis, our radiologist could not reproduce the tumour finding (Fig. 1). The patient underwent fundectomy and resection of the lower part

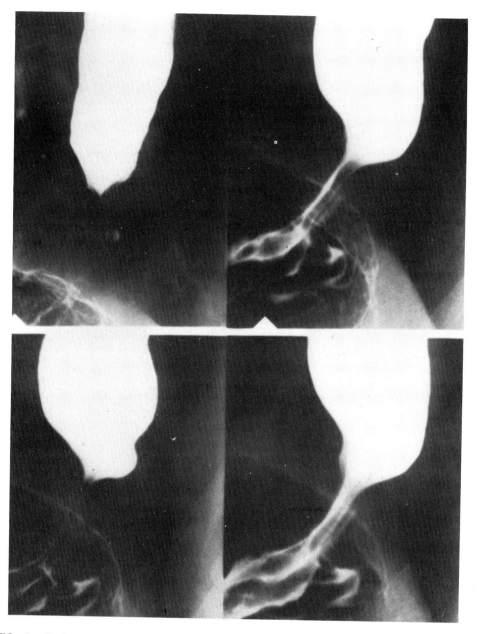

FIG. 1. Barium swallow examination of the gastro-oesophageal junction. It shows the dilated oesophagus but no hint of a tumour. (Photographs from X-ray pictures.)

of the oesophagus. The tumour had a diameter of 6 mm and the cancer was limited exclusively to the mucosa. Three months after resection the patient is still well and has no oesophageal symptoms.

The other man, age 57, had been suffering from intermittent dysphagia for 15 years. Hiatus hernia with additional reflux oesophagitis was diagnosed by X-ray barium swallow. At endoscopy erosive lesions lined the columnar-squamous epithelium border. The patient was treated with antacids for a period of 5 weeks and then a second endoscopy was performed. The oesophagus showed regular epithelium without any erosion. But Toluidine blue dyed circumscripted areas were seen at the gastro-oesophageal junction. Forceps biopsies histologically proved a squamous carcinoma of the oesophagus. At present, operative procedures are being discussed.

DISCUSSION

The endoscopic diagnosis of advanced oesophageal cancer is of little clinical interest because the prognosis is very poor. Only the diagnosis of early carcinoma cancers limited to the mucosa offers the chance of curable therapy with acceptable 5-year survival rates (3,6,7,9). Periodic and careful examination of the oesophagus in high-risk patients is necessary (4,15,16).

Sporadic reports of diagnosed early carcinomas (3,7,11–13) sparked our interest in the *in vivo* staining technique during upper GI-endoscopy. We are looking for patients at high risk to test the validity of this method. Our preliminary data since July 1981 encouraged us to continue the study and to investigate routinely additional patients. *In vivo* vital staining can supply better information about tiny but possibly malignant lesions of the oesophagus that are not visible to the naked eye (11–13).

A depressed mucosal surface associated with reddish colour change cannot easily be distinguished from normal mucosa. The use of Toluidine blue is of great value in such cases (13). This could be proved in our 40-year-old man in whom the oesophageal mucosa looked totally normal and the 59-year-old man demonstrating hiatus hernia and erosions in the distal oesophagus.

The vital staining method is not specific for tumourous changes, that is, peptic erosions, tears, fissures, and ulcers may be dyed as well. False positive results are seen, especially in Barrett's syndrome, where we found stained areas without malignant histological changes.

In general this simple and practicable technique supplies additional information for detecting dysplasia and early carcinoma. The investigation time is only slightly prolonged and patients do not suffer from any discomfort.

CONCLUSIONS

Careful endoscopic examination of the oesophagus should be done in high-risk patients. The vital staining method seems to offer some hope of detecting oesophageal carcinoma at a stage much earlier than currently realized. The method is useful in (a) defining the site of dysplasia or cancerous lesion; (b) discovering additional sites of cancer; (c) selecting relevant regions for biopsy and brush; and (d) detecting early carcinomas not visible at endoscopy.

REFERENCES

1. Appelquist, L. G., and Salmo, M. (1980): Lye Corrosion carcinoma of the oesophagus. A review of 63 cases. *Cancer*, 45:2655–2658.
2. Berenson, M. M., Riddell, R. H., Skinner, D. B., and Freston, J. W. (1978): Malignant transformation of the oesophageal columnar epithelium. *Cancer*, 41:554–561.
3. Burke, E. L., Sturm, J., and Williamson, D. (1978): The diagnosis of microscopic carcinoma of the oesophagus. *Dig. Dis.*, 23:148–151.
4. Crespi, M., Grassi, A., Amiri, G., Munos, N., Aramesh, B., and Mojtabai, A. (1979): Oesophageal lesions in northern Iran: A premalignant condition? *Lancet*, II:217–220.
5. Coordinating Group for Research on Oesophageal Cancer (1975): Studies on relationship between epithelial dysplasia and carcinoma of the oesophagus. *Chin. Med. J.*, 1:110–116.
6. Coordinating Group for Research on Oesophageal Cancer (1976): Early diagnosis and surgical treatment of oesophageal cancer under rural conditions. *Chin. Med. J.*, 2:113–116.

7. Endo, M., Kobayashi, S., Suzuki, H., Takemoto, T., and Nakayama, K. (1977): Diagnosis of early oesophageal cancer. *Endoscopy*, 2:61–66.
8. Epstein, S. S., Payne, P. M., and Shaw, H. J. (1960): Multiple primary malignant neoplasms in the air and upper food passages. *Cancer*, 13:137–142.
9. Huang, G. (1981): The oesophageal carcinoma in China—Early diagnosis and therapy. Endoscopy—Congress, Wiesbaden, West-Germany *(in press)*.
10. Larsson, L. G., Sandström, A., and Westling, P. (1975): Relationship of Plummer-Vinson disease to cancer of the upper alimentary tract in Sweden. *Cancer Res.*, 35:3308–3316.
11. Mandard, A. M., Tourneux, J., Gignoux, M., Blanc, L., Segol, P., and Mandard, J. C. (1980): In situ carcinoma of the oesophagus. Macroscopic study with particular reference to the Lugol test. *Endoscopy*, 12:51–57.
12. Miller, G., Maurer, W., Savary, M., Monnier, P., and Gloor, F. (1979): A case of oesophageal cancer limited to the mucosa and submucosa. *Endoscopy*, 3:175–177.
13. Monnier, P., Savary, M., Pasche, R., and Anani, P. (1981): Intraepithelial carcinoma of the oesophagus. Endoscopic morphology. *Endoscopy*, 13:185–191.
14. Morson, B. C. (1979): Tumours of the oesophagus. In: *Gastrointestinal Pathology*, edited by B. C. Morson and I. M. P. Dawson, pp. 33–57. Blackwell Scientific Publications, Oxford, London, Edinburgh, Melbourne.
15. Rösch, W. (1978): Gastrointestinal Karzinom—Risikogruppen. *Fortschr. Med.*, 92:102–107.
16. Teppermann, B. S., and Fitzpatrick, P. J. (1981): Second respiratory and upper digestive tract cancers after oral cancer. *Lancet*, II 8246:547–549.
17. Vaughan, C. W. (1972): Supravital staining of early diagnosis of carcinoma. *Otolaryngol. Clin. North Am.*, 5:301–302.
18. Wienbeck, M. (1978): Diagnostik und Therapie der Achalasie. *Int. Welt*, 1:392–400.
19. Wienbeck, M., Kivelitz, H., and Hanrth, R. D. (1981): Die Klinik des Oesophaguskarzinoms. *Int. Welt*, 7:285–296.

Precancerous Lesions of the Gastrointestinal Tract, edited by P. Sherlock, B.C. Morson, L. Barbara, and U. Veronesi. Raven Press, New York © 1983.

Markers of Cancer Risk in the Esophagus and Surveillance of High-Risk Groups

Kinichi Nabeya

Second Surgical Department of Kyorin University School of Medicine, Mitaka City, Tokyo 181, Japan

Nowadays, early diagnosis of patients with esophageal cancer is very difficult and the survival rate is very low. To solve this difficult problem, it is our urgent business to detect the early stage of esophageal cancer as soon as possible. However, we find reports on early esophageal cancer very occasionally in the world today (1,2,4,5,8,10–15,17,19,20) and most of them are case reports. Etiologically, Hirayama (7) reported that high incidence of esophageal cancer has a relation to the habits of smoking and drinking in Japan. Clinically, the existence of esophageal cancer patients in a family history and the presence of achalasia and corrosive esophagitis make it likely that we will observe a high incidence of esophageal cancer. We assume through the experimental study on esophageal cancer in rats that chronic stimulation helps cancer grow in the esophageal wall. We have collected only 177 cases of early esophageal cancer in Japan and made an attempt to investigate the clinico-pathologic problems in this field.

For the surveillance of high-risk groups, there are radiology, endoscopy, and biopsy including cytology as three weapons for the diagnosis of esophageal cancer, but these are still not ideal in some respects. Recently, we (16,17) have devised serial esophagogram and brushing cytology with capsule for early detection of esophageal cancer.

MATERIALS AND METHODS

The statistical analysis was done on the data from the Index of Public Welfare (6) in Japan. On the precancerous conditions of the esophagus, we have analyzed 159 consecutive esophageal cancers obtained in our department from 1974 to 1980.

In the experimental study on esophageal cancer, we used the Donryu rats 10 weeks old and administrated the feed mixing 0.25% N-methyl-benzylamin and 0.32% sodium nitrite as the carcinogens. Then we sacrificed the rats monthly until 6 months after the administration of the carcinogens and observed the cancerous change pathologically. For the clinico-pathologic analysis of early esophageal cancer, which is defined in Japan (9) as a kind of cancer whose depth of invasion should be confined to the submucosa without any metastasis, we have collected 177 cases of such cancer in Japan during the period 1966 to 1979 and analyzed the collected data statistically.

For the surveillance of high-risk groups, we have devised new methods of serial esophagram and brushing cytology with capsule. With the serial esophagogram (17), it is possible to take five serial pictures automatically at regular intervals of 1, 3, 5, 7, and 9 sec after a patient swallows barium once. The instrument for brushing cytology with a capsule (16) consists of a brush within a capsule (Fig. 1). The patient swallows the capsule into the stomach with some water (Fig. 2). About 10 min later, the capsule melts and the brush expands. Then the brush is pulled out; it scrubs the esophageal mucosa and collects cells, which are smeared onto a glass slide, fixed, stained, and observed histologically. We routinely stained it using Papanicolau's method.

RESULTS

Statistical Analysis of Esophageal Cancer in Japan

The entire population of Japan is about 100 million and the death rate for esophageal cancer is about 5,000 each year. The mortality rate from esophageal cancer among male and female is about 7.3 and 2.1, respectively, totaling 4.2 per 100,000 in Japan. In the mortality rate by age incident, it is observed that for persons over 60 years old, it increases remarkably, nearly as high as 50 per 100,000 among 70- and 80-year olds.

Every year in Japan only 20 cases of early esophageal cancer are detected. But we know from the natural history of the disease that the duration of illness, from the early stage until death, is estimated to be about 2 to 3 years. Therefore, the total number of esophageal cancer patients may amount to 15,000, of which 5,000 are going to die within one year, 5,000 with advanced cancer will expire next year, leaving 5,000 asymtomatic patients with early cancer that we are unable to detect (Fig. 3).

Precancerous Conditions of the Esophagus

Among 159 esophageal cancer patients in our department, 85.8% of 134 male patients and 32.0% of 25 female patients smoke. Drinking occurs in 81.3% of the males and 28.0% of the females, and 6.7% of the males and 56.0% of the females were negative in both.

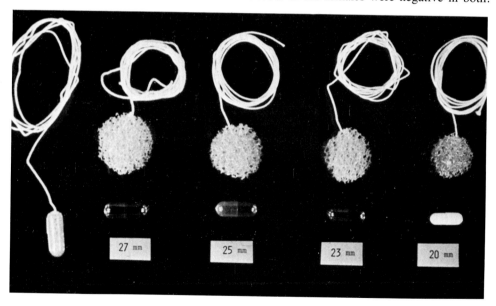

FIG. 1. Instrument for brushing cytology with capsule. Each capsule enclosing a brush of a different size, from 20 mm to 27 mm in diameter.

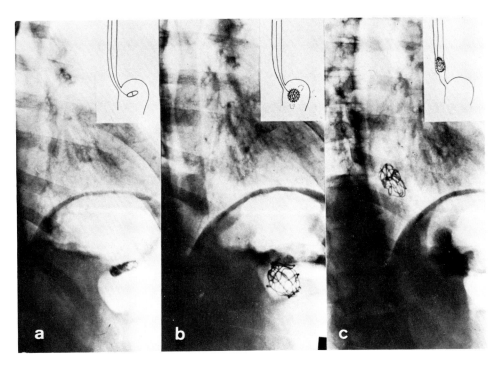

FIG. 2. X-ray findings from brushing cytology with capsule. **a:** The capsule swallowed into the stomach; **b:** capsule melts and the brush expands in the stomach; **c:** the brush scrubs the esophageal mucosa.

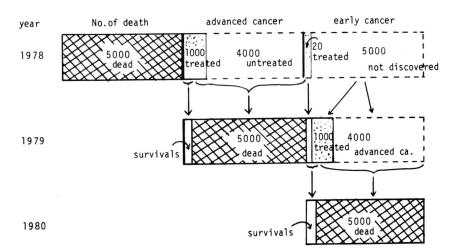

FIG. 3. Estimated number of esophageal cancer patients in Japan.

This shows the higher incidence of cancer in the group with smoking habits than in both negative groups.

According to the same study on 159 patients, a positive family history for cancer in all sites was found in 44 patients (27.7%) and 5 patients of the last group (11.4%) had a positive family history for esophageal cancer. It is clear that people with a positive family history should be considered high risk because esophageal cancer represents only 4% of all cancers in Japan.

Many esophageal diseases are considered to be predisposed towards cancer. The duration of symptoms in achalasia associated with the esophageal cancer is shown in Table 1. A greater number of years with this history is clearly correlated with a higher incidence of esophageal cancer. The location of esophageal cancer associated with achalasia is shown in Table 2. The frequency of the same location clearly indicates in many series, as in our own, a predirection for the middle esophagus; food stasis is more frequent in this portion.

Accordingly, we experienced this same condition in a 51-year-old female patient who had corrosive esophagitis since she was 3 years old because she drank caustic soda by mistake. A stenosis followed and since then, she has had a liquid oral intake. Figure 4 shows her esophagograms at ages 50 and 51 in another hospital. An advanced cancer developed at the upper side of the caustic stenotic portion 1 year later.

The influence of irradiation therapy in inducing malignant change can be suggested. This idea was confirmed when we found four cases of esophageal cancer among people who received irradiation therapy for cervical lymph node tuberculosis. Figure 5 shows such an esophagogram of a 72-year-old female patient who received irradiation therapy at the neck 20 years earlier.

Experimental Studies on Esophageal Cancer in Rats

These results are some preliminary reports of esophageal cancer growth in rats (Table 3). After 1 month, only hyperplastic change and mild dysplasia were found in the esophageal

TABLE 1. *Location of esophageal cancer associated with achalasia*

Location	No. of cases in the world	No. of cases in our dept.[a]	Total (%)
Upper esophagus	4	3	7 (7.9)
Middle esophagus	45	7	52 (58.4)
Lower esophagus	26	1	27 (30.3)
Unknown	3	0	3 (3.4)
Total	78	11	89 (100.0)

[a]Including cases of Chiba University.

TABLE 2. *Duration of symptoms in achalasia associated with esophageal cancer*

Duration (yr)	No. of cases in the world	No. of cases in our dept.[a]	Total (%)
<11	15	2	17 (19.1)
11–20	32	4	36 (40.4)
21–30	19	2	21 (23.6)
>30	10	3	13 (14.6)
Unknown	2	0	2 (2.3)
Total	78	11	89 (100.0)

[a]Including cases of Chiba University.

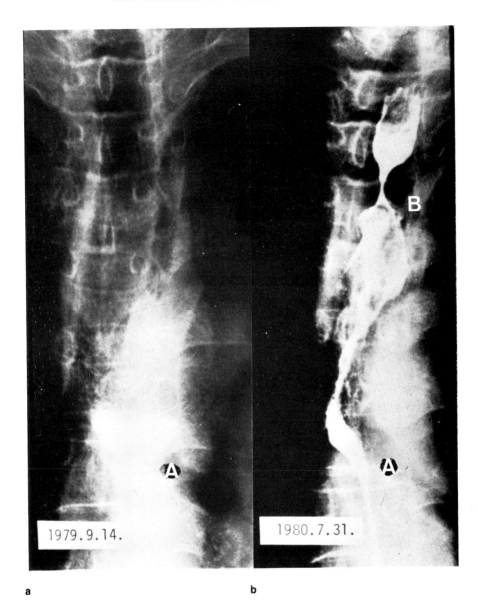

a   b

FIG. 4. X-ray findings of corrosive esophagitis. **a:** The caustic stenotic portion is observed at the lower esophagus *(A)*. **b:** An advanced cancer is developed at the upper esophagus *(B)* 1 year later.

mucosa. After 3 months, different types of polypoid lesions were observed. After 4 months, we observed a cancer lesion, which started from the basic stratum.

Clinico-pathologic Analysis of Early Esophageal Cancer

Among 177 cases of early esophageal cancer in Japan, invasion was limited to intraepithelium in 17 cases (9.6%), to lamina muscularis mucosa in 20 (11.3%), and to submucosa in 140 (79.0%).

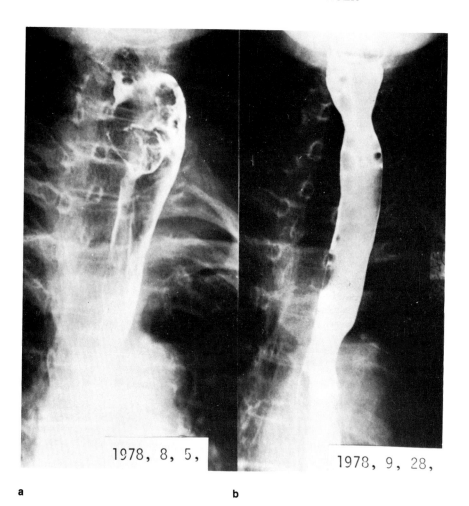

1978, 8, 5,

1978, 9, 28,

a   b

FIG. 5. X-ray findings of an esophageal cancer patient who received irradiation therapy for cervical lymph node tuberculosis. **a:** X-ray finding taken before preoperative irradiation. **b:** X-ray finding taken after preoperative irradiation. Radiation effects were remarkable and the patient is healthy 3 years after the radical operation.

According to the location of the lesion, the physiologic structures are not predirection places for early esophageal cancer. But malignant changes were almost always observed in continuous upper regions. According to the horizontal location of early esophageal cancer in the cervical esophagus (Ce), most of the cases occurred in the posterior wall (62%). In the middle esophagus (I), differences were not so relevant and more cases in the lateral walls were observed. In the lower esophagus (E), the location of the lesions were circumferentially present in a more regular fashion (Table 4).

Characteristics of the chief complaints of early esophageal cancer are a sense of stenosis and chest pain on swallowing, and dysphagia; however, depending on the type of cancer, complaints differ. There is more dysphagia in the tumorous type and more chest pain in the ulcerative type; also note that 16% showed no complaints (Table 5).

The longitudinal diameter of early esophageal cancer varied from less than 10 mm to over 80 mm. Generally, the majority of early esophageal cancerous tumors were found to have

TABLE 3. *Cancerous change of esophagus in rats with administration of carcinogens*

Types of lesion	Months after administration of carcinogens (No. of cases)				
	1 (19)	2 (21)	3 (20)	4 (22)	6 (21)
Fungoid verruca	5	3	8	5	7
Villous papilloma	12	15	17	13	10
Fibroepithelial papilloma	1	8	15	16	11
Digitating papilloma	0	0	8	15	19
Carcinoma	0	0	0	4	13

TABLE 4. *Horizontal location of lesion of early esophageal cancer[a]*

	Anterior	Right	Left	Posterior	Circumferential
Cervical esophagus (Ce) 13 cases	0%	23%	0%	62%	15%
Middle esophagus (I) 126 cases	8%	18%	12%	46%	16%
Lower esophagus (E) 38 cases	21%	13%	16%	24%	26%

[a]One-hundred seventy-seven cases collected in Japan, 1979.

TABLE 5. *Chief complaints of early esophageal cancer[a]*

Complaint	No. of cases (%)
Chest pain when swallowing	47 (26.6)
Sense of stenosis when swallowing	46 (26.0)
Dysphagia	34 (19.2)
Epigastralgia	15 (8.5)
Vomiting	4 (2.3)
Heartburn	3 (1.7)
Hematemesis	3 (1.7)
Anorexia	3 (1.7)
Fatigue	3 (1.7)
Emaciation	1 (0.6)
No complaints	28 (15.8)

[a]One-hundred seventy-seven cases collected in Japan, 1979.

a diameter of less than 30 mm (Table 6). According to the histologic findings, 90.4% are squamous cell carcinoma, the other special types are adenocarcinoma in 2.3%, adenoacanthoma in 1.7%, undifferentiated carcinoma in 1.7%, and miscellaneous carcinoma in 3.9%.

TABLE 6. *Longitudinal diameter of
early esophageal cancer[a]*

Diameter (mm)	No. of cases (%)
<11	16 (9.0)
11–20	43 (24.3)
21–30	56 (31.7)
31–40	23 (13.0)
41–50	17 (9.6)
51–60	10 (5.6)
61–70	4 (2.3)
71–80	2 (1.1)
>80	3 (1.7)
Unknown	3 (1.7)

[a]One-hundred seventy-seven cases collected in Japan, 1979.

Characteristics of these special types are considered polypoid grossly.

We broadly classified the growing type of early esophageal cancer into three types: elevated, superficial, and depressed (Fig. 6). There are only 12 cases of minute cancers and all of them were intraepithelial cancers. The intraepithelial spreading pattern of the disease

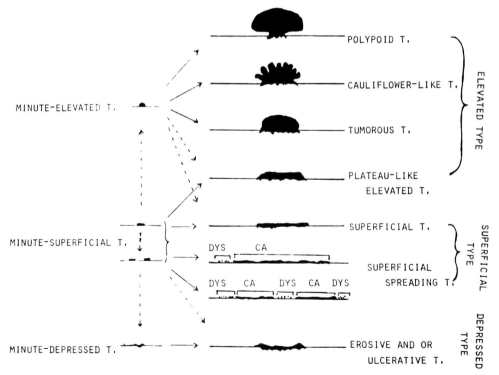

FIG. 6. Growing type of early esophageal cancer. CA: cancer. DYS: Dysplasia. (From Nabeya, ref. 15a, with permission.)

must also be considered for a better knowledge of the natural history of this condition. We also found lymphatic invasion in 25.4% and vascular invasion in 7.9%, in which cancer developed from muscularis mucosa to submucosa and distant metastasis can easily be expected. We have observed that the basal cells actually play an important role in the occurrence of squamous cell cancer. These cells can easily become dysplastic under the action of some stimulants and finally can become cancerous, whence downgrowth, upward proliferation, and/or intraepithelial spread will follow. If the lamina muscularis mucosa has been penetrated by downgrowth of cancer, lymphatic and vascular invasion does occur and the risk of distant metastasis becomes dramatically high (Fig. 7).

Follow-up results of early esophageal cancer were excellent and its 5-year survival rate was 87.9% (relative survival rate). However, it differs depending on the depth of invasion—it was better in intraepithelium (100%) and muscularis mucosa (88%) but poorer in submucosa (76%).

Method of Early Detection for Esophageal Cancer and for the Surveillance of High-Risk Groups

Figure 8 shows the serial esophagogram of a normal case. The filling picture, double-contrast picture, and relief picture can be seen in 1 sec, 3 to 5 sec, and 7 to 9 sec, respectively. Then we measured the contractibility of the maximum and minimum width of the esophageal wall (Table 7). In the case of the superficial type cancer that has invaded the submucosa, the contractibility in that region of cancer is almost the same as a normal case. But when the cancer invaded deeply into neighboring structures such as the aorta, it decreases less than 3 mm.

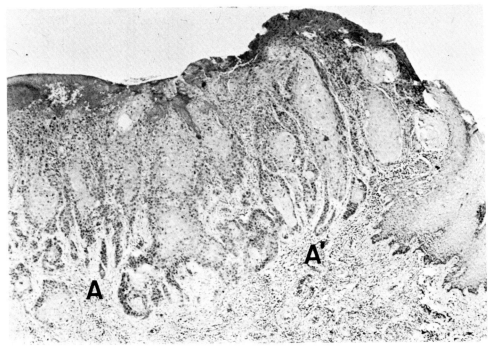

FIG. 7. The histology shows well-differentiated squamous cell carcinoma in a case of early cancer. The lamina muscularis mucosa has been penetrated by downgrowth of cancer and drop invasion is evident (*A,A'*).

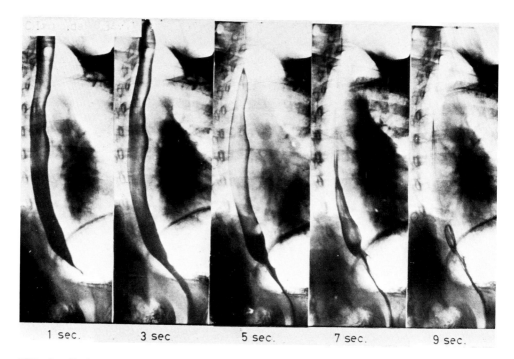

1 sec.   3 sec   5 sec.   7 sec.   9 sec.

FIG. 8. Serial esophagograms of a normal case (34-year-old female). (From Nabeya, ref. 15a, with permission.)

TABLE 7. *Depth of invasion and contractibility between minimum and maximum diameter at the cancer lesion of esophageal wall in nonirradiated cases[a]*

Depth of invasion	No. of cases	Contractibility (mm) mean value (min.–max.)
Normal	100	11.3 (6–20)
Invasion to submucosa (sm)	9	10.7 (6–17)
Invasion to muscularis propria (mp)	11	6.9 (4–12)
Doubtful invasion to adventitia (a_1)	3	6.0 (3–8)
Definite invasion to adventitia (a_2)	15	2.4 (1–6)
Invasion to neighboring structures (a_3)	14	1.7 (0–3)

[a]Examination by serial esophagograms in Kyorin University, 1980.

Next on the brushing cytology with capsule, we can collect about 100,000 cells every time from the esophageal mucosa by one brushing. Results of brushing cytology with capsule are shown in Table 8. False negative cases were 4 in 74 cases of esophageal cancer, and false positive cases were 1 in 174 cases of normal and/or benign diseases. The total diagnostic rate in 74 consecutive cancer cases was 77.0%, and it was 94.6% including class III (Table 9). Diagnosis accuracy was higher in early and serrated type cancers. Figures 9 through 13 show one such early cancer. Up to now we have utilized these methods of detecting 6 cases of early esophageal cancer in our department.

TABLE 8. *Results of brushing cytology with capsule for esophageal diseases (Kyorin University, 1980)*

Diseases	Class I	Class II	Class III	Class IV	Class V
Esophageal cancer 74 cases	0	4	13	24	33
Cardiac cancer 22 cases	0	4	0	9	9
Recurrence of esophagocardiac cancer 5 cases	0	0	3	1	1
Normal and/or benign diseases 174 cases	76	96	1	1[a]	0
Mass examination 3,436 cases	2380	1045	10	1[b]	

[a]Esophageal ulcer.
[b]Cardiac cancer.

TABLE 9. *Results of brushing cytology with capsule according to the X-ray type of esophageal cancer (Kyorin University, 1980)*

X-ray type	Class I	Class II	Class III	Class IV	Class V	Positive diagnostic rate of IV & V[a] (%)
Superficial type 8 cases	0	0	0	5	3	100.0
Tumorous type 8 cases	0	1	0	3	4	87.5
Serrated type 10 cases	0	0	0	2	8	100.0
Spiral type 40 cases	0	3	10	12	15	67.5
Funnelled type 8 cases	0	0	3	2	3	62.5
Total 74 cases	0	4	13	24	33	77.0

[a]Positive diagnostic rate including class III, IV and V is 94.6%.

DISCUSSION

Concerning the statistical analysis of esophageal cancer incidence, the ratio is only 1 to 10, but because gastric cancer yields the highest mortality cancer rate in Japan, we cannot say that the disease is very rare. Referring to the mortality rate of esophageal cancer by sex and age incident, it can be said that it is one of the geriatric diseases (3) in males.

When we speak of esophageal cancer, this includes from early to moderately to clearly advanced stages. As shown in the case of corrosive esophagitis, the duration of the illness takes only 1 to 2 years. We found that the development of esophageal cancer is much faster

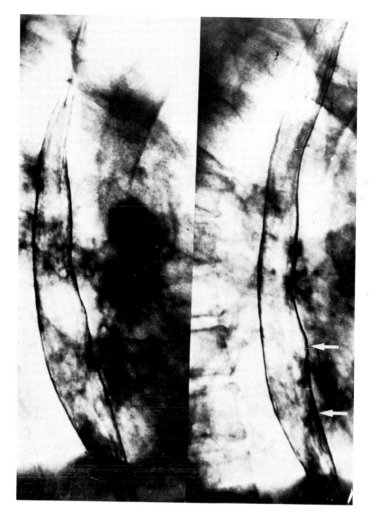

FIG. 9. Double-contrast X-ray findings of a 72-year-old male patient with early esophageal cancer. Slight roughness of the esophageal mucosa can be seen, but not so clearly.

than any other gastrointestinal cancer according to the retrospective natural history. Now it is our urgent business to detect patients in the early stages of esophageal cancer.

Etiologically, Hirayama (7) reported on the standardized mortality rate for esophageal cancer that in daily smokers is 3.26 times that of nonsmokers and in daily drinkers is 1.82 times that of nondrinkers. He has also found that there is a high cancer risk among people who usually eat a special kind of Japanese wild grass (bracken type) or who eat very hot gruel. Concerning the family history, it is worth noting that in members of the same family, location, gross, and histologic type were similar. We know also the case of a twin brother of a patient with advanced esophageal cancer. He was investigated for the disease, although asymptomatic, and early cancer was detected.

In the esophageal diseases considered to be precancerous conditions, we experienced some instances of esophageal cancer among patients who have a long history of achalasia, corrosive esophagitis, and irradiation for cervical lymph node tuberculosis. These results could be explained by chronic stimulation, which is regarded as one of the main causes of cancer

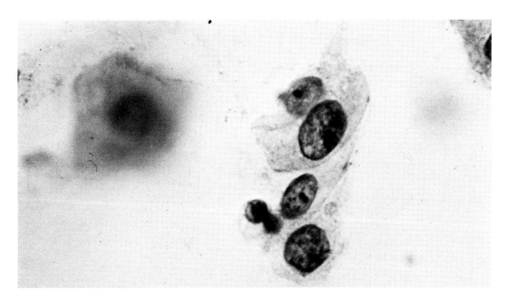

FIG. 10. The cytologic report by our brushing cytology with capsule, in which cancer cells can be seen.

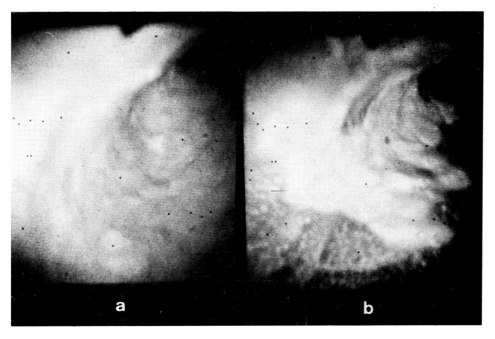

FIG. 11. Endoscopic findings. **a:** The superficial erosion at the posterior wall. **b:** The findings by Lugol dyeing method. The cancer lesion is observed more clearly not stained by Lugol dye.

development. Plummer-Vinson syndrome is thought to be a precancerous condition, but we did not see cancer cases associated with this syndrome. The preliminary results on the experimental studies of esophageal cancer in rats also stress the dangerous action of a prolonged stimulus over the esophageal mucosa.

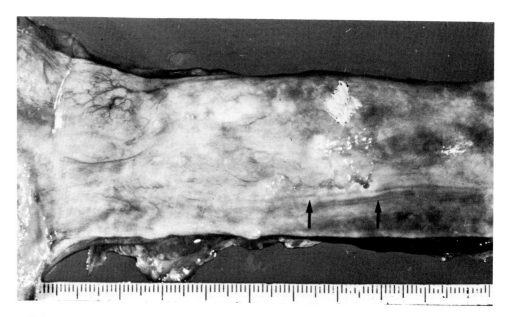

FIG. 12. Resected specimen shows the superficial erosion (20 mm ×14 mm in size).

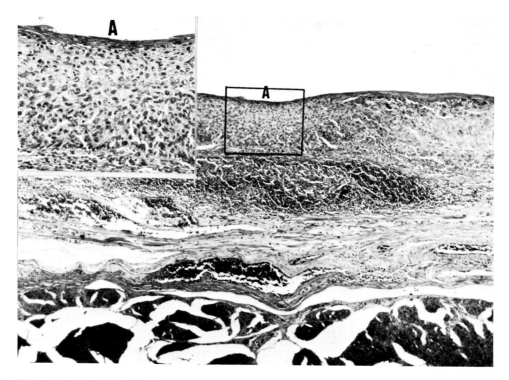

FIG. 13. The histology shows the poorly differentiated squamous carcinoma *(A)*, and the depth of invasion is limited to intraepithelium.

Concerning the horizontal location of early esophageal cancer, that data once more stress the importance of a chronic stimulus and its possible relation with carcinogenesis. In fact food first hits the posterior wall of the hypopharynx and cervical esophagus.

Regarding chief complaints, more than 16% of patients had no complaints and this was true for almost all patients with an intraepithelial cancer. Therefore, thorough examination and follow-up of high-risk patients is strongly suggested.

Generally, radiology, endoscopy, and biopsy including cytology are used for detecting esophageal cancer. With regard to the radiologic examination, Yamada et al. (19), Zernoza et al. (20), and Katayama et al. (10) reported on the value of double-contrast esophagography. Endo et al. (5), Toriie et al. (18), Miller et al. (13), and Mandard et al. (12) mentioned that the dye scattering method in endoscopy is useful in detecting early esophageal cancer. Imbriglia et al. (8) reported at first on the cytologic examination of sediment from the esophagus, and Bishop et al. (1) also reported on a case of *in situ* carcinoma detected by the cytologic method. Currently, brushing cytology is being employed for esophageal cancer. The Chinese Academy of Medical Sciences (2) reported on the excellent results obtained by using a double-lumen rubber tube with an abrasive balloon. Maimon et al. (11), Dowlatshahi et al. (4), and Mortensen et al. (14) reported the value of the combined use of endoscopy and brushing cytology, but these have not yet been perfected.

As was already mentioned, early detection is the best weapon against esophageal cancer. However, there are many difficulties in early detection. The following guidelines are suggested:

1. Mass eduction on early esophageal cancer must be promoted.
2. Patients should be seen by doctors as soon as possible.
3. Systemic examination by trained doctors must be performed to avoid misdiagnosis.
4. Mass examination (2,4) for high-risk groups, especially older males and people with a positive family history and chronic esophageal disease, should be conducted.

We are going to study mass examination (17), but many social problems remain.

Finally, our devised methods for early diagnosis do a good job in early detection of esophageal cancer. Moreover, they are easy to use and do not stress the patient. But what we need now is a better definition of the risk group in this field, because generalized screening is not possible for economic and practical reasons. Thus, more research must be done in order to better understand early cancer pathogenesis.

ACKNOWLEDGMENTS

This work was supported in part by a Grant in Aid for Cancer Research 55-S and 56-S from the Ministry of Health and Welfare. All the members of the Japanese Society for Esophageal Diseases took part in the research described herein.

REFERENCES

1. Bishop, D., Lushpian, A., and Louis, C. (1977): The cytology of carcinoma in situ and early invasive carcinoma of the esophagus. *Acta Cytol.*, 21:298–300.
2. Chinese Academy of Medical Sciences and Honan Province, the Coordinating Group for the Research of Esophageal Carcinoma (1973): The early detection of carcinoma of the esophagus. *Sci. Sin.*, 16:457–463.
3. Chinese Academy of Medical Sciences and Honan Province, Esophageal Carcinoma Research Coordinating Groups (1974): Studies on relationship between epithelial dysplasia and carcinoma of the esophagus. *Chin. Med. J.*, 11:679–681.
4. Dowlatshahi, K., Daneshbod, A., and Mobarhan, S. (1978): Early detection of cancer of esophagus along Caspian Littoral—Report of a pilot project. *Lancet*, 1:125–126.

5. Endo, M., Kobayashi, S., Suzuki, H., Takamoto, T., and Nakayama, K. (1971): Diagnosis of early esophageal cancer. *Endoscopy*, 3:61–66.
6. Health and Welfare Statistics Association (1980): *Index of Public Welfare*. Health and Welfare Statistics Association, Tokyo.
7. Hirayama, T. (1974): Prospective studies of cancer epidemiology based on census population in Japan. In: *Cancer Epidemiology, Environmental Factors*, edited by P. Bucalossi, U. Veronesi, and N. Cascinelli, pp. 3:26–35. Proceedings XI International Cancer Congress, Florence, Excerpta Medica, American, Elsevier.
8. Imbriglia, J. E., and Lopusniak, M. S. (1949): Cytologic examination of sediment from the esophagus in a case of intraepidermal carcinoma of the esophagus. *Gastroenterology*, 13:457–463.
9. Japanese Society for Esophageal Diseases (1976): Guide Lines for the Clinical and Pathologic Studies on Carcinoma of the Esophagus. *Jpn. J. Surg.*, 6:69–86.
10. Katayama, H., Nakai, A., Sakai, Y., and Matsuda, H. (1981): A radiological study of early esophageal carcinoma—with special reference to the superficial flat lesions. *Nippon Acta Radiol.*, 41:194–201.
11. Maimon, H. N., Drekin, R. B., and Cocco, A. E. (1974): Positive esophageal cytology without detectable neoplasm. *Gastrointest. Endosc.*, 5:107–111.
12. Mandard, A. M., Tourneux, J., Gignoux, M., Blanc, L., Segol, P., and Mandard, J. C. (1980): In situ carcinoma of the esophagus—Macroscopic study with particular reference to the Lugol test. *Endoscopy*, 12:51–57.
13. Miller, G., Mauer, W., Savary, M., Monnier, P., and Gloor, F. (1979): A case of oesophageal cancer limited to the mucosa and submucosa. *Endoscopy*, 3:175–178.
14. Mortensen, N. J. McC., and Mackenzie, E. F. D. (1981): Accuracy of oesophageal brush cytology: results of a prospective study and multicentre slide exchange. *Br. J. Surg.*, 68:513–515.
15. Nabeya, K. (1970): Early carcinoma of the esophagus. Stomach and Intestine, 5:1205–1213.
16. Nabeya, K., Onozawa, K., and Ri, S. (1979): Brushing cytology with capsule for esophageal cancer. *Chir. Gastroenterol.*, 13:101–107.
17. Nabeya, K., Onozawa, K., and Ri, S. (1979): Screening method for early detection of esophageal cancer. *Stomach Intestine*, 14:1325–1331.
18. Toriie, S., Kohli, Y., Akasaka, Y., and Kawai, K. (1975): New trial for endoscopical observation of esophagus by dye scattering method. *Endoscopy*, 7:75–79.
19. Yamada, A., Kobayashi, S., Kakumae, Y., Ogino, T., Ohmura, H., Ide, H., Endo, M., and Nakayama, K. (1975): Study on x-ray findings of superficial esophageal cancer. *Jpn. J. Gastroenterol. Surg.*, 8:334–342.
20. Zernoza, J., and Lindell, Jr., M. M. (1980): Radiologic evaluation of small esophageal carcinoma. *Gastrointest. Radiol.*, 5:107–111.

Precancerous Lesions of the Gastrointestinal Tract, edited by P. Sherlock, B.C. Morson, L. Barbara, and U. Veronesi. Raven Press, New York © 1983.

Carcinogenicity of Styrene Oxide on the Rat's Forestomach: An Example of the Contribution of Experimental Bioassays to the Study of Gastrointestinal Carcinogenesis

Cesare Maltoni

Institute of Oncology, S. Orsola Hospital, 40138 Bologna, Italy

Undoubtedly, in every field of medicine, the availability of proper experimental models speeds research and makes it possible to produce objective results, at the same time avoiding inadequate and often unethical trials in humans. In recent years, the demonstration that adequate long-term carcinogenicity bioassays are highly predictive for the identification and quantification of oncogenic risks to humans has brought about tremendous progress in the prevention of environmental tumours.

In the field of gastrointestinal oncology, suitable human-equivalent experimental models may be of great help in several ways, namely

1. in identifying carcinogenic factors and agents for one or more gastrointestinal segments, and in assessing the level of risk;
2. in learning about the different steps of the natural history of gastrointestinal tract tumours, and their sequence and interrelationship, with particular regard to the identification and characterization of precancerous lesions;
3. in determining the potentialities of some diagnostic methodologies;
4. and, finally, in testing the potentialities of therapeutic protocols, with particular reference to antiblastic drugs.

It is known that, in rats, the forestomach mucosa is of the same type as the oesophageal one in the same species, as well as in humans.

Epithelial tumours of the forestomach have been produced in experimental rodents (mice, rats, hamsters, and guinea pigs) by a variety of carcinogenic agents, including polycyclic hydrocarbons, nitrosamines, aromatic nitrogen compounds, and triazenes (1).

This chapter deals with the carcinogenicity of styrene oxide on the rat's forestomach. Styrene oxide is a colorless-to-pale-straw-coloured liquid. This compound is important because of its industrial production and because it is thought to be the possible active metabolite of styrene, which is one of the most highly produced monomers used in the plastics industry.

The worldwide industrial production of styrene oxide is estimated to be about 3,000 tons per year. It is used as a reactive diluent in epoxy resins to reduce the viscosity of mixed systems prior to curing, as an intermediate in the preparation of agricultural and biological chemicals, cosmetics, and surface coatings, in the treatment of textiles and fibers, and as a raw material for the production of phenylstearyl alcohol used in perfume.

TABLE 1. *Distribution of the forestomach epithelial tumours (benign and malignant)*

Group no.	Concentration	Sex	Animals (Sprague-Dawley rats, 13 weeks old at start) No. at start	Corrected no.[a]	Animals with forestomach epithelial tumors[b] No.	%[c]	Average latency time (weeks)[d]	Histotype Papillomas and acanthomas No.	%[c]	Average latency time (weeks)[d]	Squamocellular carcinomas Total No.	%[c]	Average latency time (weeks)[d]	Extension In situ No.	%[c]	Invasive No.	%[c]
I	250 mg/kg	M	40	39	19	48.7	107.7	7	17.9	109.1	16	41.0	110.9	16	41.0	8	20.5
		F	40	38	21	55.3	106.8	5	13.1	107.2	20	52.6	105.3	16	42.1	10	26.3
		Total	80	77	40	51.9	107.2	12	15.6	108.3	36	46.7	107.8	32	41.5	18	23.4
II	50 mg/kg	M	40	39	10	25.6	100.3	3	7.7	108.0	9	23.1	104.9	6	15.4	5	12.8
		F	40	37	7	18.9	121.1	2	5.4	130.0	7	18.9	121.1	7	18.9	1	2.5
		Total	80	76	17	22.4	108.9	5	6.6	116.8	16	21.0	112.0	13	17.1	6	7.9
III	Olive oil (control)	M	40	39	0	—	—	0	—	—	0	—	—	0	—	0	—
		F	40	40	0	—	—	0	—	—	0	—	—	0	—	0	—
		Total	80	79	0	—	—	0	—	—	0	—	—	0	—	0	—
Total			240	232													

[a]Alive animals after 17 weeks, when the first forestomach epithelial tumour was observed.
[b]More than 1 tumour may be present in the same animal.
[c]The percentages are referred to corrected numbers.
[d]Average time from the start of the experiment.

There have been no studies prior to the present one on the long-term general effects of styrene oxide in experimental animals, and there are no available epidemiological studies on exposed populations. The only long-term tests are two carcinogenicity studies on mice by skin application, in which no increase in the incidence of cutaneous tumours was observed (3,4).

In 1976 we started long-term carcinogenicity bioassays on styrene oxide. Early results of this experiment have been previously published (2).

MATERIALS AND METHODS

Male and female Sprague-Dawley rats, 13 weeks old, were treated by ingestion (stomach tube) with styrene oxide at the dose levels of 250 and 50 mg/kg body weight in olive oil, and with olive oil alone (controls), once daily, four to five times weekly, for 52 weeks, and then allowed to remain alive until spontaneous death. The plan of the experiment is given in Table 1. The experiment lasted 156 weeks.

During the experiment the animals were controlled every 2 weeks; they were weighed every 2 weeks during the period of treatment, and then every 8 weeks.

All the detectable gross pathological changes were recorded during the control. The animals, when moribund, were isolated in order to avoid cannibalism.

A complete autopsy was made on each animal. Histological examinations were performed on Zymbal glands, interscapular brown fat, salivary glands, tongue, lungs, liver, kidneys, adrenals, spleen, stomach, different segments of the intestine, bladder, brain, and any other organ with pathological lesions.

RESULTS

The results showed that styrene oxide is a very potent direct carcinogen for forestomach epithelium, producing a variety of benign and malignant tumours and tumour precursors. The data are shown in Tables 1 and 2.

In the forestomach of the treated animals, with or without tumours, one or more precursor lesions, that is, simple hyperplasia, acanthomatosis, and squamous dysplasia (Fig. 1), were frequently found.

Acanthomas, papillomas, and *in situ* (Fig. 2), microinvasive (Fig. 3), and invasive (Figs. 4–6) squamous carcinomas of the forestomach were observed at the two studied dose levels, with a clear-cut dose-response relationship. Invasive carcinomas often metastasize to the liver (Figs. 7, 8). More than one of these tumours may be observed in the same animal, in different parts of the organ.

It is interesting to note that precancerous lesions, benign tumours, or early carcinomas were not associated with inflammatory changes.

A very mild oedema was the only submucosal lesion found associated with some proliferative lesions; however, it was independent of the nature of the lesion itself (hyperplastic, dysplastic, or malignant).

It should be pointed out that epithelial tumours of the forestomach are rare in the colony of rats used in our laboratory. Among the historical control rats of our laboratory, kept under the same conditions and controlled and examined in the same standard way, we found the following incidence: 27 benign epithelial tumours (papillomas and acanthomas) (1.14%) out of 2,376 untreated rats; 9 benign epithelial tumours (1.40%) and 1 carcinoma (0.16%) out of 644 rats, treated by ingestion (stomach tube) with a daily dose of 0.6 to 1.2 ml olive oil, given 4 to 5 days weekly for 52 to 59 weeks.

TABLE 2. Distribution of the forestomach precursor lesions

Group no.	Concentration	Animals (Sprague-Dawley rats, 13 weeks old at start)		Animals with precursor lesions[a]			Histotype					
		Sex	No. at start	No.	%[b]	Average latency time (weeks)[c]	Simple hyperplasia		Acanthom-atosis		Squamous dysplasia	
							No.	%[b]	No.	%[b]	No.	%[b]
I	250 mg/kg	M	40	14	35.0	96.3	0	—	3	7.5	11	27.5
		F	40	12	30.0	75.2	2	5.0	4	10.0	6	15.0
		Total	80	26	32.5	86.6	2	2.5	7	8.7	17	21.2
II	50 mg/kg	M	40	5	12.5	98.0	0	—	1	2.5	4	10.0
		F	40	7	17.5	104.1	0	—	3	7.5	5	12.5
		Total	80	12	15.0	101.6	0	—	4	5.0	9	11.2
III	Olive oil (control)	M	40	1	2.5	69.0	0	—	1	2.5	0	—
		F	40	2	5.0	105.5	0	—	1	2.5	1	2.5
		Total	80	3	3.7	93.3	0	—	2	2.5	1	1.2
Total			240									

[a]More than 1 lesion may be present in the same animal.
[b]The percentages are referred to the number at start.
[c]Average time from the start of the experiment.

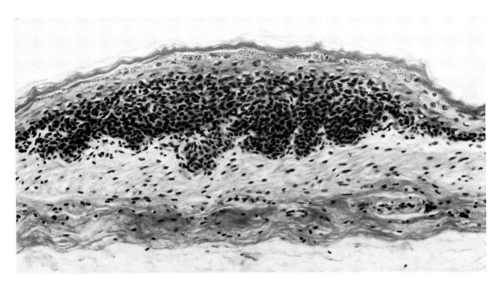

FIG. 1. Forestomach squamous dysplasia. H.-E. × 180.

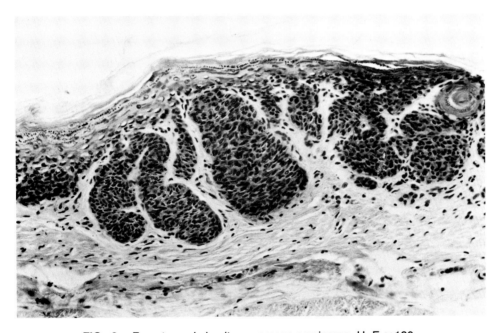

FIG. 2. Forestomach *in situ* squamous carcinoma. H.-E. × 180.

CONCLUSIONS

The results of the present experiment show that styrene oxide is a potent direct carcinogen that calls for preventive measures and for the protection of populations exposed to this compound. Moreover, in the light of these data, although the results of long-term bioassays of styrene in rats performed in our institute failed to show clear carcinogenic effects under

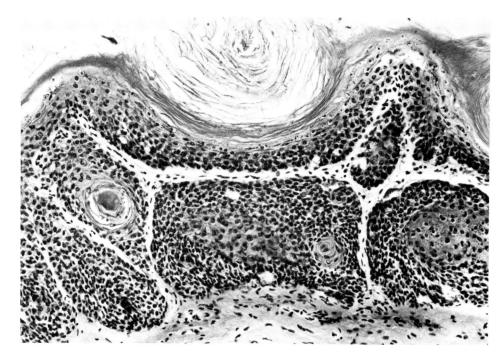

FIG. 3.   Forestomach squamous microinvasive carcinoma. H.-E. × 180.

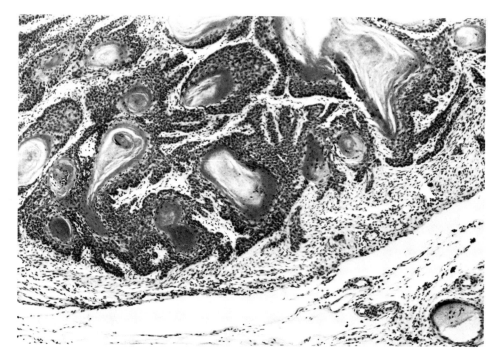

FIG. 4.   Forestomach invasive squamous carcinoma. H.-E. × 75.

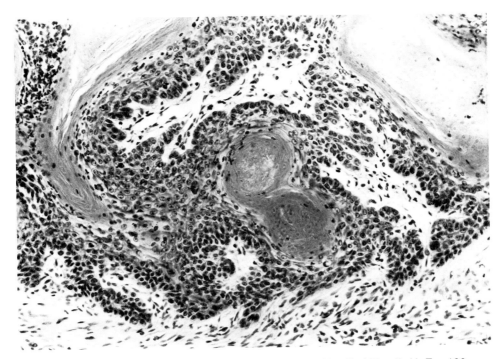

FIG. 5. Forestomach invasive squamous carcinoma (detail of Fig. 4). H.-E. × 180

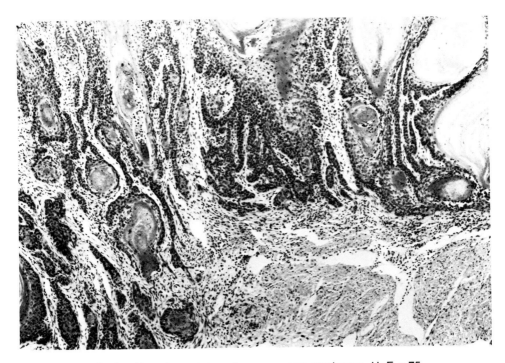

FIG. 6. Forestomach invasive squamous carcinoma. H.-E. × 75.

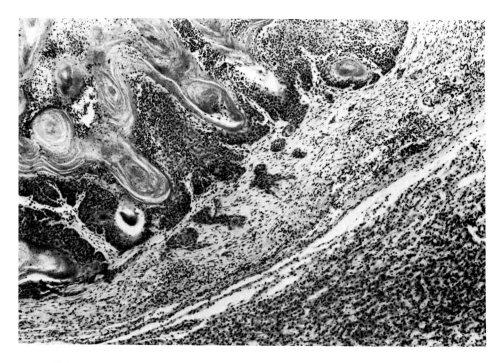

FIG. 7.   Liver metastasis of forestomach squamous carcinoma. H.-E. × 75.

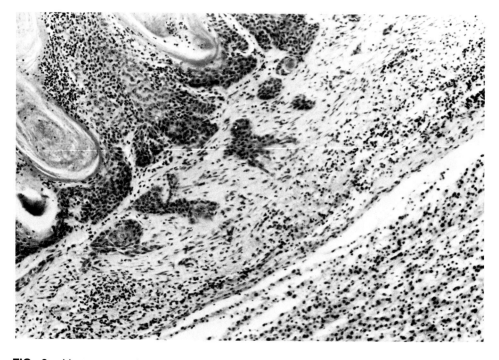

FIG. 8.   Liver metastasis of forestomach squamous carcinoma (detail of Fig. 7). H.-E. × 120.

the considered experimental conditions, the entire matter of the safety of styrene must be more carefully considered.

In consideration of the variety of the observed lesions and of their frequency, the present experimental model provides a useful tool for studying upper gastrointestinal tract carcinogenesis and proper measures of prevention, medical control, and care.

SUMMARY

Styrene oxide was administered to Sprague-Dawley rats by ingestion (stomach tube), in olive oil, at the dose levels of 250 and 50 mg/kg body weight, four to five times weekly, for 52 weeks. A high incidence of benign and malignant epithelial tumours and of tumour precursors was observed in the forestomach of tested animals at both doses, with a clear-cut dose-response relationship.

REFERENCES

1. Ivankovic, S. (1979): Site specificity of chemical carcinogens, with special reference to the upper alimentary canal. In: *Gastric Cancer: Etiology and Pathogenesis*, edited by K. J. Pfeiffer, pp. 303–355. Gerhard Witzsetrock Publishing House, New York, Baden Baden, Cologne.
2. Maltoni, C., Failla, G., and Kassapidis, G. (1979): First experimental demonstration of the carcinogenic effects of styrene oxide. Long term bioassays on Sprague-Dawley rats by oral administration. *La Medicina del Lavoro*, 70:358–362.
3. Van Duuren, B. L., Nelson, N., Orris, L., Palmes, E. D., and Schmitt, F. L. (1963): Carcinogenicity of epoxides, lactones, and peroxy compounds. *J. Natl. Cancer Inst.*, 31:41–55.
4. Weil, C. S., Condra, N., Haun, C., and Striegel, J. A. (1963): Experimental carcinogenicity and acute toxicity of representative epoxides. *Am. Ind. Hyg. Assoc. J.*, 24:305–325.

Precancerous Lesions of the Gastrointestinal Tract, edited by P. Sherlock, B.C. Morson, L. Barbara, and U. Veronesi. Raven Press, New York © 1983.

Epidemiology of Gastric Cancer: A Clue to Etiology

Jozef Victor Joossens and Jef Geboers

Division of Epidemiology, School of Public Health, University of Leuven, B-3000 Leuven, Belgium

The epidemiology of gastric cancer presents remarkable features. The most striking is the decreasing stomach cancer mortality in almost every country. This occurs almost without any medical intervention, making planned prevention programs nearly superfluous. This phenomenon results in a strong, negative time trend within each country. Large differences in mortality exist also between countries and between different regions of the same country. Lastly, there is an almost unique parallelism with stroke mortality (17,22,25).

No consensus has been reached among different research groups as to the cause of those findings. It is not the lack of etiological hypotheses; on the contrary, the sheer number of possible explanations has hampered further investigations. The confrontation of observations and hypotheses will help in unraveling the etiology of stomach cancer.

METHODS

Raw mortality data were provided, unless stated otherwise, by the World Health Organization, the National Institute of Statistics, Brussels, the Central Bureau of Statistics, The Hague and the Registrar General, London.

The 10-year age-specific mortalities were age-adjusted by the direct method for the interval 45 to 64 years using as weights numbers proportional to the total population in the given interval of England and Wales in 1951. They were equal to 599 and 457, respectively, for the 45- to 54-year and 55- to 64-year intervals. The middle-age group, 45 to 64, was selected because of the greater reliability of cancer mortality data as compared to older age groups. Stroke mortality was age adjusted 45 to 75 + for reasons previously given (22).

Linear regression was used to calculate time trends. An estimate of the percent change over a 10-year period of a mortality in a given country was calculated according to the formula $(1,000 \ b)/\bar{y}$; $\bar{y}$ stands for the mean mortality over the selected time interval and b for the slope of the regression line.

The 95% confidence interval of the regression line between two causes of mortality was calculated according to a standard formula (25). The Spearman rank correlation test (r_s) was used as a nonparametric control method (7).

TIME TRENDS OF GASTRIC CANCER

Gastric cancer is remarkable for its declining mortality in most countries (11). A temporary increase, such as in Portugal between 1955 and 1965 (Table 1), is probably due to classification errors. The behavior of gastric cancer in the United States since 1930 is illustrated

TABLE 1. *Significant[a] percent changes in gastric cancer mortality estimated over a 10-year period[b] (1955–1965)*

Rank order	Country	% Change	Rank order	Country	% Change[c]
1.	Iceland	−133	15.	Belgium	−25
2.	Finland	−57	16.	Hungary	−24
3.	Switzerland	−52	17.	England and Wales	−22
4.	Australia	−49	18.	Austria	−21
5.	Denmark	−47	19.	Czechoslovakia	−20
6.	Sweden	−45	20.	Italy	−16
7.	Norway	−44	21.	Japan	−12
8.	U.S. (all races)	−44	22.	Yugoslavia	ns
9.	Canada	−43	23.	Ireland	ns
10.	North Ireland	−36	24.	New Zealand	ns
11.	Netherlands	−35	25.	Spain	ns
12.	Scotland	−31	26.	Greece	ns
13.	France	−30	27.	Poland	ns
14.	West Germany	−27	28.	Portugal	+10

Age adjusted 45–64 years, average of both sexes.
[a]At least $p < 0.05$.
[b]See Methods.
[c]ns = not significant.

in Figs. 1 and 2 for males and females, together with a few other cancer localizations. The decline in stomach cancer mortality in the United States started probably before 1930, since the curve is very steep from the start on. The observed decrease in that country is much faster in the 1930 to 1950 period than in England and Wales (25) during the same time interval.

Illustrative time trends are also given for eight countries (males and females) in Figs. 3 and 4 from 1950 to 1954 on up to the present. The percent decline in a given country estimated over a 10-year period is in general different for the 1955 to 1965 period as compared to the 1968 to 1975–1979 period (Tables 1,2).

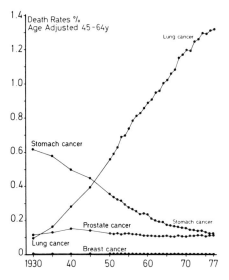

FIG. 1. Trends of different cancer localizations in U.S. males, 1930–1977. From refs. 10a and 45a.

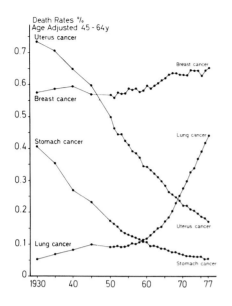

FIG. 2. Trends of different cancer localizations in U.S. females, 1930–1977.

FIG. 3. Time trends in gastric cancer mortality (males). The decrease since 1968 is fastest in Finland and Belgium and slowest in Japan and Hungary.

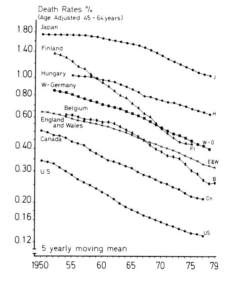

GEOGRAPHICAL EPIDEMIOLOGY OF GASTRIC CANCER

There have always been large differences in gastric cancer mortality among different countries. Gastric cancer mortality was observed in 28 countries in the first available year of the 1950 to 1961 period and similarly in 36 countries in the last available year of the 1975 to 1979 period. The data, classified into quartiles, are listed in Tables 3 and 4 for the average of both sexes. The average of both sexes was used to decrease random errors, to simplify the presentation, and also because the mortalities of each sex were significantly intercorrelated ($p < 0.0001$, $r_s = 0.91$ for 28 countries and $r_s = 0.88$ for 36 countries). Important geographical differences for stomach cancer mortality also exist within certain countries. In the United States it is more prevalent in the northern parts of North Dakota,

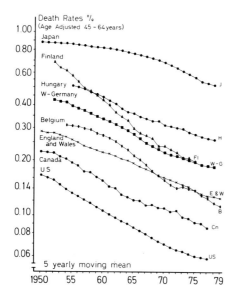

FIG. 4. Time trends in gastric cancer mortality (females). The decrease since 1968 is fastest in Finland and Belgium and slowest in Japan and Hungary.

TABLE 2. *Significant[a] percent changes in gastric cancer mortality estimated over a 10–year period[b] [(1968–(1975–1979)]*

Rank order	Country	% Change	Rank order	Country	% Change
1.	Finland	−54	19.	Poland	−31
2.	South Africa (white)	−48	20.	U.S. (all races)	−30
3.	Belgium	−46	21.	France	−30
4.	Switzerland	−45	22.	Italy	−30
5.	Norway	−44	23.	Denmark	−29
6.	Chile	−43	24.	Spain	−29
7.	Austria	−38	25.	Bulgaria	−28
8.	Japan	−38	26.	Sweden	−26
9.	Ireland	−35	27.	Hungary	−23
10.	West Germany	−34	28.	Scotland	−22
11.	Venezuela	−34	29.	Portugal	−17
12.	Netherlands	−34	30.	Greece	−16
13.	Canada	−34	31.	East Germany (DDR)	ns
14.	Israel	−33	32.	Iceland	ns
15.	Australia	−33	33.	Yugoslavia	ns
16.	New Zealand	−32	34.	North Ireland	ns
17.	Czechoslovakia	−32	35.	Malta	ns
18.	England and Wales	−32	36.	Luxembourg	ns

Age adjusted 45-64 years, average of both sexes.
[a]At least $p < 0.05$.
[b]See Methods.
ns = not significant.

Minnesota, Michigan, Texas, and Maine (31). Stomach cancer is also more prevalent in the northern parts of Italy, Belgium (18), England and Wales (20), and Japan (14). The opposite was seen in the Netherlands, at least in the 1955 to 1965 period (J. V. Joossens and J. Geboers, *unpublished data*), and in Colombia (4,6).

TABLE 3. Geographical epidemiology of gastric cancer

	1st Quartile				2nd Quartile				3rd Quartile				4th Quartile		
Rank order	Country	Year	Death rates	Rank order	Country	Year	Death rates	Rank order	Country	Year	Death rates	Rank order	Country	Year	Death rates
1.	New Zealand	58	0.21	8.	Denmark	51	0.43	15.	Northern Ireland	50	0.54	22.	West Germany	52	0.66
2.	Greece	61	0.25	9.	England and Wales	50	0.45	16.	Netherlands	50	0.55	23.	Austria	55	0.66
3.	U.S. (a.r.)	50	0.27	10.	Sweden	51	0.46	17.	Switzerland	51	0.56	24.	Czechoslovakia	53	0.75
4.	Australia	50	0.32	11.	Belgium	54	0.47	18.	Ireland	50	0.60	25.	Hungary	55	0.77
5.	Canada	50	0.35	12.	Spain	60	0.47	19.	Norway	51	0.61	26.	Iceland	61	0.80
6.	Yugoslavia	61	0.39	13.	Portugal	55	0.53	20.	Italy	51	0.62	27.	Finland	52	1.09
7.	France	50	0.41	14.	Scotland	50	0.54	21.	Poland	59	0.64	28.	Japan	50	1.30
	Mean ± SD	0.31 ± 0.08			0.48 ± 0.04				0.59 ± 0.04				0.86 ± 0.24		
	Sex Ratio Mean ♂ / Mean ♀	2.08			2.00				1.88				1.99		

Based on first available year of the 1950–1961 period. Mortality per thousand, age adjusted 45–64 years, average of both sexes.

TABLE 4. Geographical epidemiology of gastric cancer

	1st Quartile				2nd Quartile				3rd Quartile				4th Quartile		
Rank order	Country	Year	Death rates	Rank order	Country	Year	Death rates	Rank order	Country	Year	Death rates	Rank order	Country	Year	Death rates
1.	U.S. (a.r.)	77	0.09	10.	Belgium	79	0.18	19.	Ireland	75	0.27	28.	Italy	75	0.35
2.	Canada	77	0.14	11.	Greece	78	0.18	20.	Luxembourg	78	0.29	29.	Venezuela	77	0.40
3.	Australia	77	0.14	12.	Netherlands	79	0.19	21.	Finland	75	0.29	30.	Czechoslovakia	75	0.42
4.	Denmark	78	0.15	13.	South Africa	76	0.19	22.	Yugoslavia	77	0.30	31.	Bulgaria	77	0.42
5.	New Zealand	76	0.15	14.	Norway	78	0.19	23.	Spain	76	0.31	32.	Hungary	78	0.42
6.	Israel	78	0.16	15.	Malta	77	0.20	24.	Northern Ireland	77	0.32	33.	Poland	78	0.44
7.	Switzerland	78	0.16	16.	England and Wales	79	0.22	25.	Iceland	78	0.33	34.	Portugal	75	0.52
8.	Sweden	78	0.16	17.	West Germany	78	0.27	26.	Austria	78	0.33	35.	Chile	77	0.63
9.	France	76	0.17	18.	Scotland	78	0.27	27.	East Germany	76	0.34	36.	Japan	78	0.73
	Mean ± SD		0.15 ± 0.02				0.21 ± 0.03				0.31 ± 0.02				0.48 ± 0.12
	Sex Ratio Mean ♂		2.11				2.20				2.29				2.33
	Mean ♀														

Based on last available year of the 1975–1979 period. Mortality per thousand, age adjusted 45–64 years, average of both sexes.

STOMACH CANCER AND STROKE MORTALITY

Intra-country Relationship

In all countries with reliable vital statistics there is a significant within-country relationship between stomach cancer and stroke mortality over time (19,20,22,24–26). England and Wales, and the United States are given as an illustration of this phenomenon (Figs. 5, 6). In both cases there is a linear part ranging approximately over the interval 1955 to 1972. Stroke mortality is decreasing faster than gastric cancer after 1972 (Figs. 5 and 6). This is evidence for a confounding factor acting preferentially on stroke. This could be treatment of hypertension, which is now applied at the population level.

Inter-Country Relationship

There is a significant, positive, between-countries relationship between stomach cancer and stroke mortality (Fig. 7) (16,19,22,24–26): Both are low in the United States, Greece, Canada, and Sweden; both are very high in Japan, Portugal, and most East European countries. Both were high in West Germany, Finland, and Scotland. Japan is outside the 95% confidence limits in Fig. 7. This is probably due to underclassification of stroke in certain countries. This was observed in Belgium before 1968 and in Czechoslovakia before

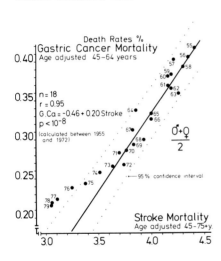

FIG. 5. The time relationship between stroke and gastric cancer mortality observed over the period 1955–1979 in England and Wales for the average of both sexes. The number next to each point is the year of observation.

FIG. 6. The time relationship between stroke and gastric cancer mortality observed over the period 1955–1977 in the U.S. for the average of both sexes. The number next to each point is the year of observation.

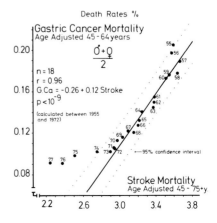

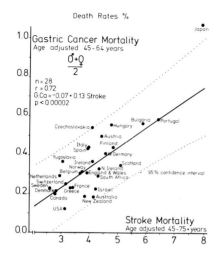

FIG. 7. The geographical relationship between stroke and gastric cancer mortality for the average of both sexes, 1965–1970. Japan was excluded from the calculation of the regression line.

1973 (22). Japan falls between those limits, when only countries with the best vital statistics are used [see Fig. 12 in Joossens (20)].

The important fact, resulting from Figs. 5 to 7, is not the presence of a strong relation between stomach cancer and stroke, which could be spurious, but the quantitative similarity of the inter- and intra-country relationships (cf. Figs. 5 and 6 with Fig. 7).

Using an equation derived from data in England and Wales over the period 1955 to 1972 (Fig. 5), it is possible to calculate stomach cancer from observed stroke mortality rates (Table 5) in countries as different as Japan, Hungary, Israel, and New Zealand.

Independence of the Stomach Cancer–Stroke Mortality Relationship

The stomach cancer–stroke relationship is independent of possible confounding factors such as linear or nonlinear time trends, lung, colon, and genital cancer, and infectious diseases. This was true for each sex (25).

Between Social Classes

There are no data available on the quantitative relationship of stomach cancer and stroke mortality between social classes, but it is well known that both mortalities are higher in lower social classes than in higher ones (3,23). This is again a positive relationship between both mortalities.

Comparison of the Degree of Decrease in Gastric Cancer and Stroke Mortality Since 1968 up to the Present

Data similar to those in Table 2, but now for stroke, have been computed. The rank and linear correlations were estimated between the 10-yearly, percent changes of gastric cancer and of stroke. The degree of change, mostly a decrease, is always a dimensionless value (see Methods); nevertheless, both parametric and nonparametric correlations remain positive and significant (Fig. 8).

PRECURSORS OF GASTRIC CANCER

Chronic atrophic gastritis and intestinal metaplasia of the stomach mucosa are well-known precursors of gastric cancer. They have been carefully studied in Japan, Finland, and Co-

TABLE 5. *Calculated gastric cancer rates from observed stroke rates, using an equation obtained for England and Wales over the years 1955 to 1972 (Fig. 5)*

Year	Japan		Hungary		Israel		New Zealand	
	Calculated	Observed	Calculated	Observed	Calculated	Observed	Calculated	Observed
1960	1.16	1.22	0.41	0.71	—	—	0.24	0.22
1961	1.18	1.22	0.50	0.68	—	—	0.28	0.26
1962	1.20	1.19	0.50	0.67	—	—	0.26	0.23
1963	1.20	1.18	0.47	0.65	—	—	0.27	0.18
1964	1.18	1.17	0.50	0.64	—	—	0.25	0.22
1965	1.20	1.15	0.54	0.58	—	—	0.27	0.18
1966	1.14	1.11	0.46	0.58	—	—	0.31	0.25
1967	1.10	1.10	0.46	0.58	—	—	0.24	0.19
1968	1.08	1.09	0.47	0.54	0.35	0.22	0.30	0.20
1969	1.07	1.04	0.48	0.52	0.41	0.22	0.29	0.18
1970	1.05	0.99	0.46	0.54	0.36	0.23	0.31	0.18
1971	0.96	0.96	0.45	0.52	0.36	0.21	0.31	0.15
1972	0.90	0.93	0.38	0.51	0.37	0.20	0.33	0.17
1973	0.88	0.90	0.40	0.48	0.34	0.19	0.34	0.18
1974	0.83	0.87	0.39	0.49	0.37	0.22	0.31	0.14
1975	0.74	0.83	0.41	0.48	0.26	0.18	0.25	0.15
1976	0.69	0.81	0.45	0.45	0.21	0.19	0.18	0.15
1977	0.62	0.77	0.43	0.44	0.23	0.16	—	—
1978	0.56	0.73	0.45	0.42	0.17	0.16	—	—

Mortality per thousand, age adjusted 45–64 years, average of both sexes. The fit is excellent for Japan between 1960 and 1974; after that one underestimates the gastric cancer rates, pointing to a confounding factor, decreasing stroke independently of the linking factor X. This confounding factor could be treatment of hypertension. The fit is less good in Hungary between 1960 and 1965; expected gastric cancer is again lower than the observed. This can be traced to improving classification of stroke, which was also observed in Belgium, Czechoslovakia, and Poland (22).

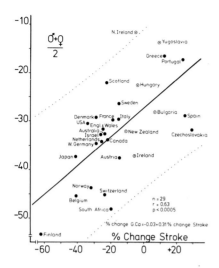

FIG. 8. Percent change in gastric cancer and stroke mortality observed for the average of both sexes from 1968 up to 1975–1979 (depending on the given country) and estimated over a 10-year period. *(Closed circles)* Countries with a significant change in both stroke and gastric cancer; *(open circles with a point)* countries with no significant change in stroke and/or gastric cancer. The relationship was calculated using all 29 points. When the nonsignificant changes were omitted ($n = 23$) a similar equation was found, not significantly different from the $n = 29$ relationship. The nonparametric Spearman rank correlation coefficient r_s was 0.62 for $n = 29$ ($p < 0.01$) and 0.54 for $n = 23$ ($p < 0.05$). When the countries are ranked according to the highest simultaneous decrease of both mortalities, i.e., the average of both changes, then Finland and Belgium rank 1st and 2nd, respectively, the U.S. ranks 14th, and Northern Ireland ranks last.

lombia (4,6,43,47). The most striking results were found in Colombia (Table 6) because of the presence of low- and high-risk areas. The localization of gastritis and of gastric cancer was in general in the antrum and the corpus (4). This is compatible with a nutritional origin of both types of morbidity. Because human beings are upright for the majority of the day, the major impact of any food factor will be strongest in the lower part of the stomach.

In pernicious anemia the situation is totally different. The chronic atrophic gastritis is now from autoimmune origin and is localized with a preference for the fundus and the corpus. Gastric cancer in cases of pernicious anemia is similarly localized (9). Another interesting feature is the equal prevalence of precursor lesions in both sexes in Finland and Colombia (4), whereas gastric cancer is more than twice as prevalent in males (cf. sex ratios in Tables 3 and 4). This is evidence for a lower susceptibility in females for getting gastric cancer.

TABLE 6. *Estimated gastric cancer incidence per 100,000 population and percent distribution (prevalence) of histologic findings of gastric biopsies: five Colombian populations, 1972–1974*

Populations	Estimated gastric cancer incidence/ 100,000 pop.[a]	No. of gastric biopsies	% Distribution		Atrophic gastritis	
			Normal	Superficial gastritis	Simple	With metaplasia
Nariño, high-risk	150	286	24.5	19.2	34.3	22.0
Nariño, low-risk	40	168	38.7	28.0	22.6	10.7
Cali, migrants from Nariño	68	45	37.8	24.4	20.0	17.8
Cali, natives	23	57	45.6	28.1	19.3	7.0
Cartegena	6	30	70.0	16.7	6.7	6.7

[a]Adjusted to the world standard population.
From Correa et al. (4), with permission.

ETIOLOGY OF GASTRIC CANCER

Many factors have been described as related to the etiology of gastric cancer. They can be separated into genetic, soil, nutrition, and social factors (Table 7). Genetic and soil factors may be important for differences among countries, but they are difficult to reconcile with what is happening within countries. It would be hard to believe that such factors could change so rapidly from year to year in the same country (Figs. 5,6). We will therefore concentrate on nutritional and social factors.

In order to explain the almost perfect parallelism between stomach cancer and stroke mortality, one can postulate the presence of one or several linking factors. Although both stomach cancer and stroke are multifactorial of origin, it is not possible that the linking mechanism should be of complex nature. The probability that the quantitative relation of both mortalities between and within countries should be identical is near 1.0 when there is only one linking factor. The more and more factors that are involved, the smaller will be

TABLE 7. *Positive etiological factors of gastric cancer and stroke*

Gastric cancer		Stroke	
Genetic:	Male sex Bloodgroup A Pernicious anemia	Genetic:	Male sex (smaller sex difference than for gastric cancer) History of hypertension and/or stroke in family
Food:	Added salt[a] Soybean sauce[a] Pickled food[a] Lard[a] Lack of fresh vegetables and fruits[a] Salted fish or meat[a] High starch[a] Low protein[a] Low fat[a] Bracken fern Added nitrates and/or nitrites Talcum in rice	Food:	Added salt[a] All kinds of salty foods[a] High caloric intake[a] Low protein[a]
Soil:	Trace elements Peaty soil Amount of NO_3 used as fertilizer Nitrates in drinking water Lack of vitamin C or other antioxidants		
Other:	Low social class[a] Lack of refrigerators[a]	Other:	Excess of alcohol Lack of refrigerators[a] Low social class[a] Contraceptive pill Cadmium, lead Stress

[a]Directly or indirectly related to salt.
Adapted from Joossens and Geboers (24), with permission.

the probability of getting similar quantitative relations between and within countries. One must therefore assume the presence of either a unique or, more probably, a predominant factor "X" linking both stomach cancer and stroke mortality in order to explain what was observed (Figs. 5,6,7,8 and Table 5). Because the possible risk factors for gastric cancer and stroke are so different, it will be easier to find a simple common factor that could be of importance for both diseases.

PROPERTIES OF THE LINKING FACTOR X

The properties of factor X can be derived from epidemiological and anatomopathological observations.

1. The amount of factor X present in the food years ago should be much higher than now, and this must be so in most of the countries mentioned.
2. X should be present at a very high to high level in the upper quartile (Tables 3,4). Among them not only Japan, Chile, Portugal, the East European countries, etc., but also Colombia and South Korea. Lower levels are expected in the lower quartile (Tables 3,4). All of them are western countries. Stomach cancer should be very uncommon in areas where factor X is not present in the food. This could be Java some years ago (8), where only one case of stomach cancer was found in 3,885 autopsies.
3. Higher social classes must have a lower intake of X than lower social classes.
4. Chronic atrophic gastritis should result from the prolonged intake of factor X and since it is ingested with the food, it should preferentially affect the antrum and corpus region of the stomach.
5. Factor X should induce hypertension, because hypertension is the major risk factor of stroke (41).

IS SALT THE LINKING FACTOR X?

The strong positive relation between stomach cancer and stroke mortality was a chance finding in 1964 (16). Looking at the etiological factors for both stomach cancer and stroke (Table 7), we can make a guess as to the identity of factor X. The working hypothesis that salt (NaCl) was factor X was presented in 1965 (16). Although many data are still lacking, a lot of evidence in favor of this hypothesis has been collected over the last 30 years.

First, salt intake should have been higher years ago than now. This decline can be unconscious, just resulting from an increased use of refrigeration techniques and from decreasing cereal intake. This was so in Switzerland (36), France (5), and possibly also the United States where decreasing salt sales have been observed. In France and in Belgium, 24-hr urinary salt excretion has been measured and found to be decreasing. In France, it came down from ± 15 g in 1947 to ± 8 g in 1975 (5). In Belgium, a vast educational campaign against salt was launched in 1968. Salt content in 24-hr urine fell from ± 15 g in 1966 to ± 9 g in 1980 (25). A similar decrease in salt was observed in Japan, coming from ± 30 g in 1937 to ± 18 g in 1965 (29).

Evolutionary and historical arguments have been given showing that life during evolution must have been without added salt (20,22). The use of salt resulted from economic pressures to preserve food in winter, when man emigrated from the tropical areas, where he originated, to colder northern areas. It is interesting to note that other techniques of food preservation, such as drying or smoking, were associated with salting, except in tropical areas. Another interesting feature is that Indians in North America did not use salt for preservation before the whites came. They used maple syrup for that purpose and to them salt was distasteful (2,34).

Refrigeration techniques were first introduced in the United States, later on in other Western countries, and more recently in East European countries. The United States was probably the only country where stomach cancer started to decline before 1930. It should be noted that stroke mortality started coming down in the United States in 1925 (1), long before any treatment of hypertension was available.

Second, the intake of salt is known to be very high in Japan (14,28,37). Stomach cancer in Japan was already linked to salt intake in 1959 (38). This was amplified later on by Hirayama (14). Salt intake, gastric cancer mortality, stroke mortality, and blood pressure are all higher in the North of Japan than in the South (14,29,37,38). Salt intake is also high in other high-prevalence gastric cancer areas: South Korea (27), Portugal (10), and Bulgaria (25). High to medium amounts were found in Scotland, Finland, and West Germany (25).

No data on 24-hr salt excretion are available from Colombia, but it was found that heavy salting of meat was nearly three times as frequent in high-risk than in low-risk areas (12). Only 2% of the population in the high-risk area (Nariño) had refrigerators, no nitrates were added to the food, and fertilizers were not used (12).

Salt intake is medium in England, the United States, New Zealand, and Belgium, at least nowadays (25). No salt was added to the food in Java according to Dungal (8).

A significant relationship was found between reported 24-hr salt excretions and observed gastric cancer mortality. This was observed in 18 pairs of data from 10 countries (25).

Third, Joossens et al. (23) found a significant difference in the salt excretion, corrected to the same amount of creatinine, between higher and lower social classes in Belgium. The higher intake in lower social groups is compatible with the observation that, at least in Belgium, all salted foods, such as bread, sausages, lard, cheese, and canned or processed foods, are in general less expensive.

Fourth, it has not been demonstrated conclusively that salt can produce atrophic gastritis. Nevertheless atrophic gastritis is extremely common in countries with a high salt intake, such as Japan (47). In general a similar pattern is observed for prevalence of gastric cancer and of atrophic gastritis [Table 6 and Siurala et al. (43)].

Experimental evidence indicates that salted, pickled food produces at least acute gastritis (30,39).

Finally, more and more evidence is becoming available linking salt intake to hypertension. Many reviews of the evidence in favor (20,22) or against (42) have been published.

Salt is probably not related to gastric cancer through carcinogenic properties. It is thought, instead, that salt, having strong osmotic properties, is caustic to the stomach mucosa. The causticity is enhanced by the fact that hypertonic gastric contents impair the emptying of the stomach (15). Once atrophic gastritis sets in, one gets a lower acidity in the stomach. This favors endogenous nitrite production (35). The latter could then combine with food constituents to powerful nitroso-carcinogens (44).

ROLE OF OTHER POSSIBLE ETIOLOGICAL FACTORS

The other most important factors from the literature are nitrate (nitrite) intake and the protective action of antioxidants such as vitamin C. Alcohol and tobacco are probably not important (13). The best arguments in favor of nitrate are data from Chile, Colombia, and Israel (4,6,40,48,49). Many inconsistencies persist, however; for example, an unknown factor had to be postulated in Colombia in order to explain what was happening in terms of atrophic gastritis (6). There are no good data available showing that nitrate intake, coming mostly from the soil, is declining in Chile. Nevertheless stomach cancer is declining very fast in Chile (Table 2).

Recently, data were published showing a significant correlation between the daily intake of nitrate and stomach cancer mortality (33). The problem is that all countries with a high nitrate intake (Japan and East European countries) have also a high salt intake. On the other hand, it is correct that nitrate intake can be lowered through lower intake of cured meat or fish, but this is again confounded by a parallel decrease in salt.

The intake of fresh vegetables has increased markedly over the last decades (46); so has the use of nitrates as fertilizer. This should theoretically produce an increase in nitrate intake, this time, however, together with a lower salt intake. A high intake of fresh vegetables has in general been found to be negatively related to stomach cancer (12,45,46).

From what is known about the epidemiology of stomach cancer and of stroke, it is difficult to make nitrate the linking factor between both types of mortality, because nothing is known about hypertensive properties of nitrates. However, it is possible that a high nitrate intake could favor the appearance of stomach cancer at the stage of atrophic gastritis, but it is not certain that atrophic gastritis could result from the relatively small amounts of nitrate ingested with the daily food, even in very high risk areas [$\pm$ 10 mmoles daily in Japan (33)].

High fat intake has generally been considered a protective factor against stomach cancer. In countries with a high fat intake and with a high colon cancer rate, such as the United States, New Zealand, Australia, and Scotland, there is less stomach cancer than expected from stroke (Fig. 7); that is, all those countries are below the regression line. One marked exception has been Finland, where a high fat intake went together with a high gastric cancer rate (Fig. 7) and a low colon cancer rate.

The protective properties of fresh vegetables and fruits have been ascribed in general to the antioxidant properties of vitamin C (32,45). It could also be due to the lack of salt in these foods. It is again not impossible that vitamin C plays a favorable role in the etiology of gastric cancer, but there are no good epidemiological data about the amount of vitamin C intake all over the world. Nothing is known of a protective action of vitamin C against stroke, making it improbable as a linking factor.

CONCLUSION

If the salt hypothesis is correct, then a simple and nonexpensive method will be available to reduce the prevalence of gastric cancer and by the same token that of stroke (Figs. 7,8). Since stroke is also an important determinant of all causes of mortality, a fall in the latter can be expected, together with decreasing stomach cancer rates.

The experience in Belgium with a reduction in salt intake at the population level has been satisfactory (compare Belgium in Tables 1 and 2). Gastric cancer, stroke, and all causes of mortality were decreasing faster in Belgium than in any other Common Market country [Fig. 8 and Joossens (21)].

In conclusion it can be said that the present evidence favors the role of salt in the etiology of gastric cancer. Many more data are nevertheless necessary in order to ascertain this. In the first place, data on salt excretion in Chile, Colombia, and many East European countries are needed. Similarly more data on time trends of salt excretion from different countries are necessary. Careful monitoring of salt excretion is therefore mandatory. Techniques for the collection and analysis of 24-hr urines have been described in detail (26).

SUMMARY

The epidemiology of gastric cancer highlights several interesting phenomena. First, the decreasing mortality rate of stomach cancer observed in most countries; second, the wide range in gastric cancer mortality rates observed in different countries all over the world or in different regions of the same country; and third, the strikingly similar behavior of gastric cancer and stroke mortality. Quantitative similarity of the relationship, existing between both mortalities within and among countries, is exemplified. Stroke, as well as gastric cancer mortality, is higher in lower social classes. A further argument for the linking of both mortalities is the significant correlation between 10-yearly percent changes of stroke and similar changes of gastric cancer mortality, observed since 1968. From these facts it can be derived that the factor determining gastric cancer must also influence stroke. Hence the notion of a linking factor X.

The properties of this factor X, linking both mortalities, are described. Evidence is given for a food factor, namely, salt (NaCl), as being the predominant linking factor X.

Nitrates and/or nitrites could be active at the stage of chronic atrophic gastritis produced by the lifetime ingestion of food, hypertonic from its salt content, hence caustic. Similarly the protective action of vitamin C could be important at that stage. The Belgian experience with an educational campaign aimed at salt reduction at the population level was satisfactory. This campaign was started in 1968. Measured 24-hr salt excretion levels fell from ± 15 g in 1966 to ± 9 g in 1980. Concomitant with this, a decrease in gastric cancer, stroke, and all causes of mortality was observed. This decrease was faster than in any other Common Market region.

Monitoring of salt excretion in different countries, especially in Chile, Colombia, and East European countries is most important. The same should be done in different years in the same country and in different regions of the same country, as in the northern and southern parts of Colombia, England and Wales, and Italy. Epidemiological studies, concerning the frequency of atrophic gastritis, should be started in the latter two countries. It should also be verified if atrophic gastritis and stomach cancer are nearly absent in no added salt regions, for example, certain parts of South America.

ACKNOWLEDGMENTS

This work was aided by grants from the FWGO, Brussels, and the ASLK, Brussels. J. Smisdom-Rongy and A. Menten-Mellaerts made the graphs and typed the manuscript. The photographs were made by V. Noppen and R. Roels. L. Cooreman and G. De Vadder of the Faculty Campus Library were of great help in the bibliographic research. The Nationaal Instituut voor Statistiek, Brussels (P. Van Landeghem, A. Dillaerts, M. Luyckx-Draelants, and M. Portaels) gave us the regional data on gastric cancer in Belgium and together with the Ministry of Public Health they provided us with the mortality data of Belgium from 1977 to 1979. To all of them our most sincere thanks.

REFERENCES

1. Acheson, R. M. (1966): Mortality from cerebrovascular disease in the United States. In: *Cerebrovascular Disease Epidemiology, Public Health Monograph 76*, edited by K. Kost, pp. 23–40. DHEW, Washington, D.C.
2. Barger, A. C. (1982): Discussion of "Nutrition and hypertension." In: *Blood Pressure Measurement and Systemic Hypertension*, edited by H. A. Snellen, A. J. Dunning, and A. C. Arntzenius, pp. 169–176. Medical World Press, Breda.
3. Clemessen, J. (1965): *Statistical Studies in Malignant Neoplasms*. Munksgaard, Copenhague.
4. Correa, P., Cuello, C., Duque, E., Burbano, L. C., Garcia, F. T., Bolanos, O., Brown, C., and Haenszel, W. (1976): Gastric cancer in Colombia. III. Natural history of precursor lesions. *J. Natl. Cancer Inst.*, 57:1027–1035.
5. Cottet, J. (1981): Evolution de la consommation du sel en France. *Bull. Acad. Roy. Med. Belg.*, 136:556–565.
6. Cuello, C., Correa, P., Haenszel, W., Gordillo, G., Brown, C., Archer, M., and Tannenbaum, S. (1976): Gastric cancer in Colombia. I. Cancer risk and suspect environmental agents. *J. Natl. Cancer Inst.*, 57:1015–1020.

7. Diem, K., and Lenter, C., editors (1976): *Scientific Tables*, 7th edition, p. 181. Ciba-Geigy Ltd., Basel.
8. Dungal, N. (1958): Cancer in Iceland. In: *Cancer*, edited by R. W. Raven, pp. 262–271. Butterworth, London.
9. Elsberg, L., and Mosbeck, J. (1979): Pernicious anemia as a risk factor in gastric cancer. *Acta Med. Scand.*, 206:315–318.
10. Forte, J. A. G., Miguel, J. M. P., and de Padua, F. (1979): Salt in the primary prevention of arterial hypertension (Portuguese). In: *Hypertensão Arterial*, edited by J. Nogueira de Costa and J. Braz Nogueira, pp. 103–109. Merck, Sharp and Dohme, Lisbon.
10a. Gordon, T., Crittenden, M., and Haenszel, W. (1961): Cancer mortality trends in the United States. In: *End Results and Mortality Trends in Cancer*, NCI Monograph Number 6, pp. 131–350, DHEW, Washington, D.C.
11. Haenszel, W. (1958): Variations in incidence of and mortality from stomach cancer, with particular reference to the United States. *J. Natl. Cancer Inst.*, 21:213–262.
12. Haenszel, W., Correa, P., Cuello, C., Guzman, N., Burbano, L. C., Lores, H., and Muñoz, J. (1976): Gastric cancer in Colombia. II. Case-control epidemiologic study of precursor lesions. *J. Natl. Cancer Inst.*, 57:1021–1026.
13. Higginson, J. (1966): Etiological factors in gastrointestinal cancer in man. *J. Natl. Cancer Inst.*, 37:527–545.
14. Hirayama, T. (1967): The epidemiology of cancer of the stomach in Japan with special reference to the role of diet. In: *Proceedings of the 9th International Cancer Congress, Tokyo, 1966, UICC, Monograph Series 10*, edited by R. J. C. Harris, pp. 37–48. Springer-Verlag, Berlin.
15. Hunt, J. N., and Pathak, J. D. (1960): The osmotic effects of some simple molecules and ions on gastric emptying. *J. Physiol.*, 154:254–269.
16. Joossens, J. V. (1965): The riddle of cancer mortality (Dutch). *Verh. Kon. Vlaam. Akad. Geneesk. Belg.*, 27:489–545.
17. Joossens, J. V. (1973): Salt and hypertension, water hardness and cardiovascular death rate. *Triangle*, 12:9–16.
18. Joossens, J. V. (1979): Food pattern and mortality in Belgium. In: *Polyunsaturated Fatty Acids and Cardiovascular Diseases*, edited by Z. M. Bacq and J. V. Joossens, pp. 133–161, *Acta Cardiol. (Suppl.)*, XXIII.
19. Joossens, J. V. (1980): Trends in cardiovascular mortality. In: *Prevention and Treatment of Coronary Heart Disease and Its Complications*, edited by J. Lequime, pp. 12–36. Excerpta Medica, Amsterdam.
20. Joossens, J. V. (1980): Dietary salt restriction. The case in favor. In: *The Therapeutics of Hypertension*, edited by J. I. S. Robertson, G. W. Pickering, and A. D. S. Caldwell, pp. 243–250. Academic Press and Royal Society of Medicine, London.
21. Joossens, J. V. (1980): Recent mortality trends. (Editorial) *Acta Clin. Belg.*, 35:65–70.
22. Joossens, J. V. (1980): Stroke, stomach cancer and salt. A clue to the prevention of hypertension. In: *Epidemiology of Arterial Blood Pressure*, edited by H. Kesteloot and J. V. Joossens, pp. 489–508. Martinus Nijhoff Medical Division, The Hague.
23. Joossens, J. V., Claessens, J., Geboers, J., and Claes, J. (1980): Electrolytes and creatinine in multiple 24-hour urine collections (1970–1974). In: *Epidemiology of Arterial Blood Pressure*, edited by H. Kesteloot and J. V. Joossens, pp. 45–63. Martinus Nijhoff Medical Division, The Hague.
24. Joossens, J. V., and Geboers, J. (1981): Nutrition and gastric cancer. *Proc. Nutr. Soc.*, 40:37–46.
25. Joossens, J. V., and Geboers, J. (1981): Nutrition and gastric cancer. *Nutr. Cancer*, 2:250–261.
26. Joossens, J. V., Willems, J., Claessens, J., Claes, J., and Lissens, W. (1971): Sodium and hypertension. In: *Nutrition and Cardiovascular Diseases*, edited by F. Fidanza, A. Keys, G. Ricci, and J. C. Somogyi, pp. 91–110. Morgagni Edizioni Scientifiche, Rome.
27. Kesteloot, H., Park, B. C., Lee, C. S., Brems-Heyns, E., Claessens, J., and Joossens, J. V. (1980): A comparative study of blood pressure and sodium intake in Belgium and in Korea. *Eur. J. Cardiol.*, 11:169–182.
28. Komachi, Y., Iida, M., Shimamoto, T., Chikayama, Y., Takahashi, H., Konishi, M., and Tominaga, S. (1971): Geographic and occupational comparisons of risk factors in cardiovascular diseases in Japan. *Jpn. Circ. J.*, 35:189–207.
29. Komachi, Y., and Shimamoto, T. (1980): Salt intake and its relationship to blood pressure in Japan. Present and past. In: *Epidemiology of Arterial Blood Pressure*, edited by H. Kesteloot and J. V. Joossens, pp. 395–400. Martinus Nijhoff Medical Division, The Hague.
30. MacDonald, W. C., Anderson, F. H., and Hashimoto, S. (1967): Histological effect of certain pickles on the human gastric mucosa: a preliminary report. *Can. Med. Assoc. J.*, 96:1521–1525.
31. Mason, T. J., McKay, F. W., Hoover, R., Blot, W. J., and Fraumeni, Jr., J. F. (1975): *Atlas of Cancer Mortality for U.S. Counties (1950–1969)*. DHEW (NIH), No. 75-780, Washington, D.C.
32. Mirvish, S. S. (1975): Blocking the formation of N-nitroso compounds with ascorbic acid in vivo and in vitro. *Ann. NY Acad. Sci.*, 258:175–180.
33. National Research Council (1981): *The Health Effects of Nitrate, Nitrite and N-Nitroso Compounds*. National Academy Press, Washington, D.C.
34. Nearing, H., and Nearing, S. (1950): *The Maple Sugar Book*. Galahad Books, New York.

35. Ruddell, W. S., Bone, E. S., Hill, M. J., Blendis, L. M., and Walters, C. I. (1976): Gastric-juice nitrite. A risk factor for cancer in the hypochlorhydric stomach. *Lancet*, 2:1037–1039.

36. *Salines Suisses du Rhin Réunies: La Situation du Sel Iodé en Suisse (1978).* Schweizerhalle, Switzerland.

37. Sasaki, N. (1964): The relationship of salt intake to hypertension in the Japanese. *Geriatrics*, 19:735–744.

38. Sato, T., Fukuyama, T., Suzuki, T., Takayagani, J., Murukami, T., Shiotshuki, N., Tanaka, R., and Tsuji, R. (1959): Studies of the causation of gastric cancer. 2. The relation between gastric cancer mortality rate and salted food intake in several places in Japan. *Bull. Inst. Public Health*, 8:187–198.

39. Sato, T., Fukuyama, T., Urata, G., and Suzuki, T. (1959): Studies of the causation of gastric cancer. 1. Bleeding in the glandular stomach of mice by feeding with highly salted foods, and a comment on salted foods in Japan. *Bull. Inst. Public Health*, 8:10–13.

40. Shubal, H. L., and Gruener, N. (1972): Epidemiological and toxicological aspects of nitrates and nitrites in the environment. *Am. J. Public Health*, 62:1045–1052.

41. Shurtleff, D. (1974): Some characteristics related to the incidence of cardiovascular disease and death. In: *The Framingham Study*, Section 30. DHEW (NIH), No. 74-599, Washington, D.C.

42. Simpson, F. O. (1979): Salt and hypertension: a sceptical review of the evidence. *Clin. Sci.*, 57:463S–480S.

43. Siurala, M., Isokoski, K, Varis, K., and Kekki, M. (1968): Prevalence of gastritis in a rural population. Bioptic study of subjects selected at random. *Scand. J. Gastroenterol.*, 3:211–223.

44. Tatematsu, M., Takahashi, M., Fukushima, S., Hananouchi, M., and Shirai, T. (1975): Effects in rats of sodium chloride on experimental gastric cancers induced by N-methyl-N'-nitro-N-nitrosoguanidine or 4-nitroquinoline-1-oxyde. *J. Natl. Cancer Inst.*, 55:101–106.

45. Weisburger, J. D. (1979): Mechanism of diet as a carcinogen. *Cancer*, 43:1987–1995.

45a. World Health Statistics Annual. Volume 1:Vital Statistics and Causes of Death (1962–1980). WHO, Geneva.

46. Wynder, E. L., Kmet, J., Dungal, N., and Segi, M. (1963): An epidemiological investigation of gastric cancer. *Cancer*, 16:1461–1496.

47. Yoshitoshi, Y. (1967): Gastritis: incidence and pathogenesis of gastritis. In: *Proceedings of the 3rd World Congress of Gastroenterology, Tokyo, 1966*, pp. 179–185. Congress Publication, Tokyo.

48. Zaldivar, R. (1977): Epidemiology of gastric and colo-rectal cancer in the United States and Chile with particular reference to the role of dietary and nutritional variables, nitrate fertilizer pollution and N-nitroso compounds. *Zbl. Bakt. Hyg., I. Alt. Orig. B*, 164:193–217.

49. Zaldivar, R., and Wetterstrand, W. H. (1978): Nitrate nitrogen levels in drinking water of urban areas with high- and low-risk populations for stomach cancer: an environmental epidemiology study. *Z. Krebsforsch.*, 92:227–234.

Precancerous Lesions of the Gastrointestinal Tract, edited by P. Sherlock, B. C. Morson, L. Barbara, and U. Veronesi. Raven Press, New York © 1983.

Precancerous Changes of the Stomach from the Aspect of Dysplasia of the Gastric Mucosa—Histological Study

Takeo Nagayo

Aichi Cancer Center, Research Institute, Chikusa-ku, Nagoya, Japan 464

It is not easy to completely understand precancerous change of the stomach, since, unlike cases of obvious carcinoma or of animal experiments, concrete bases for recognition of these changes are hardly established and our knowledge regarding them has to be based greatly on our experiences.

DEFINITION OF PRECANCEROUS CHANGE

Before going into detail, the definition of precancer of the stomach must be clarified. The term precancer should be classified into two different concepts—precancerous condition and precancerous change. Precancerous condition is a clinical term indicating that the condition is in higher risk for the development of cancer than any other condition. In the stomach, the large polyp, especially with adenomatous structures, the very chronic or callus-like ulcer, and chronic atrophic or atrophic-hypertrophic gastritis, including pernicious anemia, can be cited as examples. Ménétrier's disease, the remnant stomach long intervals after surgery especially in the area of anastomosis and chronic ulcer scar can also be included in this category. All these diseases are characterized by chronic existence.

On the other hand, precancerous changes are recognizable only by histological examinations. Owing to the criteria of this strict sense, the term is used only for histological findings and not for clinical ones. However, it is certain that all the precancerous changes are found in the lesions of precancerous condition and not in healthy mucosa.

HISTOLOGICAL CRITERIA AND HISTOLOGICAL NATURE OF DYSPLASIA RELATED TO PRECANCEROUS CHANGES

Histologically, several types and several grades of precancerous changes can be seen on the gastric mucosa. To understand these changes, the concept of "dysplasia" seems to be indispensable.

It was agreed in the WHO Expert Committee on "Precancerous Conditions of the Stomach," which was held in London in 1978 [the report of this meeting was published elsewhere (5,12)], that for lesions related to precancerous changes, the term dysplasia was most suitable and it was defined as changes having the following three histological features:

1. cellular atypia
2. abnormal differentiation
3. disorganized mucosal architecture.

As in cases of squamous epithelia, dysplasia was classified into three grades—mild, moderate, and severe—according to the severity of the changes. In general, grades of the three histological features run parallel, but this is not always the case: there are some dysplastic lesions, in which cellular atypia is relatively slight in spite of prominent structural disorganization and vice versa.

The dysplasia has a histological and biological nature different from that of hyperplasia or neoplasia. Hyperplasia is simply an overgrowth of epithelia composing the gastric mucosa without prominent cellular and structural atypia, whereas neoplasia shows autonomous and invasive cell growth with apparent cellular and structural abnormalities. From these aspects, dysplasia is situated between these two changes and has its own histological characteristics. It must be pointed out, however, that some types of hyperplasia may change to dysplasia and certain types of dysplasia may transform into neoplasia in the course of their development (Fig. 1).

MATERIAL AND METHODS

Among 16,606 cases of the stomach, which were resected surgically at Aichi Cancer Center Hospital or Yokoyama Hospital during the period of 27 years from 1953 to 1979, 115 cases (0.7%) of an isolated lesion with dysplastic changes were observed. They were found in the mucosa apart from the main lesion of cancer or of peptic ulcer, mostly the former. Owing to the limitation of surgical intervention, the solitary dysplastic lesions were only 40 cases, of which 31 cases (77.5%) showed broad-based mucosal elevations with flat surface (Table 1).

There were many cases of dysplastic changes in or adjacent to the cancerous mucosa. These cases were very important for the histogenesis on development of gastric cancer but were omitted from the statistics, owing to uncertainty of their number.

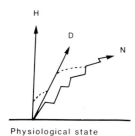

Physiological state

FIG. 1.   Relationship between hyperplasia (H), neoplasia (N), and dysplasia (D).

TABLE 1. *Materials used in this study*

Dysplastic lesions	No. of cases
In or adjacent to cancer	Many
Apart from cancer or ulcer	115
Alone	40
Elevated type	31
Hollowed type	9
(focal atrophy or erosion)	

From 16,606 cases of resected stomachs (1953–1979).

When dysplastic changes were found in the resected stomachs by routine histological examinations, the size, shape, and nature of the lesions were confirmed by step-section. Beside hematoxylin-eosin staining, special staining such as Alcian-blue-PAS (pH 2.5), Azan-Mallory, Elastica Van Gieson, or Silver staining were supplemented for many cases. For more detailed study, the mitotic epithelial cells in the dysplastic lesions were counted by the aid of microphotographs and their frequency and pattern of distribution were examined.

HISTOLOGICAL FINDINGS OF DYSPLASIA

Findings of cellular atypia are summarized as follows:

1. Dense distribution of hyperchromatic, slender, and elongated nuclei in the tall columnar epithelia.
2. Irregular arrangements of the nuclei leading to pseudostratification.
3. Increased nucleocytoplasmic ratio.
4. Diversity of the nuclei.
5. Disturbances of cellular polarity.

The first is seen when the atypical epithelia show the nature of intestinal metaplasia and the others are common in both metaplastic and nonmetaplastic epithelia.

Abnormal differentiation can be noticed by one or more of the following changes:

1. Decrease in the number of cells with secretory granules or of goblet cells.
2. Disappearance of maturing cells on the surface of the mucosa.
3. Atrophy of pyloric glands, leading to appearances of intestinal metaplasia and/or pseudopyloric gland formation of the fundic glands.
4. Loss of Paneth cells or their irregular distribution.
5. Increase in the layer of generative cells.

Disorganized mucosal architecture is characterized by one or more of the following changes:

1. Irregularities in the form and structure of foveolae, such as elongation, distortion, dilatation, branching, or fusion.
2. Cystic dilatation of the glands with or without irregular contour.
3. Diffuse or sporadic glandular heterotopia with or without proliferative change.
4. Irregular running of muscularis mucosae and/or fibrosis or scar formation at the base of the lesion.
5. Loss of smoothness or regularity of the mucosal surface.

HISTOLOGICAL FEATURES OF EACH GRADE OF DYSPLASIA

Mild Dysplasia

Mild dysplastic changes are visible both on elevated or depressed lesions. In both types, they are characterized by darkly stained, atypical, and metaplastic foveolar epithelia on the surface layer of the affected mucosa. Arrangement of the slender, elongated, and hyperchromatic nuclei is dense but relatively well preserved in the lower half of the columnar epithelia. Usually the number of goblet cells is few and Paneth cells are not visible. These slightly atypical foveolar epithelia are almost always accompanied by glandular cysts in the deeper layer of the lesion. In general, the number and size of the cysts are small and their shape is regular—round or oval.

Some elevated lesions with mild dysplastic change result from an overgrowth of "gastritis verrucosa" developed confluently in certain limited areas of the mucosa (Fig. 2).

Mild dysplastic change may be seen occasionally on depressed lesions. Darkly stained foveolar tubules show diffuse intestinal metaplasia with decreased number of goblet cells. From the histological and structural similarity of these tubules to regenerative ones, this lesion may be diagnosed as incomplete regeneration following deep erosion (Fig. 3).

Moderate Dysplasia

Changes of moderate dysplasia are also observable on both elevated and depressed lesions, but are more frequent in the former. Grades of cellular atypia of foveolar tubules are more

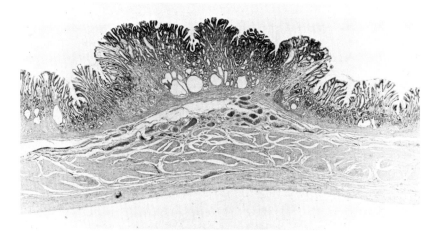

FIG. 2. Elevated lesion with mild dysplasia. The lesion is considered to be resulted from overgrowth of "gastritis verrucosa."

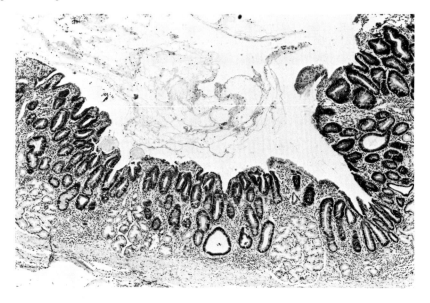

FIG. 3. Depressed lesion with mild dysplasia. The lesion may be a result of incomplete epithelial regeneration following deep erosion.

pronounced than those of mild dysplasia, as indicated by a slightly piled-up arrangement of slender, hyperchromatic nuclei, and a decrease in the number of goblet cells, which sometimes disappear altogether. In some cases, the number of Paneth cells is increased and their distribution is often irregular.

These atypical tubules, however, scarcely occupy the whole layer of the affected mucosa, leaving nonatypical pyloric or pseudopyloric glands in its lower half, and cystically dilated glands found there are often multiple and their shape is, more or less, deformed. Thus architecture of the mucosal lesion is disturbed.

The "borderline lesion" with broad-based mucosal elevation is a typical example of this grade. The upper half of the flat elevated lesion is composed diffusely of atypical and metaplastic foveolae; cystic dilatation of the glands in the lower half are numerous and their shape is various. Some glandular cysts are replaced by atypical and metaplastic epithelia (Fig. 4).

Even in the depressed lesion, moderate dysplasia can be seen. The lesion is composed entirely of atypical metaplastic tubules, some of which are irregularly dilated and distorted, but no fusion of the neighboring tubules can be seen. On the surface of the lesion, erosive changes are superimposed. Disorganized mucosal architecture is relatively slight in this lesion (Fig. 5).

Severe Dysplasia

Findings of cellular atypia, abnormal differentiation, and disorganized mucosal architecture are more obvious in this grade, even though the grades are not always run parallel. Most atypical tubules are composed of tall columnar epithelia with intestinal metaplasia, but unlike cases of mild or moderate dysplasia, some tubules or glands, especially in the deeper part of the lesion, may take the form of cuboidal or flat epithelia.

Abnormal differentiation of mucosae is characterized by the imbalance of the epithelial components: elongation of foveolae and atrophy or disappearances of pyloric or fundic glands.

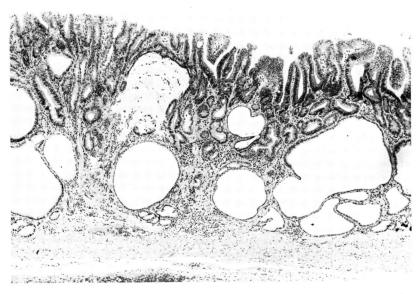

FIG. 4. Broad-based mucosal elevation with moderate dysplasia. The changes show both structurally and cytologically so-called borderline-lesion.

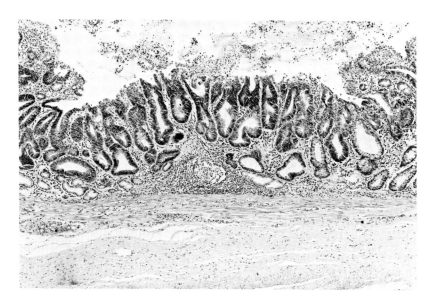

FIG. 5. Depressed lesion with moderate dysplasia. The lesion is composed of atypical and metaplastic tubules with structural abnormality.

Disorganized mucosal architecture is also more marked than with mild or moderate dysplasia, and such change is most frequently and most easily recognizable by cystically dilated glands with irregular contour.

Despite these severe cellular and structural changes, obvious evidence of malignancy (pleomorphism and random distribution of the nuclei, loss of cellular polarity, fusion or taching of the neighboring glands, sprouting of the small glands to the neighboring stroma, etc.) are not visible in this lesion.

As a whole, the broad-based mucosal elevation shows the typical picture of moderate dysplasia, but in a part of the lesion, downgrowth of the atypical epithelial glands is visible. By higher magnification of this part (shown in the lower half of Fig. 6), these growing

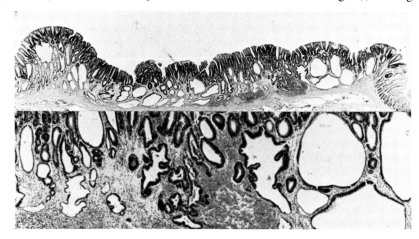

FIG. 6. Broad-based mucosal elevation with severe dysplasia. Most of the lesion shows the change of moderate dysplasia, but in a part, growing glands have cyst-papillary structure, suspicious of adenocarcinoma.

glands are composed of cuboidal epithelia with higher nucleocytoplasmic ratio and have a cyst-papillary structure suspicious of adenocarcinoma. From these findings, this case is diagnosed as severe dysplasia quite close to malignant transformation.

Figure 7 shows another type of severe dysplasia. The whole layer of the elevated lesion is composed of tortuously-elongated and metaplastic tubules and glands, indicating clearly a disorganized mucosal architecture. Irregularly dilated and disoriented glands, seen in the deeper layer of the lesion, are covered by nonmetaplastic, cuboidal epithelia and some of them are replaced by downward growth of the metaplastic ones. Cellular atypia suggestive of malignancy, however, is not visible in the epithelia.

Foveolar tubules composed of columnar epithelia are hyperplastic, metaplastic, and proliferative, but cellular and structural atypia of these tubules are not so prominent. However, cystically dilated glands seen in the deeper layer of the mucosa are quite deformed and some of them show irregularly directed branching. These glands are composed of small cuboidal cells with little cytoplasm, doubtful of commencement of malignancy (Fig. 8).

DIFFERENCES IN HISTOLOGY BETWEEN SEVERE DYSPLASIA AND INCIPIENT PHASE OF CANCER

Severe dysplasia is sometimes very difficult to differentiate from incipient cancer or cancer very close to the state of carcinoma *in situ*, but the latter can be distinguished from dysplasia by (a) pleomorphism and disturbance in arrangement of the nuclei; (b) more increased nucleocytoplasmic ratio (except for mature signet-ring cell); (c) loss of cellular differentiation and polarity; (d) random shape and disoriented structure of the tubules or glands; (e) invasive or infiltrative growth of epithelia into the surrounding tissues; (f) abrupt transition or serrated border of the epithelial tissues to the surrounding one; (g) cord-like structure, budding, or cluster formation of the small glands composed of flat or cuboidal epithelia; (h) disturbed epitheliostromal relationship; (i) occupation of the whole layer of the mucosa by malignant tissues in the central area of the lesion; and (j) rough or ragged surface of the affected mucosa.

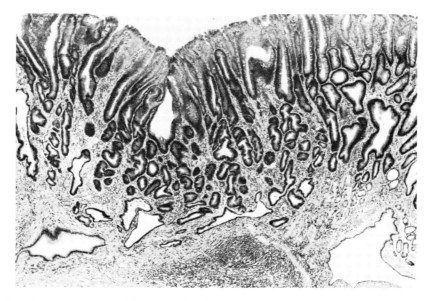

FIG. 7. Elevated mucosa with severe dysplasia. Disorganized mucosal architecture is quite prominent, in spite of relatively slight cellular atypia.

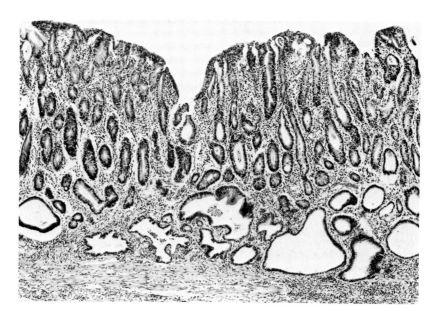

FIG. 8. Mucosa with severe dysplasia. In deeper layer of the mucosa, irregularly deformed glands composed of small cuboidal cell with little cytoplasm, doubtful of malignancy, are seen.

Finding (g) is characteristic for cases of well-differentiated adenocarcinoma (intestinal-type carcinoma in Lauren and Järvi's classification), (h) is seen only in cases of poorly differentiated adenocarcinoma (diffuse-type carcinoma), and the others are common in both types.

When incipient cancer or intramucosal cancer with *in situ*-like appearances still have the following histological findings, they might be considered as cancer developed through the course of dysplasia: (a) Tubules composed of atypical epithelia are seen sporadically or fragmentally on the central upper half zone of the adenocarcinomatous lesion. (b) Cystically dilated and nonmalignant glands or their remnants are seen in the central deeper layer of the cancerous lesion.

The upper half of the atrophic mucosa is composed diffusely of well-differentiated tubular adenocarcinoma without prominent invasion, the higher magnification of which is shown in the lower half of Fig. 9. In the deeper layer of the mucosa, many cystically dilated, nonmalignant glands covered by cuboidal or flat epithelia are seen and some of them are replaced by malignant epithelia. On the basis of these findings, this cancerous lesion is considered to be preceded by severe dysplasia (Fig. 9).

The atrophic mucosa is occupied diffusely by moderately differentiated adenocarcinoma and in the lower half it is irregularly dilated. A high-power view of the center of the mucosa (lower half of Fig. 10) reveals infiltrative growth of the small cancerous glands composed of cuboidal cells. In both sides of the lowest layer of the atrophic mucosa, nonmalignant and cystically dilated glands are still visible. With these features, the case was diagnosed as cancer preceded by dysplasia.

HISTOGENESIS ON DEVELOPMENT OF GASTRIC CANCER

On the basis of the findings described above, it can be said that certain types of gastric cancer—both elevated and depressed—develop through a stage of severe dysplasia. But it

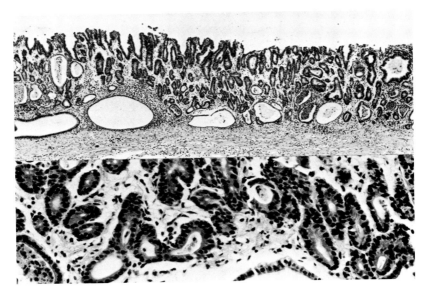

FIG. 9. Cancerous atrophic mucosa preceded by dysplasia. Upper half of the mucosa is occupied diffusely by adenocarcinoma; in the deeper layer, cystically dilated, nonmalignant glands replaced by malignant epithelia remain.

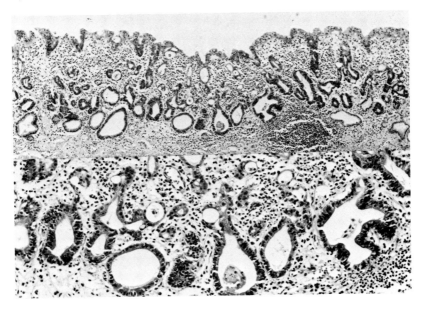

FIG. 10. Cancerous atrophic mucosa preceded by dysplasia. In center of the atrophic mucosa, infiltration of small cancerous gland is visible. In lowest layer, however, nonmalignant and cystically dilated glands are still visible.

is, by no means, always the case, since most of the gastric mucosa in and around the minute cancers—less than 5 mm in diameter—merely show atrophy of the proper gastric glands with or without intestinal metaplasia, and dysplastic changes as defined in this paper cannot be recognized.

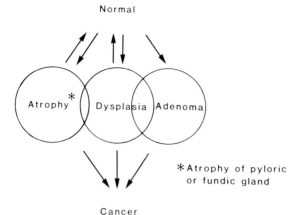

FIG. 11. Histogenesis on the development of gastric cancer.

On the other hand, there are enough reports that gastric polyps with the histology of tubular, tubulopapillary, or villous adenoma often coexist with adenocarcinoma, and thus we have histological evidence of high risk of malignant transformation from adenomatous polyps.

The course of development of gastric cancer can be summarized as shown in Fig. 11, even though the real frequency of each course is still uncertain. It must be added that atrophy and atrophic dysplastic mucosa and adenoma and proliferative dysplastic mucosa share common histological features to some extent.

DISCUSSION

As shown in the figures accompanying this chapter, mild dysplasia does not necessarily progress into higher grades of dysplasia and may recover to the normal state in not a few instances, whereas this possibility is hardly expected in cases of moderate dysplasia from the aspects of their disorganized mucosal structure. However, evidence indicating that lesions with moderate dysplasia are destined to become malignant is insufficient and needs further investigation. On the contrary, on the basis of the findings described above, severe dysplasia can be assumed as precancerous changes in the strict sense of the terminology.

In the literature, there are a few reports using the terminology *dysplasia of the stomach.* Concerning the possible precursor for the development of gastric cancer, Grundmann (1) classified the dysplastic lesions into low grade and high grade and commented the latter as "in full awareness of their fluent transition into the intestinal type of early gastric cancer." Using studies on cell kinetics, karyometry, and histochemistry, Oehlert (10) classified dysplasia into grades I, II, and III, and as characteristic findings of dysplasia III, he pointed out the following changes: "Unwandlung der kryptenartigen Foveolae gastricae," "mehrreihigen Epithel mit deutlicher Kernpolymorphie, vergrösserten Nukleoren und zytoplasmatischer Basophelie mit völlingen Verlust der Schleimbildung."[1] He also commented on the possible reversibility or presistence of the lesion without transition into early cancer. Ming (4) denoted dysplasia of gastric epithelia as "deviation from the histological feature of the normal stomach, both structurally and cytologically" and classified it into four grades: grades I and II are in benign conditions; III and IV are seen in severe atrophic gastritis, adenoma, or mucosa bordering adenocarcinoma. In conclusion, he said that "Grade IV

---

[1]"Change of gastric foveola into crypt-like structure," "piled-up epithelia with evident sign of nuclear pleomorphism, increased nucleoli, and cyto plasmic basophilia with complete loss of mucous formation."

dysplasia, exhibiting prominent cellular pleomorphism, is occasionally difficult to differentiate from carcinoma." Schade (11) also described the borderline lesion of the stomach and concluded that the histological findings, such as heaped-up, multinucleated epithelia with absence of goblet cells, are good guides for the diagnosis of intraepithelial neoplasm. Recently Johansen (3) described dysplasia as "malignant change without convincing evidence of invasion" and said that "there are some highly differentiated tumor, distinction of it from severe grade of dysplasia is very difficult."

In Japan, papers using the term *dysplasia* are very few but papers using other synonymous terms such as *atypical epithelium, atypical epithelial hyperplasia*, or *borderline lesion* are numerous. Among them, Sugano et al. (13) and Nakamura et al. (9) reported the atypical lesions in full detail with ample description and microphotographs. Ten years ago, the author (6–8) also reported histological features of the borderline lesion. Other than these elevated and atypical lesions, the report by Iwanaga and colleagues (2) seems to be most noteworthy from the viewpoint of this chapter. Iwanaga et al. found 12 cases of superficial gastric cancer, all of which were accompanied in the submucosa by diffuse and heterotopic glandular cysts.

At the present time, we still have no objective indicator for knowing precancerous change of the stomach. Thus we have to rely on subjective interpretation of the examiners for its diagnosis. It is, therefore, unavoidable that histological criteria of the precancerous lesion do not coincide completely with each investigator. It is necessary for us to define more clearly the histological, cytological, and biological nature of gastric epithelial dysplasia.

SUMMARY

Precancerous changes of the stomach were defined as changes recognizable only by histological examination of clinically detectable lesions and were classified into three groups—adenoma, atrophy, and dysplasia.

Dysplasia of gastric mucosa was characterized by three histological features: (a) cellular atypia, (b) abnormal differentiation, and (c) disorganized mucosal architecture. It was graded into three categories: mild, moderate, and severe.

Each grade and each type of dysplasia were described with some examples, and emphasis was put on histological differences between severe dysplasia and mucosal cancer nearly to the state of carcinoma *in situ*. It is concluded that some types of gastric cancer develop through changes of severe dysplasia.

ACKNOWLEDGMENTS

The author thanks Drs. E. Yamada, T. Kasugai, and T. Suchi of Aichi Cancer Center Hospital and H. Yokoyama, Y. Yokoyama, and I. Yokoyama of Yokoyama Hospital for providing the materials and encouragement of the study. This study was supported in part by a grant-in-aid for cancer research from the Ministry of Education, Science and Culture of Japan.

REFERENCES

1. Grundmann, E. (1975): Histologic types and possible initial stages in early gastric carcinoma. *Beitr. Pathol.*, 154:256–280.
2. Iwanaga, T., Koyama, H., Takahashi, Y., Taniguchi, H., and Wada, A. (1975): Diffuse submucosal cysts and carcinoma of the stomach. *Cancer*, 36:606–614.
3. Johansen, A. (1981): *Early Gastric Cancer*. Bispebjerg Hospital, Copenhagen. p. 15.
4. Ming, S. C. (1979): Dysplasia of gastric epithelium. *Front. Gastrointest. Res.*, 4:164–172.
5. Morson, B. C., Sobin, L. H., Grundmann, E., Johansen, A., Nagayo, T., and Serck-Hanssen, A. (1980): Precancerous conditions and epithelial dysplasia in the stomach. *J. Clin. Pathol.*, 33:711–721.

6. Nagayo, T. (1971): Histological diagnosis of biopsied gastric mucosa with special reference to that of borderline lesions. *Gann Monogr.*, 11:245–256.

7. Nagayo, T. (1980): Dysplastic changes of the digestive tract related to cancer. *Acta Endoscopica*, 10:69–80.

8. Nagayo, T. (1981): Dysplasia of the gastric mucosa with regard to its precancerous nature. *Gann*, 72:813–823.

9. Nakamura, K., Sugano, H., Takagi, K., and Fuchigami, A. (1966): Histopathological study on early carcinoma of the stomach: Criteria for diagnosis of atypical epithelium. *Gan.*, 57:613–620.

10. Oehlert, W., Keller, P., Henke, M., and Strauch, M. (1975): Dysplasien der Magenschleimhaut. *Dtsch. Med. Wschr.*, 100:1950–1956.

11. Schade, R. O. K. (1974): *The Borderline Between Benign and Malignant Lesions in the Stomach: Early Gastric Cancer*, edited by E. Grundmann, H. Grunze, and S. Witte. Springer-Verlag, Berlin, Heidelberg, New York.

12. Serck-Hanssen, A. (1979): Precancerous lesions of the stomach. *Scand. J. Gastroenterol. (Suppl.)*, 54:104–105.

13. Sugano, H., Nakamura, K., and Takagi, K. (1971): An atypical epithelium of the stomach. A Clinicopathological entity. *Gann Monogr.*, 11:257–269.

Precancerous Lesions of the Gastrointestinal Tract, edited by P. Sherlock, B.C. Morson, L. Barbara, and U. Veronesi. Raven Press, New York © 1983.

Histochemistry of Mucins and Carcinogenic Sequence: A Study of Some Gastric and Colorectal Lesions

*Walter Grigioni, **Mario Miglioli, *Donatella Santini, *Michele Vanzo, *Alessandro Piccaluga, and **Luigi Barbara

*Departments of *Histopathology and **Gastroenterology, University of Bologna, Policlinico S. Orsola, Bologna, Italy*

The morphological changes found in colonic and gastric mucosa during the carcinogenic sequence have been the subject of several studies. Moreover, during the last few years, several histochemical techniques have been used to find quantitative and qualitative variations in the pattern of mucin secretion (1,3,8,9,12).

If these changes would arise before the morphological alterations identifiable with normal hematoxylin-exosin (H.-E.) stains, they could be used as an early marker of precancerous situations.

Filipe and Branfoot (2) described some morphological and histochemical changes in the mucosa adjacent to primary adenocarcinomas and in some precancerous lesions and conditions of the colorectal mucosa (1,2,4,7,10). They suggest that this type of mucosa, called "transitional," is indicative of a premalignant change (2,4). Using the High Iron Diamine–Alcian Blue (HID/AB) (pH 2.5) technique (12), also in the absence of any microscopic features of malignancy, this type of mucosa shows a prevalence of sialomucins, whereas the mucin in normal colonic mucosa is predominantly sulphomucin positive stained (1,2). As in gastric mucosa, where sulphomucins are occasionally found, their presence would indicate a specific preneoplastic change (1,6,7).

Therefore, if the cancerogenic sequence is related to a qualitative modification of mucin production, the histochemical techniques would be useful in the detection of early malignancy and in the assessment of the malignant potential of precancerous lesions. We have tested these hypotheses both in the colon and in the stomach.

MATERIALS AND METHODS

One hundred polyps of the colon-rectum were selected: 20 were hyperplastic, 20 juvenile, and 60 adenomatous. Fifty specimens obtained from the mucosa surrounding cancers in ulcerative colitis (U.C.) were also examined.

The adenomatous polyps (tubular, villous, and tubulovillous) were of different size and degree of dysplasia. Similarly, high and low grades of dysplasia were present in U.C. specimens. All the lesions were located in the left colon. Furthermore, 50 hyperplastic polyps, 10 adenomatous polyps, 200 specimens of mucosa with intestinal metaplasia (I.M.)

from 20 early gastric cancers (E.G.C.), and 50 specimens of mucosa with I.M. from 20 unselected advanced gastric cancers (A.G.C.) were collected.

The hyperplastic polyps were removed endoscopically and the adenomatous ones were obtained from surgical specimens, so that in the latter cases the surrounding mucosa was also examined. The age range of the cancer patients was 60 to 70 years.

The I.M. present both in E.G.C. and A.G.C. was classified as scattered or diffuse. Following histological and cytological criteria, the cancers were classified as well differentiated and poorly differentiated; the E.G.C.'s were macroscopically classified according to the Japanese Society for Gastroenterological Endoscopy.

The colonic and gastric specimens were fixed in 10% buffered formol saline for a standardized time to avoid alterations of the mucins. Each section was stained with hematoxylin and eosin, Alcian blue-PAS at pH 2.5, Masson's trichrome, and the HID/AB at pH 2.5 (12).

In the colonic mucosa, semiquantitative estimate of the proportion of mucins was made by separating goblet cells with prevalent production of sulphomucins from those in which there was a balance between sialo- and sulphomucins and those with predominance of sialomucins.

In the stomach, the presence of sulphomucins in I.M. was estimated semiquantitatively as light staining (s-IM +), intense staining (s-IM + +), and no staining (s-IM −).

RESULTS

Fifty percent of the colonic polyps showed an altered mucin production, compared with normal colonic mucosa.

Sialomucins were predominant in 30% to 35% of the cases, whereas a balance between sialo- and sulphomucins was present in 16.6% to 20% of the cases.

However, the change in mucin secretion was similar in the three types of polyps (Table 1, Fig. 1). In the adenomatous polyps of the colon, the mucin variations were not related to the histological features, to the size of the polyps, or to the degree of dysplasia (Figs. 2–4).

The same degree of dysplasia often showed different patterns of mucus. Mucin production decreased along with the increase in severity of dysplasia. In the neoplastic polyps with severe dysplasia, mucins were often observed in traces. A similar pattern was observed in dysplastic mucosa of U.C. patients (Fig. 1).

The mucin production of the hyperplastic polyps of the stomach was similar to the normal gastric epithelium. Sialomucins in traces were present only in some cystic glands and in some focal areas of I.M. In no case were sulphomucins detected.

TABLE 1. *Mucin production in neoplastic and nonneoplastic colonic polyps*

	Hyperplastic polyps (20) (%)	Juvenile polyps (20) (%)	Neoplastic polyps (60) (%)
Predominance of sulphomucins	8 (40)	7 (35)	20 (33.3)
Predominance of sialomucins	7 (35)	7 (35)	18 (35)
Balance between sulpho- and sialomucins	4 (20)	4 (20)	10 (16.6)
Mucin in traces	1 (5)	2 (10)	12 (20)

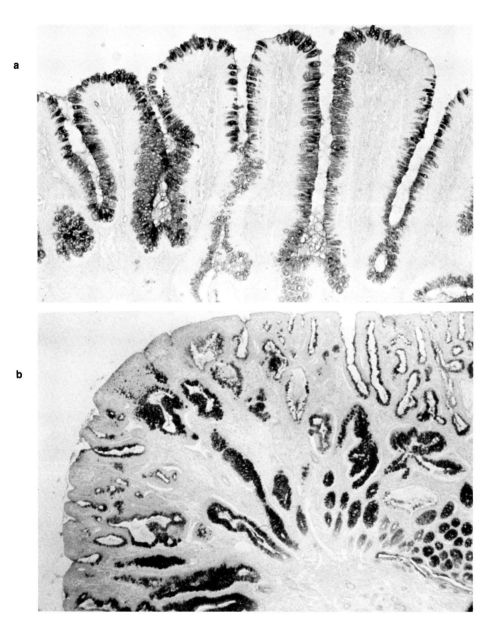

FIG. 1. *(above and following page)* Equivalence of type of mucin production in different types of colonic polyps and in ulcerative colitis associated dysplasia. **a:** Hyperplastic polyp. **b:** Juvenile polyp.

In only 7 of 10 adenomatous polyps of the stomach were small amounts of apical sulphomucins observed (Fig. 5). In these cases sulphomucins were also found in the metaplastic surrounding mucosa (s-IM+) (Table 2). In a high percentage of E.G.G.'s (80%) I.M. in the absence of sulphomucins was detected (s-IM−) (Fig. 6a). In 20% of the E.G.C.'s, in which sulphomucin positive I.M. was present, this was diffuse, the adenocarcinoma was well differentiated and of the elevated type; the lack of sulphomucins was associated

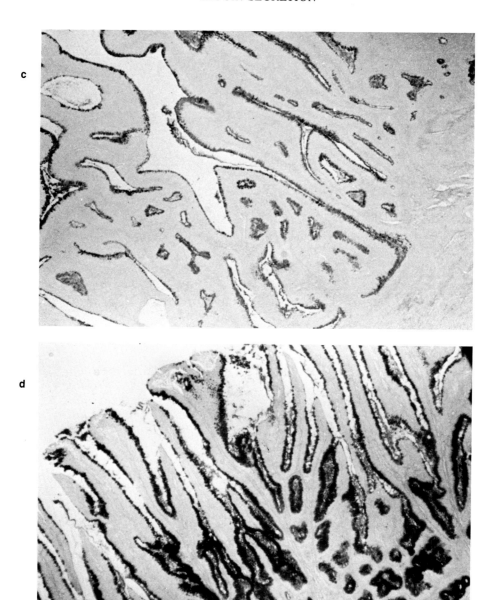

FIG. 1. *(continued)*   **c:** Neoplastic polyp. **d:** Epithelial dysplasia in ulcerative colitis.

with scattered I.M. and poorly differentiated carcinoma either of the depressed or flat type (Table 3).

The mucosa surrounding A.G.C. very often showed s-IM+ and this depended neither on the diffusion of the I.M. nor on the differentiation of the carcinoma (Table 4, Fig. 6b).

DISCUSSION

In the mucosa of the colon, the goblet cells secrete sulphated mucins, though a small number of sialomucin positive goblet cells can be found, mainly in the right colon (1,2,9).

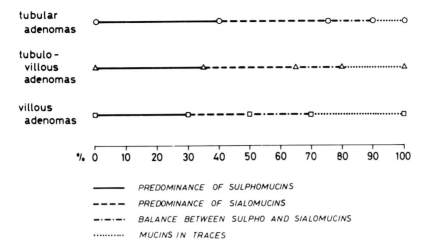

FIG. 2. Relationship between hystology and mucin, neoplastic colonic polyps.

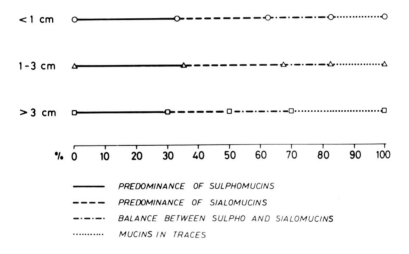

FIG. 3. Relationship between polyp size and mucin, neoplastic colonic polyps.

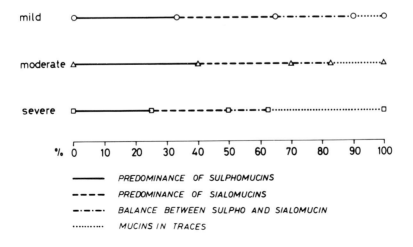

FIG. 4. Relationship between degree of dysplasia and mucin, neoplastic colonic polyps.

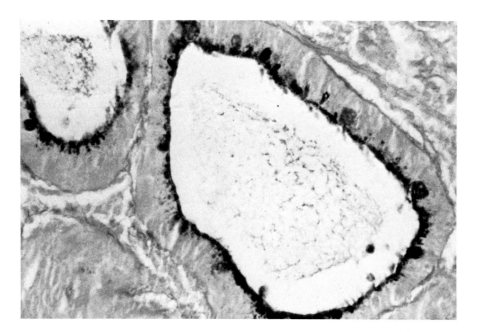

FIG. 5. Small amounts of apical sulphomucins in some glands of an adenomatous gastric polyp.

TABLE 2. *Mucin production in gastric adenomas and in surrounding mucosa (10 cases)*

	No. of cases	s – IM+ in surrounding mucosa	s – IM– in surrounding mucosa	Absence of IM in surrounding mucosa
s – IM+	7 (70%)	6 (86%)	1 (14%)	—
s – IM+ +	—	—	—	—
s – IM–	1 (10%)	—	1	—
Absence of IM	2 (20%)	—	—	2

s – IM, intestinal metaplasia with sulphomucins; s – IM+, light staining HID; s – IM+ +, intense staining with HID; s – IM–, intestinal metaplasia without sulphomucins.

According to some authors, the predominance of sialomucins might represent an early stage of carcinogenesis (2,4,7,10). As in the stomach, where sulphomucins are not found or are present only in traces, their presence would indicate an early carcinomatous change of the cells (5–7).

Therefore, the modification in mucin secretion would be useful in the detection of early malignancy and in the assessment of the malignant potential of precancerous lesions.

Our results seem in contrast with this hypothesis. In fact, in our series, the hyperplastic juvenile and adenomatous polyps of the colon with verified different cancerogenic potential, showed a similar variation in mucin secretion. Besides, in the neoplastic polyps the variation of mucus production was not related to the histological type, to the size of the polyp, or to the degree of dysplasia; these are useful morphological criteria for the assessment of malignant

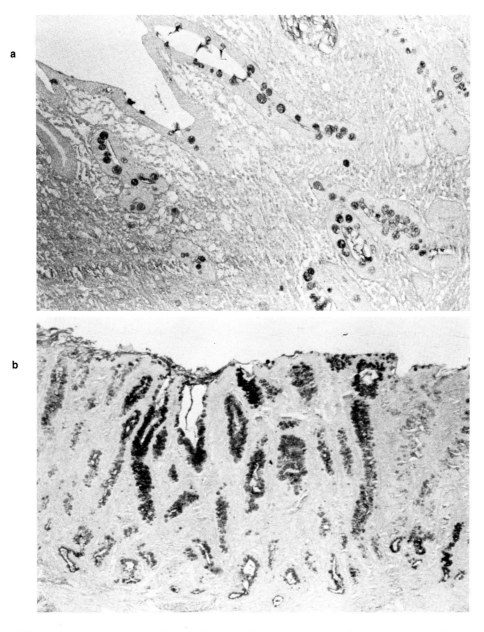

FIG. 6. **a:** Intestinal metaplasia without sulphomucins surrounding an early gastric cancer. **b:** Sulphomucin positive intestinal metaplasia surrounding an advanced gastric cancer.

potential of neoplastic polyps of the colon. The dysplasia in U.C. patients leads us to the same conclusion.

Our results about the mucin production of the adenomatous gastric polyps and of the I.M. associated to E.G.C. suggest that the lack of sulphomucins in the I.M. of a high percentage of E.G.C.'s casts doubt on the use of sulphomucins as a marker of risk for gastric carcinoma.

TABLE 3. *Sulphomucins histological and macroscopical types of carcinomas and diffuse or scattered intestinal metaplasia (20 EGC; age range 60–70)*

| | No. of cases | I.M. | | Histological types[a] | | Macroscopical type |
		Diffuse	Scattered	Diff.	Undiff.	
s − IM +	4 (20%)	4	—	4	—	4 elevated
s − IM + +	—	—	—	—	—	—
s − IM −	16 (80%)	2 (12.5%)	14 (87.5%)	1 (6.25%)	15 (93.75%)	14 (87.5%) depressed, 2 (12.5%) flat

[a]Differentiated and undifferentiated.
s − IM +, light staining with HID; s − IM + +, intense staining with HID; s − IM −, intestinal metaplasia without sulphomucins.

TABLE 4. *Sulphomucins histological types and diffuse or scattered intestinal metaplasia (20 advanced gastric cancer; age range 60–70)*

	No. of cases	Diffuse I.M.	Scattered I.M.	Diff. CA	Undiff. CA
s − IM +	13 (65%)	4 (31%)	9 (69%)	3 (23%)	10 (77%)
s − IM + +	6 (30%)	6	—	6	—
s − IM −	1 (5%)	—	1	—	1

s − IM +, light staining with HID; s − IM + +, intense staining with HID; s − IM −, intestinal metaplasia without sulphomucins.

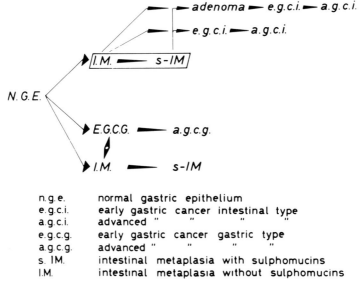

n.g.e.	normal gastric epithelium
e.g.c.i.	early gastric cancer intestinal type
a.g.c.i.	advanced " " " "
e.g.c.g.	early gastric cancer gastric type
a.g.c.g.	advanced " " " "
s. IM.	intestinal metaplasia with sulphomucins
I.M.	intestinal metaplasia without sulphomucins

FIG. 7. Postulated mechanism of progression from normal gastric epithelium to advanced gastric cancer.

The s-IM+ is frequently associated with advanced neoplastic lesions; s-IM+ is also associated with adenomatous polyps and with some types of EGC which arise from metaplastic epithelium.

A possible explanation for s-IM+ and s-IM− is that it might represent two stages of the same evolution sequence (11), so that in gastric adenomas and in E.G.C.'s arising in metaplastic areas, the preexisting I.M. is usually detected in an advanced stage, and therefore sulphomucin positive.

Alternatively, when E.G.C.'s and exceptionally gastric adenomas arise from gastric non-metaplastic epithelium, I.M, if present, might represent an associated finding simultaneous to the neoplastic lesion or due to it (Fig. 7).

In these latter situations the presence of s-IM− should be due to the earliest stage of the metaplastic process.

This hypothesis agrees with the low prevalence of s-IM+ in E.G.C.'s of the gastric type and its presence in a high percentage of A.G.C.'s of both intestinal and gastric types.

Therefore, our results do not support the role of some histochemical analysis of mucus production in the detection of early malignancy and in the assessment of the malignant potential of preneoplastic gastric and colonic lesions.

REFERENCES

1. Filipe, M. I. (1979): Mucins in the human gastrointestinal epithelium: A review. *Invest. Cell. Pathol.*, 2:195–216.
2. Filipe, M. I., and Branfoot, A. C. (1976): Mucin histochemistry of the colon. In: *Current Topics in Pathology*, edited by E. Grundmann and W. H. Kirsten, vol. 63, pp. 143–178. Springer Verlag, Berlin, Heidelberg, New York.
3. Gad, A. (1969): A histochemical study of human alimentary tract mucosubstances in health and disease. 1. Normal and tumours. *Br. J. Cancer*, 23:52–63.
4. Greaves, P., Filipe, M. I., and Branfoot, A. C. (1980): Transitional mucosa and survival in human colorectal cancer. *Cancer*, 46:764–770.
5. Jass, S. R. (1980): Role of intestinal metaplasia in the histogenesis of gastric carcinoma. *J. Clin. Pathol.*, 33:801–810.
6. Jass, S. R., and Filipe, M. I. (1979): A variant of intestinal metaplasia associated with gastric carcinoma: a histochemical study. *Histopath.*, 3:191–199.
7. Jass, S. R., and Filipe, M. I. (1980): Sulphomucins and precancerous lesions of the human stomach. *Histopathology*, 4:271–279.
8. Kalevi, K. L., Mäkelä, V., and Lilius, C. (1971): Carbohydrate-rich compounds in the colonic mucosa of man. II. Histochemical characteristics of colonic adenocarcinomas. *Cancer*, 27:128–133.
9. Mäkelä, V., Kalevi, K. L., and Lilius, C. (1971): Carbohydrate-rich compounds in the colonic mucosa of man. I. Histochemical characteristics of normal and adenomatous colonic mucosa. *Cancer*, 27:120–127.
10. Montero, C., and Segura, D. I. (1980): Retrospective histochemical study of mucosubstances in adenocarcinomas of the gastrointestinal tract. *Histopathology*, 4:281–291.
11. Sippone, P., Seppälä, K., Varis, K., Hjselt, L., Ihanaki, T., Kekki, M., and Siurala, M. (1980): Intestinal metaplasia with colonic-type sulphomucins in the gastric mucosa: its association with gastric carcinoma. *Acta Pathol. Microbiol. Scand.*, Sect. A, 88:217–224.
12. Spicer, S. S. (1965): Diamine methods for differentiating mucosubstances histochemically. *J. Histochem. Cytochem.*, 13:211–234.

Precancerous Lesions of the Gastrointestinal Tract, edited by P. Sherlock, B.C. Morson, L. Barbara, and U. Veronesi. Raven Press, New York © 1983.

Comparative Morphologic and Morphometric Analysis of the Borderline Lesion of the Antral Mucosa of the Stomach

J. F. Riemann,   H. Schmidt, and   *P. Hermanek

*Departments of Medicine and *Surgical Pathology, Division of Surgery, University of Erlangen-Nuremberg Medical School, Erlangen, Federal Republic of West Germany*

Borderline cases between benign and malignant growth in the stomach are sometimes extremely difficult to decide and to judge correctly. A large number of papers published during the last years indicate the existence of diverging opinions concerning the applicable criteria forming the basis for this decision. For this reason, various research teams utilized a classification into different degrees of dysplasia, considering both the severity of the cytological and structural changes of the epithelium as well as a possible reversibility of the disorder (6).

The term *borderline lesion* in the stomach was coined by Nagayo (1971) (7). This expression covers a particular type of proliferation of the epithelium in conjunction with a severe cellular atypia (1). Other authors stick to the terminology *severe dysplasia* or *dysplasia III* not necessarily always implying a transition into carcinoma (4,6,8).

Very few studies on ultrastructural peculiarities of these borderline lesions have been published so far (10). This chapter is intended to present our ultrastructural observations and findings in such changes where in two cases the transition of a borderline lesion into a fully matured intestinal carcinoma was observed (both patients had refused surgical intervention).

When viewed through the endoscope, the borderline lesion is seen as a shallow, elevated polypoidal lesion of the gastric mucosa (9). Since the macroscopical appearance of this disturbance is already so evident and fairly characteristic in comparison to either inflammatory or cancerous lesions, except for early gastric carcinoma type I, inspection by the naked eye allows diagnosing of suspicious conditions. Final confirmation of the diagnosis, however, is achieved via biopsy or endoscopically executed polypectomy.

MATERIAL AND METHODS

In the course of routine endoscopic inspection of the upper digestive tract in 7 patients, a borderline lesion located always in the prepyloric antrum was diagnosed. The lesion was removed by means of a diathermally heated loop and the specimen obtained submitted to routine histological examination and to electron microscopic studies.

Histologically in all cases a proliferation was found in the area of the glandular neck with severe atypical appearance of the cells in the region of the superficial glandular epithelium of the mucosa of the antrum.

For electron microscopy, individual miniature rectangular blocks measuring 2 mm by 3 mm were cut from the ectomized specimen, fixed in 2.5% glutaraldehyde solution first and then in 1% osmium tetroxide.

Following these preliminary steps, the blocks were dehydrated in a graded series of alcohol and embedded in EPON 812 synthetic epoxy resin. The semithin sections prepared by means of an LKB brand ultramicrotome were stained with Azur-II-methylene blue to permit topographical localization of the ultrathin cuts to be obtained selectively later. Preselecting the initial cuts for regions of particular interest proved to be an opportunity for a backup confirmation of the initial histological diagnosis.

Regions from which ultrathin cuts were subsequently prepared were accordingly selected from the semithin sections showing a particularly characteristic appearance. Contrast in the ultrathin cuts was enhanced using uranyl acetate and lead citrate. The final sections were investigated in an electron microscope model, ELMISKOP 1 A made by Siemens Corporation.

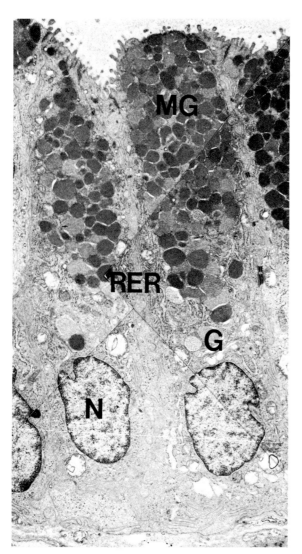

FIG. 1. Electron micrograph of a normal cell of antral mucosa. MG, Mucin granules; G, Golgi complex; RER, rough endoplasmic reticulum; N, nucleus. × 6,400 (Montage).

Tissue samples of normal mucosa of the antrum (10 cases), biopsies of reactive dysplasia I and II from the edge of a gastric ulcer (20 cases), and carcinoma of the intestinal cell type (10 cases) were used for comparison.

Morphometric analysis was carried out using a manual optic processing system (MOP). This technique allows calculation of a variety of data such as we measured—area and circumference of the cell, the nucleus and the nucleolus, area of mucin granules, number of desmosomes, mitochondria, and length of endoplasmic reticulum.

From each case, 20 electron micrographs were taken at random; however, only epithelial cells were used stretching from the luminal side to the basement membrane.

RESULTS

Normally the mucosa of the antrum shows uniform cells exhibiting a specific architecture (Fig. 1). The apical pole of the individual cell is evenly filled with mucoid granules of varying osmiophilia, the nucleus of the cell is situated in the lower third of the cell. At a typical location above the nucleus, a clearly distinguishable Golgi complex is found as well as formed rough endoplasmatic reticulum (RER). The basal membrane is undisturbed.

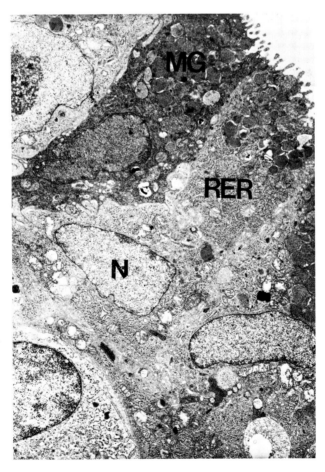

FIG. 2. Ultrastructural pattern of antral cells in reactive dysplasia (benign gastric ulcer). See legend to Fig. 1 for abbreviations. × 5,400.

Compared with these regular conditions, a significantly decreased number of mucoid granules can be noted in cases of moderate reactive dysplasia within a benign ulcer (Fig. 2). The polarity of the cell is maintained however. The structure of the nuclei of the cells is similar to the one seen in normal cells. There is a slight reduction in mucoid granules.

In the cases of the borderline lesion, the cells exhibit an entirely different appearance (Fig. 3). In addition to a noticeable shift in the relation "nucleus versus cytoplasma," favoring the nucleus, and an increase in the number of nucleoles, the polarity of the cell is found to be suspended. Furthermore, almost no more mucoid granules can be detected inside the cells. The number of mitochondria is significantly increased, the RER can, however, hardly be demonstrated anymore. In all seven cases of borderline lesion investigated, a particularly striking feature is sometimes grotesque bulges of the luminar surface of the cells in the form of so-called bubbles or blips (Fig. 4). These manifestations are bulges of the cytoplasmic structures into the lumen, containing predominantly free ribosomes. In some cases, these bulges show a smooth border, but they may also exhibit a population of coarse, plump microvilli developed to various extents and may be attached with a sort of stem to the surface. Finally, cytoplasmatic inclusions, for example, mucin granules, may occur. Intestinal cell type carcinoma is likewise distinguished by a complete loss of cell polarity, by a very large flapped nucleus (2) with multiple nucleoles, and by an architecture of the cytoplasma similar to the structure found in borderline lesions.

The ultrastructural cell profile based on different areas demonstrates the significant shift

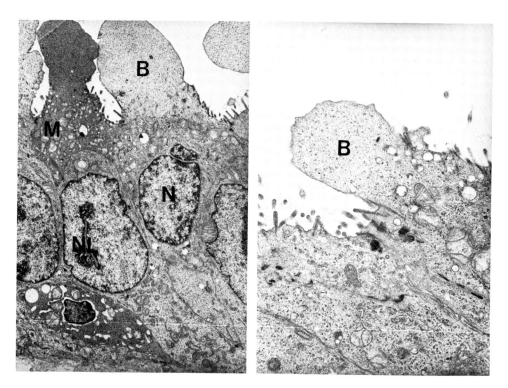

FIG. 3.   Left: Ultrastructure of typical cells in cases of borderline lesion. B, Luminal bulging; M, mitochondria; N, nucleus; NL, nucleolus; note increase in mitochondria and reduction of RER. × 4,300. **Right:** Higher power of a smooth surfaced luminal bulge (B) in borderline lesion. Note the nearly complete absence of RER. × 9,850.

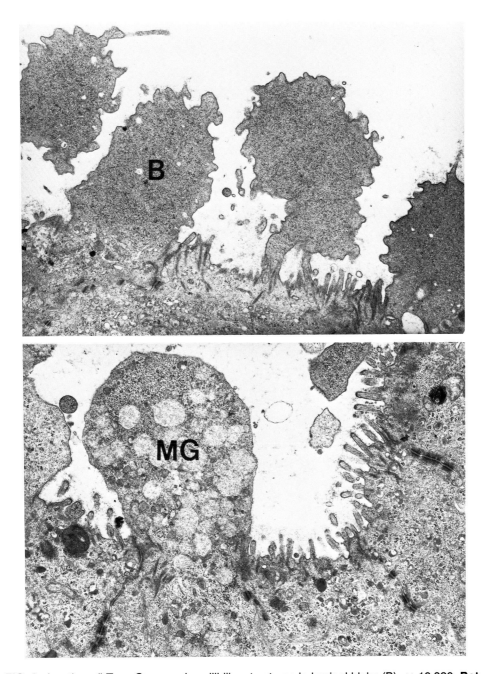

FIG. 3. *(continued)* **Top:** Coarse microvilli-like structures in luminal blebs (B). × 12,320. **Bottom:** Cytoplasmatic inclusions like mucin granules (MG) in enorm bubble on the luminal surface. × 12,320.

(Fig. 5) towards an increase in nucleus and nucleolus area, but a reduction in mucoid granules.

A close relationship between borderline lesion and carcinoma (Fig. 6) also exists in regard to number of desmosomes, mitochondria, and length of endoplasmic reticulum. As expected

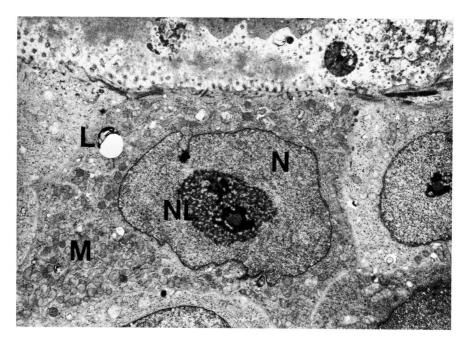

FIG. 4. Ultrastructural aspect of a cancer cell in intestinal type gastric carcinoma. M, Mitochondria; N, nucleus; NL, nucleolus; L, lysosome. ×6,400.

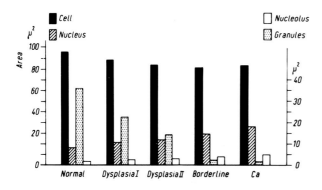

FIG. 5. Ultrastructural cell profile in different diseases. Antral mucosa of the stomach.

FIG. 6. Ultrastructural cell profile in different diseases. Antral mucosa of the stomach.

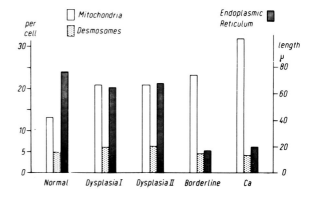

(Fig. 7), a clear tendency can be shown towards an increase in the ratio of nucleus-cytoplasma as well as nucleus-nucleolus. At least there is a slight decrease in the ratio circumference/area (Fig. 8) in regard to nucleus and cell.

DISCUSSION

Comparative morphometrical investigations of ultrastructural parameters of normal cells and cancer cells from various organs have repeatedly been carried out in the past (5,11,12). With respect to different parameters such as nucleus/plasma ratio, nucleolus/nucleus ratio, ratio of circumference of nucleus versus area of the nucleus and number of cytoplasmatic structures, these studies proved that quite characteristic and significant differences do exist. Ultrastructural characteristics of gastric adenocarcinoma have been defined (3) and proved to coincide with our observations.

Our results demonstrate that on the ultrastructural level the borderline lesion of the stomach as a recognized precancerous lesion occupies a middle position between normal cells and cancer cells. Morphometrical data, however, show this precancerosis, based on the fundamental structure of the cell, to have a clear tendency to the intestinal cell type carcinoma of the stomach. The electron micrographs of our series are pointing in the same direction. Reduction of RER runs parallel to the significant decrease in number of mucin granules. This finding is typical for a progressive loss of differentiation of the mucus-forming cells. The process is additionally emphasized by a pleomorphia and an atypical distribution pattern of the secretion granules in the cytoplasm. The transposition of the Golgi complex towards a basal cell fraction, which is seen frequently in cases of borderline lesion and carcinoma, underscores the beginning of depolarization, respectively a depolarization of the cell structure, which has already taken place. In addition to the phenomena mentioned, a decrease in number of desmosomes, a remarkable reduction in interdigitations, and a lysosomal activity, which is particularly increased in carcinoma cells, are seen. These changes likewise correspond to the increasing loss of differentiation of the cells.

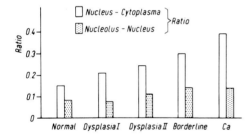

FIG. 7.   Ultrastructural cell profile in different diseases. Antral mucosa of the stomach.

FIG. 8.   Ultrastructural cell profile in different diseases. Antral mucosa of the stomach.

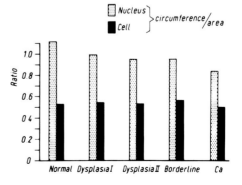

The striking feature of a change in the appearance of the surface in cases of borderline lesion with the club-like bulges of the cells at the apical pole was not observed in normal cells. In cases of reactive dysplasia they were seen sporadically only, but comparatively extremely infrequently. Bulges of this type described are known from gastric carcinoma cells as we also saw in our series. In this context it may be asked if this manifestation constitutes an increased neoplastic potency of the cell directed towards the apical pole of the cell, since an expansion in the basal direction is impossible as long as the basal membrane is still mostly intact. In gastric carcinoma this direction of expansion probably reverses, since in carcinomas an infiltrative growth results after penetration of the basal membrane.

In our opinion the borderline lesion shows some characteristic morphological peculiarities, which allow proving the borderline lesion as a manifestation of its own in comparison with a reactive dysplasia. The transition of a borderline lesion into an intestinal cell type carcinoma exhibiting similar phenomena which has been observed in two cases, demonstrates that these changes might be interpreted after all in the sense of a final step towards differentiation into malignant neoplasia (J. F. Riemann et al., *unpublished data*).

ACKNOWLEDGMENT

J. F. Riemann's work was supported by the Wilhelm-Sander Foundation, Neustadt (Donau), West Germany.

REFERENCES

1. Elster, K. (1974): A new approach to the classification of gastric polyps. *Endoscopy*, 6:44–47.
2. Ghadially, F. N. (1980): *Diagnostic Electron Microscopy of Tumours.* Butterworths, London, Boston, Sydney, Wellington, Durban, Toronto.
3. Goldman, H., and Ming, S. C. (1968): Fine structure of intestinal metaplasia and adenocarcinoma of the human stomach. *Lab. Invest.*, 203–210.
4. Grundmann, E. (1975): Histologic types and possible initial stages in early gastric carcinoma. *Beitr. Pathol.*, 154:256–280.
5. Meyer-Arendt, J. R., and Humphreys, D. M. (1972): Quantitative morphology of cancer cells. *Acta Histochem.*, 44:41–48.
6. Morson, B. C., Sobin, L. H., Grundmann, E., Johansen, A., Nagayo, T., and Serck-Hanssen, A. (1980): Precancerous conditions and epithelial dysplasia in the stomach. *J. Clin. Pathol.*, 33:711–721.
7. Nagayo, T. (1971): Histological diagnosis of biopsied gastric mucosae with special reference to that of borderline lesions. *Gan. Monogr. Cancer Res.*, 11:245–256.
8. Oehlert, W., Keller, P., Henke, M., and Strauch, M. (1975): Die Dysplasien der Magenschleimhaut. Das Problem ihrer klinischen Bedeutung. *Dtsch med Wochenschr.*, 100:1950–1956.
9. Rösch, W., and Frühmorgen, P. (1980): Endoscopic treatment of precanceroses and early gastric carcinoma. *Endoscopy*, 12:109–113.
10. Sugano, H., Nakamura, K., and Takagi, K. (1971): An atypical epithelium of the stomach. A Clinicopathological Entity. *Gan. Monogr. Cancer Res.*, 11:257–269.
11. Uchida, Y., Roessner, A., Stahl, K., Schlake, W., Blanke, G., Rühland, D., Themann, H., and Grundmann, E. (1977): Development of tumors in the glandular stomach of rats after oral administration of carcinogens. *Z. Krebsforsch.*, 89:87–98.
12. Wiernik, G., Bradbury, S., Plant, M., Cowdell, R. H., and Williams, E. A. (1973): A quantitative comparison between normal and carcinomatous squamous epithelia of the uterine cervix. *Br. J. Cancer*, 28:488–499.

Precancerous Lesions of the Gastrointestinal Tract, edited by P. Sherlock, B.C. Morson, L. Barbara, and U. Veronesi. Raven Press, New York © 1983.

Chronic Atrophic Gastritis as a Precursor of Cancer

Pelayo Correa

Department of Pathology, Louisiana State University Medical Center, New Orleans, Louisiana 70112

HISTORICAL NOTE

Evidence gathered from several scientific fields has led to the hypothesis that the clinical manifestations of most gastric cancers are only a late event of a biologic phenomenon initiated many years before (6). The study of gastric lesions linked to eventual development of gastric cancer probably started approximately a century ago when Kupfer (14) described islands of intestinal glands ("heterotopia") in the gastric mucosa. Schmidt (23), as many other investigators after him, soon challenged Kupfer's interpretation of the findings and proposed that the intestinal islands represented metaplastic regeneration triggered by chronic atrophic gastritis (CAG).

The link between these lesions and gastric cancer came from epidemiologic observations in southeast Asia, where Bonne and co-workers (1) in 1938 reported that Chinese immigrants had a high frequency of gastric carcinoma and atrophic gastritis with "goblet cell metaplasia," whereas both lesions were infrequent in native Malays. Jarvi and Lauren (12) in 1951 pointed out that carcinomas originating in stomachs with such lesions had histologic characteristics similar to those of the intestinal tumors. Morson (19) in 1955 described small carcinomas originating in areas of intestinal metaplasia (I.M.) and reviewed the evidence suggesting a causal link between metaplasia and carcinoma. Several investigators reviewed the evidence linking CAG and I.M. and concluded that I.M. was part of the histologic spectrum of chronic gastritis (18).

CAG has been used as a marker of gastric cancer risk in certain rural areas of Colombia where gastroscopy studies of the general population have been instrumental in linking cancer risk with environmental factors (6). The study of risk factors related to cancer has, therefore, been complemented with the study of risk factors of precursor lesions, which offers the advantage of shortening the time lag between carcinogenic events and assessment of risk. Repeated biopsies in individuals with CAG have shown that they are at much greater risk of developing carcinoma than others without such lesions (21,24).

It should be emphasized that CAG is related only to one histologic type of gastric cancer: the so-called intestinal type. The diffuse type of gastric cancer, as a rule, is not preceded by the gastric lesions under consideration (7). It has been noted for many years that there is much variation in the proportional representation of the several types of intestinal cells in metaplasia. Some foci resemble small intestinal mucosa, others resemble large intestine

(17). Heilman and Hopken (10) have reported a closer association of the latter type with gastric carcinoma. The distinction between types of metaplasia has been carried to the histochemical field and enzymes characteristic of both types of intestine have been identified in metaplastic foci. Differences in mucous secretion have also been found and correlated with marker enzymes. This has led to the distinction between complete and incomplete metaplasia, according to the degree of phenotypic expression of small intestinal enzymes and mucus (17).

There have been some difficulties concerning the terminology of cancer precursors. Part of the controversy is semantic and arises because the meaning of the term is understood according to the needs of the users. For the clinicians concerned with each individual patient's diagnosis and therapeutics needs, the term *precancerous* means "obligate antecedents of invasive carcinoma" (13). This interpretation of the term often leads to a pragmatic decision: if the lesion "inevitably" becomes cancer, all attempts to remove the lesion should be made; if it only "sometimes" becomes cancer, no immediate therapeutic measures are usually warranted (22). On the other hand, researchers interested in better understanding the cellular alterations that precede invasive neoplasia use the term to describe morphologic and chemical cellular alterations that begin at the earlier phases of the process, even if in many cases they do not lead to invasive cancer (16). These semantic difficulties were recognized by Stout (25), who in 1932 wrote in his introduction to *Human Cancer*, referring to the term *precancerous*, "In some ways it has been an unfortunate term because it has connoted in many minds an inevitable sequence of events. Such, of course, is very far from the truth. By precancerous, therefore, is meant simply a condition which may be associated with development of cancer." For the purposes of epidemiology and primary prevention of cancer, Stout's definition is more applicable and is, therefore, adopted for our purposes. Several similar terms have been used in the medical literature in an effort to avoid this semantic confusion: *precancerous* and *premalignant* frequently lead to misinterpretation and, because of that, the terms *antecedent* and *precursor* have been used to encompass lesions that might precede cancer chronologically but do not inevitably lead to it (2,9). In epidemiologic terms these lesions are statistically associated with cancer in interpopulation comparisons. Since, in our opinion, the term *precursor* better fits the latter concept, we have preferred it in our discussion.

For practical purposes precursor lesions are generally divided in two categories:

1. Less-advanced lesions share their morphologic characteristics with other benign processes and do not involve the proliferation of cell clones with neoplastic phenotypes. Such is the case of the inflammatory, hyperplastic, atrophic, and metaplastic lesions of the cervix, stomach, and bronchus.

2. More-advanced lesions include abnormal clones, are considered dangerous if untreated, and are usually called dyplasias.

TEMPORAL RELATIONSHIPS

CAG and I.M. have been investigated extensively in autopsy material and in surgically resected specimens (5). Both sets of data show that the disease appears in younger individuals as multiple small independent foci, which can be detected in the second decade of life in the lower portion of the lesser curvature and around the corpus-antrum junction. With advancing age it spreads to other areas of the mucosa covering first the antrum, then the corpus, and lastly the fundus. The lesions appear earlier and cover more extensive areas at a given age in populations at high cancer risk, as compared with those at low cancer risk.

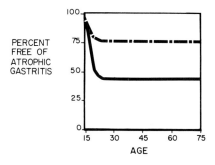

FIG. 1. Depletion curve showing the proportion of persons in the community expected to be free of atrophic gastritis at any given age in populations at high *(solid line)* and low *(broken line)* cancer risk.

It thus appears that CAG starts as clinically insignificant foci, which expand and coalesce and which in a period of 20 years or more bring about enough atrophy of the gastric mucosa to become clinically manifest.

The area covered by CAG, as well as the intensity of the lesions, increase with age. The initiation of CAG, however, appears to occur mostly around the second and third decade. Figure 1 shows the depletion curve for CAG, representing the proportion of individuals free of the disease at a given age. By age 30 most of the individuals who will eventually develop CAG already have histologic evidence of the disease whether they live in a low-risk or a high-risk environment. The proportion of individuals entering the CAG cycle is, of course, much greater in high-risk environments.

MODEL OF PROGRESSION

The idea that CAG advances in extension and severity with time has been born out of observations in biopsy and autopsy materials. Biopsies of individuals at different ages, as well as repeated biopsies in the same individuals, provide information on specific moments of the evolution of the biological process. From such fragmentary information we can speculate about the spectrum covered by the disease, as described in the following paragraphs. It should be clearly understood that the connection between the different "stages" of the process is attained only through logical inference as a substitute for direct observations. The conclusions are, therefore, open to different interpretations.

CAG entails chronic inflammation and atrophy and there is some difference of opinion as to how the transition from a normal stomach to CAG takes place. Some investigators are of the opinion that this transition is independent of acute gastritis, among other reasons because most of us have episodes of acute gastritis that never lead to chronicity. That does not, however, exclude the possibility that chronic gastritis may have begun as repeated episodes of acute gastritis. Since atrophy calls for previous cell death and cell death usually elicits inflammation, we take the position that chronic gastritis may be the result of repeated acute injuries. Foci of acute inflammation are frequent in a background of CAG. Most acute gastritis are completely resolved by the main defense mechanisms: the mucous barrier and the regeneration capacity of the mucosa. Chronic gastritis may indicate that these defense mechanisms become insufficient to cope with repeated acute injuries.

The full spectrum of lesions from normal mucosa to cancer will be too extensive to illustrate adequately. The following stages can be identified in the gastric mucosa:

1. Superficial gastritis. This consists of infiltration by lymphocytes, plasma cells, and polymorphonuclear leukocytes located in or around the epithelium of the gland neck or the lamina propria of the superficial half of the mucosa (Fig. 2). The lesion is frequently

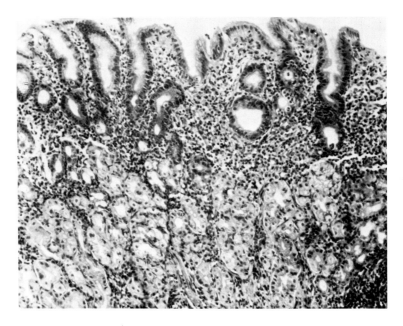

FIG. 2.   Superficial gastritis. Inflammatory infiltrate in the upper lamina propria.

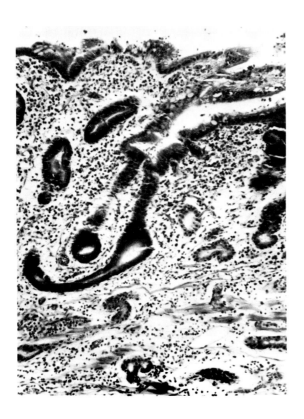

FIG. 3.   Chronic atrophic gastritis. Loss of gastric glands, regeneration, and inflammatory infiltrate.

associated with regenerative changes of the surface and gland neck epithelium characterized by increased nucleocytoplasmatic ratio and large plump nuclei.

2. CAG. This consists of loss of normal gastric glands. There is hypertrophy and elongation of gland necks (Fig. 3). Infiltration by plasma and lymphocytes may be present.

3. Mature I.M. The original gastric glands are replaced by straight, short, tubular crypts of regular size and shape lined by alternating absorptive and goblet cells (Fig. 4). The nuclei are round, homogeneous, and located at the base of the cell. The lamina propria shows variable numbers of lymphocytes and plasma cells. The affected mucosa is considerably thinner than the normal gastric mucosa. Metaplastic changes can be observed in glands deep in the mucosa or in the surface (foveolar) cells.

4. Dysplasia. Irregularities of glandular architecture and nuclear atypia characterize the advanced phases of the precursor state. The architectural abnormalities may be of two types. One type consists of hyperplastic epithelial changes resulting in intraluminal epithelial folds and branching glands (Fig. 5). The other type results in new tubular lumens resembling adenomatous proliferation (Fig. 6). The first type is usually seen in the superficial part of the mucosa and in the foveolar epithelium. It has been called hyperplastic dysplasia (7) or foveolar dysplasia (20). Both types may vary in degree from mild to severe. In severe dysplasia the epithelium may be indistinguishable from carcinomatous cells still bound by the basement membrane of the gland. The term *carcinoma in situ* has been applied to this lesion, but it is not recommended because it leads to confusion with invasive "superficial"

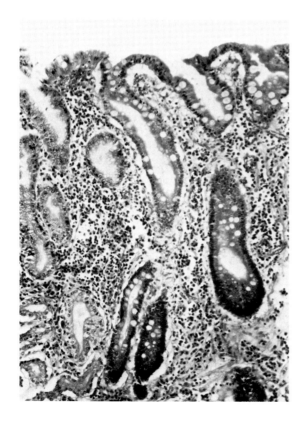

FIG. 4. Intestinal metaplasia. Gastric glands replaced by straight tubular structures lined by goblet and absorptive cells.

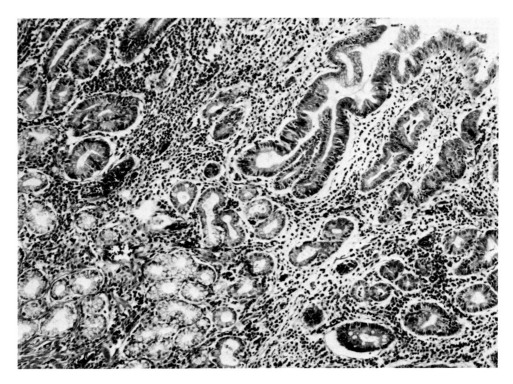

FIG. 5. Hyperplastic dysplasia. Dysplastic glands develop tortuous lumens with intraluminal folds.

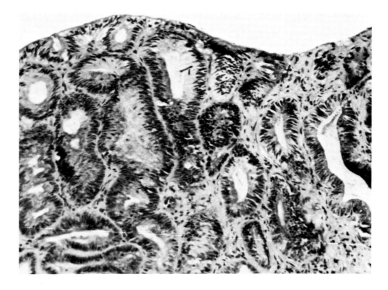

FIG. 6 Adenomatos dyplasia. Dysplastic glands arranged in closely packed tubules with crowded hyperchromatic nuclei.

carcinomas. Large goblets are infrequent, but small intracytoplasmatic mucus droplets can be seen in Alcian blue stain. The nuclei are elongated, hyperchromatic, and piled up, with prominent pseudostratification.

In most specimens dyplastic lesions are seen in the flat mucosa. Occasionally the glands proliferate and a mass protrudes into the lumen forming an adenomatous polyp. More dysplastic polyps have a papillary arrangement characteristic of villous adenomas.

Specimens with small carcinomas usually show them to be surrounded by intestinal metaplasia and dysplasia. Histochemical studies show that most metaplastic glands in the immediate vicinity of small carcinomas are of the "incomplete" type, suggesting that loss of enzymes is a marker of more advanced dysplasia (17).

NATURAL HISTORY OF CHRONIC GASTRITIS

There is epidemiologic evidence that strongly suggests that gastric cancer risk is influenced by events taking place early in life. Migrants from high-risk countries to the United States maintain the high-risk characteristics of their country of origin (8). This prolonged latency period probably reflects the chronicity of atrophic gastritis. During these years a complex spectrum of signs and symptoms can be observed. Many patients with histologic proof of gastritis do not have clinical complaints (6,24) and others have only vague symptoms such as postprandial fullness and belching. In the intermediate stages of the process many patients have signs and symptoms of peptic ulcer, frequently proven by X-rays and treated by surgical or medical means. Such ulcers are usually located in the area of the incisura angularis and are surrounded by severe I.M. The ulcer represents weakening of the mucosa by atrophy and metaplasia in the presence of normal acid pepsin secretion coming from uninvolved mucosa hyperstimulated by excessive gastrin. This type of peptic ulcer is, therefore, part of the clinicopathologic complex of CAG. As the patients become older and more areas of the mucosa become atrophic, the acid pepsin secretion diminishes and the ulcer heals.

There are indications that the progression of lesions just described varies markedly in different individuals. One such indication is the fact that autopsy and biopsy studies show similar prevalence of CAG and I.M. for both sexes (5,24). The same type of study shows that the prevalence of dysplasias in previously metaplastic mucosa is higher in males, apparently indicating stronger promoting forces in that sex (7). Similar excessive frequency is observed for gastric cancer in males, again apparently indicating more effective promotion.

There have been several reviews of the symptomatology and physiopathology of chronic gastritis (3,4,15,26) and the reader is referred to those publications for a detailed presentation of the subject.

There are marked interpopulation differences in the frequency of chronic gastritis througout the world. The type of gastritis just described predominates in the same populations having a high incidence of gastric cancer: Japan, the Andean part of Latin America, northern and eastern Europe, etc. This coincidence in geographic distribuiton points to environmental influences predisposing to both diseases. The diet in such populations is usually high in salt and fiber and low in fat and antioxidants. For these reasons, this type of gastritis has been referred to as environmental chronic gastritis (ECG).

A second type of gastritis has been referred to by Strickland and Mackay (26) as type A gastritis. It is characterized by diffuse involvement of the corporal mucosa, reduced acid secretion, circulating parietal cell antibodies, and eventually impaired absorption of vitamin B_{12}. It thus seems to form part of the pernicious anemia complex.

A third type of chronic gastritis accompanies peptic ulcers of the duodenum or the pylorus. They are predominantly antral, usually without atrophy, occasionally with small foci of I.M. They usually have evidence of acid-pepsin hypersecretion.

Alcoholic gastritis is well recognized by clinicians but its anatomic substratum is not well defined. Old descriptions of the histopathology of alcoholic gastritis were done in populations in which other forms of gastritis, including ECG, were frequent. Alcoholism per se has not been found to correlate positively with gastric cancer in populations of high risk, such as Japan and Colombia. On the other hand, wine drinking has been identified as a risk factor in certain areas of France (11).

Type A (autoimmune) and multifocal atrophic gastritis of antrum and corpus (ECG) are statistically associated with gastric carcinoma. Hypersecretory gastritis has not been associated with cancer. The role of alcoholic gastritis as a possible precursor has not been established.

EPILOGUE

Accumluated evidence from clinical and epidemiologic studies indicates that before gastric cancer develops most patients go through a lengthy and complex series of mucosal changes, which constitute the precursor status. This status can be divided into 3 main phases: (a) inflammation and atrophy, (b) metaplasia, and (c) dysplasia. Phase 2 probably represents a mutation or a similar transformation, since new "daughter" cells, strange to the normal stomach, replace the original gastric epithelium. Phase 3 probably represents promotional forces that result in progressive quantitive changes acting on a previously mutated epithelial cell. Phases 2 and 3 therefore fit the 2 classical phases of carcinogenesis: initiation and promotion. Phase 1, however, is not clearly defined in the experimental carcinogenesis models.

Given the epidemiologic evidence for an etiologic role of atrophic gastritis, it seems appropriate that a new phase should be added to carcinogenesis models: the phase of pre-disposition. In the case of humans, gastritis may predispose one to carcinogenesis in a number of ways. It may act by modifying the microenvironment in a way that favors the *in situ* formation of carcinogens. This may be accomplished by allowing bacterial proliferation that reduces nitrate to nitrite and provides a highly reactive molecule capable of nitrosating compounds to carcinogens. Chronic gastritis may also predispose one to cancer by increasing the mitotic rate and supplying an increased number of replicating cells that may receive the impact of mutagens found in the microenvironment.

If the gastric precursors status were to be used as a model for human carcinogenesis, it would emphasize the changes that take place before initiation by genotoxic agents that induce mutations. It would also provide a morphologic substratum for the different phases of carcinogenesis, including predisposition, initiation, and promotion.

ACKNOWLEDGMENT

The work described herein was supported by grant no. P01-CA-28842 from the National Cancer Institute of Health U.S.P.H.S.

REFERENCES

1. Bonne, C., Hartz, P. H., Klerks, J. V., Postuma, J. H., Redsma, W., and Tjokronegoro, S. (1938): Morphology of the stomach and gastric secretion in Malays and Chinese and the different incidence of gastric ulcer and cancer in these races. *Am. J. Cancer*, 33:265–279.

2. Burdette, W. (1970): *Carcinoma of the Colon and Antecedent Epithelium.* Charles C. Thomas, Springfield, Illinois.
3. Chatterjee, D. (1976): Idiopatic chronic gastritis. *Surg. Gynecol. Obstet.*, 143:986–1000.
4. Correa, P. (1980): The epidemiology and pathogenesis of chronic gastritis. Three etiologic entities. *Front. Gastrointest. Res.*, 6:98–108.
5. Correa, P., Cuello, C., and Duque, E. (1970): Carcinoma and intestinal metaplasia of the stomach in Colombian migrants. *J. Natl. Cancer Inst.*, 44:297–306.
6. Correa, P., Haenszel, W., Cuello, C., Archer, M., and Tannenbaum, S. (1975): A model for gastric cancer epidemiology. *Lancet*, 2:58–60.
7. Cuello, C., Correa, P., Zarama, G., López, J., Murray, J., and Gordillo, G. (1979): Histopathology of gastric dysplasias. Correlations with gastric juice chemistry. *Am. J. Surg. Pathol.*, 3:491–500.
8. Haenszel, W. (1961): Cancer mortality among the foreign-born in the United States. *J. Natl. Cancer Inst.*, 26:37–132.
9. Haenszel, W., Correa, P., Cuello, C., Guzmán, N., Burbano, L., Lores, H., and Muñoz, J. (1976): Gastric cancer in Colombia. II. Case-control epidemiologic study of precursor lesions. *J. Natl. Cancer Inst.*, 57:1021–1026.
10. Heilman, K. L., and Hopken, W. W. (1979): Loss of differentiation in intestinal metaplasia in cancerous stomach. A comparative morphology study. *Pathol. Res. Pract.*, 164:249–258.
11. Hoey, J., Montvernay, C., and Lambert, R. (1981): Wine and tobacco: risk factors for gastric cancer in France. *Am. J. Epidemiol.*, 113:668–674.
12. Jarvi, O., and Lauren, P. (1951): On the role of heterotopias of the intestinal epithelium in the pathogenesis of gastric cancer. *Acta Pathol. Microbiol. Scand.*, 29:26–44.
13. Koss, L. (1975): Precancerous lesions. In: *Persons at High Risk of Cancer*, edited by J. Fraumeni, pp. 85–102. Academic Press, New York.
14. Kupfer, C. (1883): Fetschrift. *Arz. Verein Munch*, p. 7.
15. Lambert, R. (1972): Chronic gastritis. *Digestion*, 7:83–126.
16. Lipkin, M. (1977): Growth kinetics of normal and premalignant gastrointestinal epithelium. In: *The University of Texas System Cancer Center M.D. Anderson Hospital and Tumor Institute 29th Annual Symposium on Fundamental Cancer Research*, pp. 569–589. Williams and Wilkins.
17. Matsukura, N., Kawachi, T., Sugimura, T., Ohnuki, T., Higo, M., Itabashi, M., Hirota, T., and Kitasha, H. (1980): Variety of phenotypical expression of intestinal marker enzymes and mucin in human stomach intestinal metaplasia. *Acta Histochem. Cytochem.*, 13:499–507.
18. Michalany, J. (1959): Metaplasia intestinal da mucosa gastrica. *Rev. Assoc. Med. Brasil*, 5:25–36.
19. Morson, B. (1955): Carcinoma arising from areas of intestinal metaplasia in the gastric mucosa. *Br. J. Cancer*, 9:377–385.
20. Morson, B. C., Sobin, L. H., Grundman, E., Hohansen, A., Nagayo, T., and Serk-Hansen, A. (1980): Precancerous conditions and epithelial dysplasia in the stomach. *J. Clin. Pathol.*, 33:711–721.
21. Muñoz, N., and Matko, I. (1972): Histologic types of gastric cancer and its relationship with intestinal metaplasia. *Recent Results Cancer Res.*, 39:99–105.
22. Rosai, J., and Ackerman, L. V. (1978): The pathology of tumors: Part I: Precancerous and pseudomalignant lesions. *CA*, 28:331–342.
23. Schmidt, A. (1896): Untersuchungen uber des mensliche Magenepithel unter normalen und pathologischen Werhaltnissen. *Virchows Arch. [Pathol. Anat.]*, 143:477–508.
24. Siurala, M., Varis, K., and Wiljasalo, M. (1966): Studies of patients with atrophic gastritis: a 10-15 years follow-up. *Scand. J. Gastroenterol.*, 1:40–48.
25. Stout, A. P. (1932): *Human Cancer.* Lea and Febiger, Philadelphia, p. 18.
26. Strickland, R. G., and Mackay, I. R. (1973): A reappraisal of the nature and significance of chronic atrophic gastritis. *Dig. Dis.*, 18:426–440.

*Precancerous Lesions of the Gastrointestinal
Tract*, edited by P. Sherlock, B.C. Morson,
L. Barbara, and U. Veronesi. Raven Press,
New York © 1983.

Atrophic Gastritis

R. Cheli and A. Giacosa

Department of Gastroenterology, Ospedale S. Martino, 16132 Genova, Italy

Atrophic gastritis is a histopathologic condition characterized by parenchymatous atrophy, with metaplasia of surface epithelium as well as of the residual glandular component, and by an increase of inflammatory cells in the chorion.

ENDOSCOPIC FINDINGS

Various appearances on gastroscopy were originally interpreted as gastritis, but since it has been possible to correlate these findings with histologic data it became clear that the gastroscopic picture is often misleading.

The endoscopic appearance of atrophic gastritis is more reliable when compared with different types of gastritis. Atrophic gastritis is endoscopically characterized by thin, smooth, flat, gray-rose or pale colored mucosa (4,11) (Fig. 1). A specific finding is a bluish (venous) or red (arterial) vascular network, with polymorphous distribution: the vascular visualization

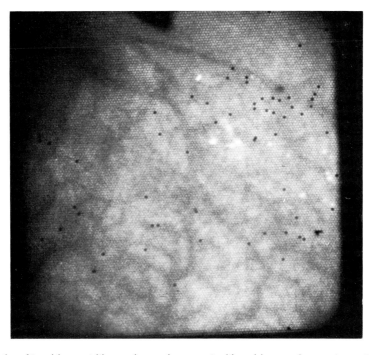

FIG. 1. Atrophic gastritis: endoscopic aspect with evidence of vascular network.

155

is considered a consequence of atrophy of mucosal structures and therefore of decreased thickness of the mucosal layer. This aspect is generally diffuse: other possible aspects are represented by opaque, whitish areas in which vascular vessels may be observed, indicating that atrophic gastritis may appear as a patchy process (27). These whitish areas may be associated with an endoscopically normal mucosa or with congestive aspects, as well as with erosive-hemorrhagic phenomena.

Sometimes, and particularly in the presence of severe and diffuse atrophic phenomena, pearly areas may be observed, as found in case of pernicious anemia (60).

HISTOLOGIC FINDINGS

In atrophic fundic gastritis, surface epithelium is reduced in height, is very poor in mucous content, and often is interrupted by erosions (9). A frequent finding is goblet cells as well as enterocyte-like cells, with evidence of a brush border: both these data demonstrate the presence of intestinal metaplasia (9) (Figs. 2,3). On histochemical study, the surface epithelium reveals

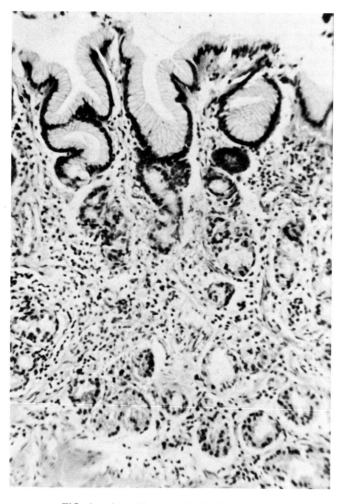

FIG. 2.   Atrophic gastritis. H.-E., × 120.

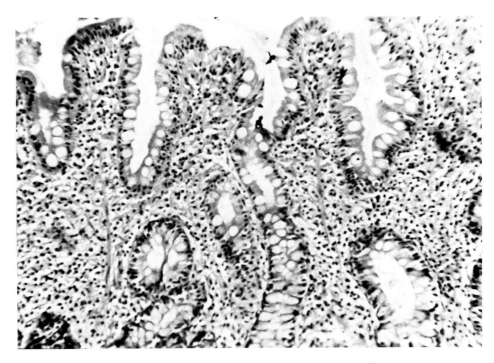

FIG. 3. Atrophic gastritis with relevant intestinal metaplasia. H.-E., × 120.

a marked decrease of PAS positive mucosubstances—that is, the neutral ones—with the presence of acid mucopolysaccharides for carboxylic groups and for sulphomucins. Foveolae are usually elongated and tortuous, frequently assuming finger-like aspects.

Glandular tissue is markedly reduced or even entirely disappeared: in this regard, as far as fundic mucosa is concerned, parietal cells are the last cellular component to disappear. In the residual glandular tubuli, as well as in surface epithelium, metaplastic cells may frequently be observed. A further alteration is constituted by epithelial dysplasia, whose main features are cellular atypia, abnormal cellular differentiation, and disorganised mucosal architecture (61). Dysplasia is found in about 10% of cases with atrophic gastritis, with prevalence of the mild type, characterized by epithelial cells with slender, elongated, and hyperchromatic nuclei, the arrangement of which is dense but well preserved (19).

In the surface epithelium, lymphocyte infiltrate is markedly increased (41). In the chorion, inflammatory cells are diffusely distributed, and their number is significantly increased, with prevalence of the plasmacellular component (9,41) (Figs. 2,3). Connective tissue is thickened (though not in all cases), with frequent evidence of collagenous elements. Muscularis mucosae often appears hyperplastic, with degenerative phenomena, fragmentation of fibercells, and inflammatory cell infiltrates. A particular pattern rarely visualized is represented by atrophic hyperplastic gastritis, in which the above-described phenomena are associated with hyperplasia of the superficial layer, with finger-like protruding structures simulating villi (9) (Fig. 4).

Atrophic gastritis of the antral mucosa (the gastric area within 3 to 5 cm from the pylorus) (79) reproduces histological patterns that overlap the fundic ones, except for the specific parenchymatous characters, which differentiate the two areas. Therefore antral antrophic

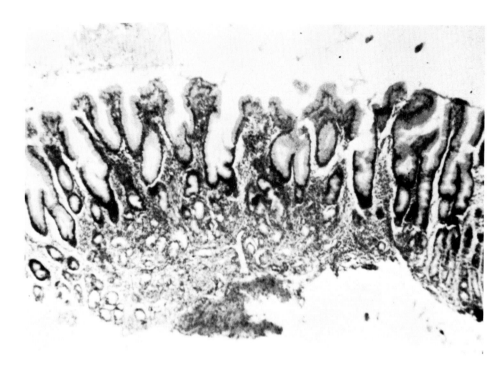

FIG. 4. Atrophic hyperplastic gastritis. H.-E., × 60.

gastritis is characterized by reduced mucosal thickness, marked and diffuse inflammatory cell infiltrate, and a great reduction of the glandular component, with severe reduction of endocrine cells and in particular of G cells (9).

As far as histomorphological patterns are concerned, some authors describe as an autonomous entity a particular condition called gastric atrophy, which differs from atrophic gastritis for the higher degree of atrophic and metaplastic phenomena and for the lower inflammatory cell infiltrate (50,59). Even though this distinction is classical knowledge in gastroenterology, in our opinion this terminology appears questionable, and in agreement with other authors (78) it has to be abandoned, since it does not represent a true morphological content (20). In effect, the inflammatory cell count does not reveal significant differences in the two conditions from both the qualitative and quantitative point of view (20). Moreover, the two aspects may be alternatively present in the same patient at different times (78), and lastly, the severity of the epithelial lesions is quite variable, but in any case insufficient to allow a differential diagnosis (20).

CYTOLOGIC FINDINGS

Cytologic smears are of specific interest and a valuable aid in the diagnosis of atrophic gastritis, thus representing a technical tool that is complementary to gastric histology (6,12,62).

In the cytologic smears of atrophic gastritis patients, inflammatory cells, particularly lymphocytes, are numerous though not consistently present. Groups of mucous cells and of goblet cells are frequently noted and interpreted as a manifestation of metaplasia (12).

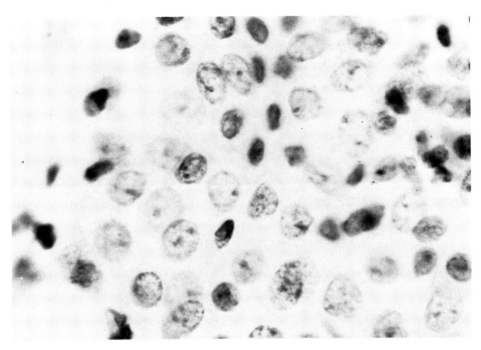

FIG. 5. Gastric smears in atrophic gastritis: prevalence of "pale cells" (Papanicolaou, × 600).

The surface mucosal cells often have cytoplasmic changes that consist primarily of vacuolization: these cells are specifically called "pale cells" (6,12) (Fig. 5). They show evident nuclear alterations characterized by increased nuclear size and anisokaryosis rarely associated with an altered nuclear/cytoplasmic ratio. The nuclear structure has a pattern of chromatin bands and chromocenters and clear spaces between the bands. The nuclear hypochromasia results in the pale appearance of the chromatin. Prominent nucleoli are frequently present (12).

The nuclear alterations reported above are of great importance, since they constitute a sufficiently specific marker of atrophy and are interpreted as indicative of maturation disorders (62).

GASTRIC SECRETORY FINDINGS AND GASTRINEMIC BEHAVIOUR

The characteristic secretory finding of atrophic gastritis is represented by achlorhydria or severe hypochlorhydria, which do not respond even to maximal pentagastrin stimulation (7,10,15). These findings are the obvious expression of the disappearance or at least of the marked decrease of fundic parietal cells (9).

The gastrinemic levels are related to gastric secretion by means of an inverse correlation, with evidence of serum increase in the fasting state and after meals (42). This increase is interpreted as due to the alteration of the physiological negative feedback mediated by antral pH (18).

Hypergastrinemia is particularly relevant when fundic atrophy is associated with normal patterns of antral mucosa, as in pernicious anemia (Table 1) (42). This hormonal increase

TABLE 1. *Parietal cell index (PI), maximal acid output (MAO), and gastrinemia (fasting and after meal) in subjects with normal gastric mucosa or with atrophic gastritis*

Cases	Histology Fundus	Histology Antrum	PI	HCl MAO (mEq/hr)	Gastrinemia Fasting (pg/ml)	Gastrinemia After meal (pg/ml)
13	N	N	425 ± 82	14.7 ± 9.3	65 ± 28	100 ± 21
12	N	A	385 ± 56	20.3 ± 2.3	70 ± 26	93 ± 15
5	S	A	342 ± 73	17.5 ± 2.1	60 ± 17	110 ± 24
4	P	A	102 ± 6	2.5 ± 1.2	76 ± 14	95 ± 22
15	A	N	9.9 ± 0.9	0	515 ± 186	1640 ± 325
7	A	S	47 ± 6	1.2 ± 0.5	155 ± 36	250 ± 42
5	A	A	87 ± 8	1.6 ± 0.8	80 ± 24	108 ± 16

N, Normal mucosa; S, superficial gastritis; P, preatrophic gastritis; A, atrophic gastritis.

is smaller or even absent when chronic atrophic funditis is accompanied by different damage of the antral parenchyma, owing to the decrease of hormonal source, that is, of the antral G cell mass (Table 1) (42).

This wide variability limits the physiopathological concept of Strikland and McKay (71), who considered just a type A and a type B atrophic gastritis, respectively constituted by isolated fundic atrophic gastritis (type A) and prevalence of antral atrophic gastritis (type B). This schema appears to be too dogmatic and does not correspond to reality.

IMMUNOLOGIC ASPECTS

The immunologic problem constitutes a relatively recent aspect of atrophic gastritis. In this regard, the possible serological finding of parietal cell antibodies (APA) and of anti-intrinsic factor antibodies (IFA) have to be considered (37,38,56).

APA, beside being observed in 5% of the asymptomatic population with normal gastric mucosa, reveal a progressive increase directly related to the severity of gastritis in up to 60% of patients with atrophic fundic gastritis; this percentage is even higher when patients with pernicious anemia are taken into account (37,38,56). The latter condition corresponds to the A type atrophic gastritis, which is strictly localized in the fundus, according to Strickland and McKay (71), the B type being characterized by the rare APA finding and by the prevalence of antral atrophic gastritis.

An important question regards the meaning of APA: "Do they represent a primitive pathogenetic factor or a consequence of the cellular damage that follows the inflammatory phenomenon, also considering the correlation between the presence of antibodies, their concentration, and the severity of the gastritis process (37,38,56)?"

Although definitive proofs are lacking, the aspecificity of autoantibodies (they may also be found in autoimmune thyroiditis, in Sjögren's disease, in Addison's disease, etc.) and the increase of their titre, which is proportional to mucosal damage, suggest that they do not represent a primary factor in the development of atrophic gastritis. These considerations permit us to hypothesize that the gastritic phenomenon may well be initiated by environmental factors and subsequently maintained by autoimmune phenomena, especially in a genetically determined group (77).

As far as IFA are concerned, two antibodies have been demonstrated: one blocks the interaction of vitamin B_{12} with intrinsic factor, and the second combines with the vitamin B_{12}/intrinsic factor complex (5). According to Samloff et al. (64) and Fujimura (38), IFA of the first type are present in the 70% to 73% of pernicious anemia patients, whereas the second type is observed in 30% to 43% of them. In atrophic gastritis without pernicious anemia, blocking IFA are never observed, and it is very rare to find the second type of IFA (precipitating IFA) (1).

ETIOPATHOGENESIS

In the past much of the literature seemed to indicate various single factors as responsible for atrophic gastritis: but recent experiences did not confirm the former results (18). In particular, the comparison of data pertaining to chronic alcoholics (21) as well as to heavy smokers (39) with the data pertaining to abstemious or nonsmoking controls does not reveal significant differences, except for the antral mucosa.

Also the role of acute intake of drugs is denied, since the induced damages are ephemeral and constituted by congestive-erosive phenomena, instead of true chronic inflammatory alterations (22). Similarly, after chronic consumption of drugs there is a prevalence of acute lesions (8). Confirmatory data implicating an etiologic role to alimentary acute errors are also lacking.

There is increasing interest in the possible genetic factor involved in some cases of atrophic gastritis. Recent observations demonstrate a significant increase in atrophic gastritis in first-degree relatives of patients with atrophic gastritis whether or not associated with pernicious anemia (73,74). In general, members of the same family tend to show a similar behaviour as far as morphology, function, and immunology of gastric mucosa are concerned (74). As a matter of fact, this genetic factor could act, from the pathogenetic point of view, as a predisposing background, favouring the intervention of multiple additional factors of immunological, biological, and environmental type. In this regard the possible pathogenetic role of an *autoimmune mechanism* mediated by APA and IFA has been previously described (37,38,56).

Great importance is attributed also to the *duodenogastric biliary reflux*, initially described by Schindler (65) and Lambling (51) and subsequently confirmed by the experiences of Davenport (29): this factor becomes truly important when it is constant, or at least frequent, and quantitatively relevant. Our recent experience indicates a high frequency of atrophic antral gastritis in patients with duodenogastric reflux in comparison with control groups; fundic lesions are less frequent and less severe than the antral ones (17).

Surely the possible intervention of other factors have to be considered in gastritis development: the lifelong administration of ordinary food, multiple acute dietary errors, thermic, environmental, psychical, and medicamentous agents, and infectious diseases may all be involved.

In conclusion, a multifactorial pathogenesis is hypothesized for the development of atrophic gastritis, with involvement of specific conditions such as genetic background and some pathogenetic mechanisms such as the immunological behaviour in atrophic funditis or duodenogastric reflux in atrophic antritis.

CLINICAL SIGNIFICANCE OF ATROPHIC GASTRITIS

Some clinical experiences tend to implicate dyspeptic troubles as an expression of chronic gastritis. However, this observation may be made *a posteriori*, since the same symptomatic troubles may be also observed in the absence of gastric inflammatory phenomena.

In a previous monograph by Fieschi and Cheli (35), the careful clinical evaluation of atrophic gastritis patients selected from a group of dyspeptics revealed a high frequency of epigastric postprandial pain (50%) or of epigastric discomfort (80%). Less represented were regurgitation (50%) and nausea (40%); the incidence of ulcer-like symptoms was very low (20%), as was vomiting (20%) and pyrosis (4%) (35). Appetite was often depressed, although in some cases it appeared normal or even increased. An almost constant symptom was the sensitivity to the ingestion of specific foods such as fried fats, which was accompanied by a prompt rise of epigastric pain (35).

Among symptoms concerning general well-being, alteration of cenaesthesia was frequent (70%), with asthenia (35%) and weight loss (40%) (35). As far as hemorrhage is concerned, Schindler (65) described the occurrence of the phenomenon in 7.3% of patients with atrophic gastritis; Moutier and Cornet (60) found it in 10.2%.

These data are not confirmed by our experience, since relevant hemorrhagic phenomena were never observed in our cases of atrophic gastritis (35).

Biopsy experience in the past has also excluded an absolute correlation between gastritis and dyspepsia. Doig and Wood (33) investigated 112 patients with gastritis and found a history of epigastric pain or discomfort related to meals only in 45% of cases. Therefore, a new problem concerning the occurrence of atrophic gastritis in asymptomatic patients was realized. Initial data on this account were provided by Henning in 1959 (45) and by Heinkel and Henning in 1964 (44).

Recently this matter was reviewed by our own group in collaboration with a group of Hungarian colleagues: In this way it was possible to verify at the same time the frequency of atrophic gastritis in asymptomatics and in different ethnic groups (25). This prospective study demonstrated a high frequency of atrophic gastritis in both groups, with a prevalence in Hungarians (37%) when compared with Italians (22%) (25). A similar behaviour was noticed for intestinal metaplasia, which was observed in 24% of the Hungarians and in 11% of the Italians (25). This difference was closely related to age, since the incidence of atrophic gastritis and of intestinal metaplasia in patients less than 60 years was similar in the groups studied; above 60 years of age the incidence of both pathological conditions was significantly higher in the Hungarians (25). Therefore, atrophic gastritis does not always represent a clinical condition, but rather an anatomofunctional situation.

Obviously this statement must be accepted with the benefit of particular exceptions, such as some clinical conditions in which atrophic gastritis represents a more or less constant finding. As a matter of fact, pernicious anemia and, even if at a lesser extent, sideropenic anemia and chronic rosacea may be included in this group (3,16,23,53,54). In these cases fundic atrophic gastritis represents a constant condition, or at least a frequent phenomenon, so that it can be considered a diagnostic datum.

EPIDEMIOLOGY

Many considerations limit the possibilities for a proper epidemiologic evaluation of atrophic gastritis. In effect, the diagnosis of atrophic gastritis may be confirmed just by histologic data: when we consider in particular asymptomatic gastritis, we come to the conclusion that clinical indications are not helpful. Subsequently, atrophic gastritis cannot find anatomo-pathological events, since autopsy studies are not mandatory for atrophic gastritis patients. Furthermore, autopsy material cannot be conveniently utilized because of autolysis.

Therefore, epidemiology of atrophic gastritis is still today a difficult matter to deal with, since the disease is frequently observed and generally evaluated as *a posteriori*, that is, on the basis of histobiopsy data; as a consequence, the studied samples are not always expressive of the general population.

A further epidemiologic remark always obtained from biopsy information, concerns the close relationship with age: the greater the age, the higher the percentage of atrophic gastritis (25,66,75). This is in agreement with a long-term follow-up biopsy examination, which illustrates the dynamic concept of chronic gastritis, showing that generally superficial and preatrophic gastritis represent intermediate steps in the development of atrophic gastritis. According to Siurala's data, the mean time required for the realization of this process is 18 years (66,67). In this evolutionary process we differentiate superficial gastritis (inflammatory cell infiltrate limited to the area between superficial epithelium and parenchyma, with normal glandular component), preatrophic gastritis (inflammatory infiltrate extending through the entire thickness of the parenchyma, which is reduced in size; initial appearance of metaplasia), and atrophic gastritis (9).

A further important point is obtained by the evaluation of the biopsy site. It has been well known for a long time (32,57) that antral gastritis is much more frequent than fundic gastritis. According to Strickland and McKay (71), the atrophic antritis/atrophic funditis ratio is 4 to 1.

After having examined these initial considerations, we now need to consider some epidemiological data. Siurala et al. (66) performed a biopsy control of fundic mucosa by means of tube biopsy in randomly selected inhabitants of a Finnish rural commune. The series was representative of the whole population as regards sex, age, and occupational distribution. Gastritis was found in 53% of the studied cases, being atrophic in 28%. As previously mentioned (66), the prevalence rate of atrophic gastritis increased linearly with age, with constant percentual value computed to $1.25 \pm 0.19\%$ per year. On the contrary the prevalence of superficial gastritis remained unchanged, thus suggesting a dynamic equilibrium between subjects developing superficial gastritis and those changing into atrophic gastritis (66).

More recently Villako et al. (75) examined the state of antral and fundic mucosa by gastroscopic biopsies in randomly selected subjects of a rural Estonian district. Fundic atrophic gastritis was found in 20% of the cases and antral atrophic gastritis in 29%. In both fundic and antral mucosa, the prevalence of atrophic lesions increased with age, confirming previous experiences worked out in the Finnish population (66), even though limited to the fundic mucosa.

A comparative epidemiological evaluation performed in 1980 in a group of Italian and Hungarian asymptomatic subjects revealed atrophic gastritis in 22% of the Italians and in 37% of the Hungarians, with an increase in atrophic gastritis incidence with advancing age in both groups (Fig. 6) (25).

When specific clinical conditions are considered, the strong correlation between pernicious anemia and fundic atrophic gastritis with normal antral mucosa (3,33,54,55) becomes clear. Atrophic gastritis in chronic hypochromic anemia (Cheli et al., 62%; Davidson and Markson, 43%; Badenoch et al., 40%) (2,16,30) and in chronic rosacea is also frequent (23).

Further considerations come *a posteriori* from clinical experience. Confirming numerous data in the literature, in gastric ulcer of the lesser curvature we observed antral atrophic gastritis in 25 of 50 cases (50%) and fundic atrophic gastritis in 17 (34%) of 50; both the fundic and antral lesions were strictly related to the age of patients (Table 2) (40). In prepyloric ulcer (22 cases) we found 10 patients with atrophic antritis (45%), whereas atrophic fundic gastritis was never observed (Table 2) (40).

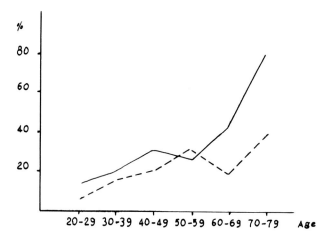

FIG. 6. Age distribution of atrophic gastritis in Italian and Hungarian asymptomatic subjects. *Solid line*: Hungarian; *broken line*: Italian.

TABLE 2. *Antral and fundic atrophic gastritis in gastric ulcer of the lesser curvature and in prepyloric ulcer*

		Fundus				Antrum			
		Normal		Atrophic gastritis		Normal		Atrophic gastritis	
	Cases	*n*	(%)	*n*	(%)	*n*	(%)	*n*	(%)
Gastric ulcer of lesser curvature	50	11	(22)	17	(34)	6	(12)	25	(50)
Prepyloric ulcer	22	16	(72)	0		4	(18)	10	(45)

In advanced gastric cancer many authors describe a high incidence of atrophic gastritis (14,48,53,63). In our experience, out of 52 cases of gastric cancer, atrophic gastritis was found in 18 (34%) (24). Out of 90 cases of early gastric cancer Johansen (49) found atrophic funditis in 48% of the cases and atrophic antritis in 96%. Elster et al.'s (34) research showed that histobiopsy findings of gastric mucosa in cases with early gastric cancer are correlated with Laurén's (52) classification of gastric cancer, considering an intestinal and diffuse cancer type. Out of 151 cases of early gastric cancer of the intestinal type Elster et al. (34) found 65 cases (43%) with atrophic gastritis; among the 122 with early gastric cancer of the diffuse type just 15% had atrophic gastritis. In extragastric pathological conditions, the frequency of atrophic gastritis does not seem to be particularly relevant, when compared with asymptomatic controls (9).

Among patients with biliary diseases we could demonstrate 10 cases of atrophic gastritis out of 41 with cholecystopathy without lithiasis, 2 out of 17 with cholecystolithiasis, and 7 out of 15 with previous cholecystectomy (13). Also in this case the relationship between obtained data and age of patients is strict, and the importance of biliary diseases in atrophic gastritis development is denied.

ATROPHIC GASTRITIS AND GASTRIC CANCER

Evidence for a close relation between atrophic gastritis and the development of gastric cancer has been reported by numerous investigators (48,53,63). Riegler and Kaplan (63), Jenner (48), and Magnus (53) found that pernicious anemia patients with atrophic gastritis and intestinal metaplasia had an increased incidence of gastric carcinoma. As previously reported, other evidence for the suggestion that atrophic gastritis plays a role in the development of gastric carcinoma was based on the frequent association of gastric cancer with atrophic gastritis (Guiss and Stewart, 97%; Cheli et al., 82%) (14,43).

These reports led to the follow-up observation of patients with prior evidence of atrophic gastritis. Siurala et al. (68,69) followed 116 patients with atrophic gastritis by means of two annual examinations, for a period of 15 years, and found that 9 of these patients had developed gastric carcinoma (68,69). None of the subjects with initially normal gastric mucosa or with superficial gastritis subsequently developed a carcinoma.

Walker et al. (76), in a follow-up study of 40 patients with atrophic gastritis, found 4 cases of gastric carcinoma after 9 to 21 years. This 10% incidence is in close agreement with Siurala et al.'s observations (68,69).

A further study of our own was made on 363 patients, whose initial biopsies revealed preatrophic gastritis in 69 and atrophic gastritis in 36 (24). The follow-up study of these patients 11 to 18 years after initial examination revealed 114 deceased, with 65 cases of preatrophic or atrophic gastritis. The cause of death was gastric carcinoma in 9 of these 65 patients, that is, in 13% (24).

The correlation between atrophic gastritis and gastric cancer could additionally be proved considering that our figures demonstrate an overall mortality for cancer of 29% in the group with atrophic gastritis and of 30.6% in the subjects with normal gastric mucosa or superficial gastritis, with gastric cancer localization in 47% of the former group and with absence of gastric cancer in the latter one (24). The comparative study of gastric cancer death rates in the Italian and Hungarian populations showed a significant prevalence in the Hungarians above 50 years, thus supporting the hypothesis that an ethnic group with a high gastric cancer rate has a higher prevalence of atrophic gastritis (24).

Evidence in support of the concept that atrophic gastritis constitutes a precursor to gastric carcinoma was also obtained by gastric acid secretory studies. Histamine-resistant achlorhydria as a reflection of atrophic alterations of gastric mucosa was frequently noted prior to the development of the malignant neoplasms (26,47). According to Hitchcock et al. (46) the incidence of gastric carcinoma was four to five times greater in achlorhydric patients than in the normal population. Therefore, the evolutionary study clearly demonstrates that patients with initial histologic findings of atrophic gastritis have a predilection for the development of gastric carcinoma.

In this possible evolutive process, time represents an essential parameter: the mean time interval between the first histobiopsy study and the cancer diagnosis is 15 years according to Siurala et al. (68,69) and is 8 years in our experience (24). In effect, Findley et al. (36), following a group of 100 patients with atrophic gastritis, did not observe gastric cancer in any of the cases reexamined within a 5-year period. However, it remains undetermined how long the gastritic process had existed in these patients before their first examination.

Moreover, the precise role of atrophic gastritis in the pathogenesis of gastric carcinoma remains obscure. Of interest in this respect are the studies of Nieburgs and Glass (62). In pernicious anemia these authors demonstrated a systemic cellular maturation disorder in blood and in epithelial cells, with interest of gastric mucosa. They found also that nuclear alterations due to altered cellular differentiation could be observed in gastric malignant tumor cells as well as in those of pernicious anemia (62). Similar disorders of cell differentiation were observed in atrophic gastritis even in the absence of anemia. These observations led the two authors to hypothesize a relationship between the alterations of atrophic gastritis and those of gastric carcinoma.

The interest in finding the biological key that could explain the phenomenon gave rise to numerous additional considerations: the first concerns the meaning of epithelial metaplasia. Cells with intestinal characteristics are observed in some cases of normal gastric mucosa towards the bottom of gastric pits, that is, in the area associated with proliferation and cell renewal (77). Morson (58) has shown that atrophic gastritis with diffuse intestinal metaplasia in the epithelial districts is found in over 90% of cases of gastric cancer. Immunological (31), histochemical (70), and electron microscopic studies (72) demonstrated that almost all gastric cancers have a relevant proportion of cells with characteristics of intestinal epithelium. In atrophic gastritis the increase in cellular turnover is marked and the tendency to produce intestinal type cells is high; in these conditions cancer may be expected to develop.

More recently, growing interest is dedicated to the dysplastic phenomena that might occur in atrophic gastritis. In particular the cytological and structural alterations typical of the most severe types of dysplasia indicate that the change is irreversible and has the potential to progress, sooner or later, into mucosal cancer (61).

In our experience severe gastric dysplasia is a very rare finding in subjects with atrophic gastritis as well as in its relationship with intestinal metaplasia (19). Therefore, speaking from a statistical point of view, it seems difficult to propose a relevant role for dysplasia in the atrophic gastritis–cancer sequence.

In conclusion, besides the significant data provided by clinical and follow-up studies, the biological interpretation of the relationship between atrophic gastritis and gastric cancer remains unsolved.

POSSIBLE DETECTION OF ATROPHIC GASTRITIS

The importance of atrophic gastritis and intestinal metaplasia in gastric cancer development, as verified by follow-up studies, makes the surveillance of this condition mandatory. The first step to be achieved is the need for identifying atrophic gastritis, and this is a problem that may hardly be solved. Atrophic gastritis in effect is an anatomopathological condition accompanied by precise secretory impairment, but just partly associated with clinical expressions. Therefore, a broad study of atrophic gastritis has to be considered impossible.

Also the statistical and epidemiologic criteria are not helpful: as a matter of fact, we know that this pathological picture is found in more than 1 out of 4 asymptomatic subjects older than 40 years (25). As a consequence, it is well understood why preventive research may not find reasonable application in such a wide population. Thus, reference parameters may be identified in morbid conditions revealing a high incidence of atrophic gastritis (such as pernicious anemia, sideropenic anemia, and rosacea), and it is possible that at least a part of the cases complaining of dyspepsia may reveal an anatomopathological substratum of atrophic gastritis (9,16,23).

Obviously, even more selective and, in a word, "specific" indications may be derived from the analysis of laboratory data, as achlorhydria, hypergastrinemia, and, at least from a hypothetical point of view, creatorrea. In these cases the diagnostic identification of atrophic gastritis is mandatory.

But which procedures must be followed to obtain diagnostic confirmation? As previously stated, histology is the fundamental element for a correct diagnostic approach; therefore, screenings have to be done in gastroenterology units and have to be based on multiple perendoscopic biopsies, which involve fundic as well as antral mucosa.

Also, cytology may add diagnostic confirmation through the visualization of cells with pale nuclei or of goblet cells. This method is not evident in all the cases and shows data that may only be indirect markers of atrophy. Furthermore, the attempt of evidencing achlorhydria by means of tubeless methods represents a prediagnostic stage, certainly not effective for the high number of false positive and false negative findings (28).

Histology remains, therefore, the only fundamental element for correct and sure diagnostic demonstration: its realization is mandatory in the groups indicated by the experience *a posteriori* as having a high frequency of atrophic gastritis.

These are the possible guidelines for the modern diagnostic assessment of atrophic gastritis.

REFERENCES

1. Ardeman, S., and Chanarin, I. (1966): Intrinsic factor secretion in gastric atrophy. *Gut*, 7:99–103.
2. Badenoch, J., Evans, J. R., and Richards, W. C. D. (1957): The stomach in hypochromic anemia. *Br. J. Haematol.*, 3:175–180.
3. Baldini, M., and Cheli, R. (1957): Le alterazioni anatomiche e funzionali dello stomaco negli anemici. *Minerva Med.*, 48:322–325.
4. Banche, M., and Verme, G. (1971): L'endoscopia delle gastriti croniche. *Recent Prog. Med.*, 51:121–129.
5. Bernier, G. M., and Hines, J. D. (1967): Immunologic heterogeneity of auto-antibodies in patients with pernicious anemia. *N. Engl. J. Med.*, 277:1386–1391.
6. Bigotti, A., and Crespi, M. (1976): Citopatologia e citodiagnostica (Apparato digerente). In: *Trattato di citologia e citodiagnostica*, edited by C. Cavallero, pp. 387–412. Marrapese, D.E.M.I., Rome.
7. Burhol, P. G., and Myren, J. (1968): Gastritis and gastric secretion. In: *The Physiology of Gastric Secretion*, pp. 626–641. Universitäts Vorlaget, Oslo.
8. Caruso, I., and Bianchi Porro, G. (1980): Gastroscopic evaluation of antiinflammatory agents. *Br. Med. J.*, I:75–81.
9. Cheli, R. (1966): *La biopsie gastrique par sonde*. Masson, Paris.
10. Cheli, R. (1971): La biopsia nella diagnosi delle gastriti croniche. *Recent Prog. Med.*, 51:130–143.
11. Cheli, R. (1975): Gli aspetti endoscopici delle gastropatie. Le gastropatie da famaci. *Abstract book of: Corso di aggiornamento in gastroenterologia*. Montecatini Terme.
12. Cheli, R., Carli, C., and Ciancamerla, G. (1974): Cytology of the gastric mucosa in the development of chronic gastritis. *Am. J. Dig. Dis.*, 19:161–166.
13. Cheli, R., Celle, G., Dodero, M., and Orlando, G. (1959): Reperti bioptici e comportamento secretorio della mucosa gastrica nella patologia biliare. *Epatologia*, 5:211–220.
14. Cheli, R., Dodero, M., and Celle, G. (1961): Aspetti anatomofunzionali della mucosa fundica in soggetti con carcinoma gastrico. *Rass. Ital. Gastroenterol.*, 5:176–180.
15. Cheli, R., Dodero, M., and Celle, G. (1962): The anatomic basis of the gastric secretion. *Am. J. Dig. Dis.*, 7:922–926.
16. Cheli, R., Dodero, M., Celle, G., and Vassalotti, M. (1959): Gastric biopsy and secretory findings in hypochromic anemias. *Acta Haematol.*, 22:1–11.
17. Cheli, R., Giacosa, A., and Molinari, F. (1981): Chronic atrophic gastritis and duodenogastric reflux. *Scand. J. Gastroenterol. (Suppl.)*, 16 (67):125–127.
18. Cheli, R., and Giacosa, A. (1980): Le gastriti croniche. In: *La mattia peptica*, edited by L. Barbara and G. Bianchi Porro, pp. 215–239. Medis, Milan.
19. Cheli, R., and Giacosa, A. (1982): Dysplasia and chronic gastritis of the fundic and antral mucosa. In: *Abstracts of World Congress of Gastroenterology*. Stockholm.
20. Cheli, R., and Giacosa, A. (1983): Atrophic gastritis and gastric atrophy: dogma or reality? *Gastrointest. Endosc. (in press)*.
21. Cheli, R., Giacosa, A., Marenco, G., Canepa, M., Dante, G. L., and Ghezzo, L. (1981): Chronic gastritis and alcohol. *Z. Gastroenterol.* 9:1–5.
22. Cheli, R., Molinari, F., and Giacosa, A. (1981): *Drug Induced Gastric Lesions*. Piccin, Padoa.

23. Cheli, R., Moretti, G., Dodero, M., Celle, G., and Orlando, G. (1959): Bioptic findings and secretory behaviour of the gastric mucosa during some dermatoses. *Gaz. Med. Portug.*, 12:147–150.
24. Cheli, R., Santi, L., Ciancamerla, G., and Canciani, G. (1973): A clinical and statistical follow-up study of atrophic gastritis. *Am. J. Dig. Dis.*, 18:1061–1066.
25. Cheli, R., Simon, L., Aste, H., Figus, I. A., Nicolo', G., Bajtai, A., and Puntoni, R. (1980): Atrophic gastritis and intestinal metaplasia in asymptomatic Hungarian and Italian populations. *Endoscopy*, 12:105–108.
26. Comfort, M. W., Butsch, W. L., and Eustermann, G. B. (1937): Observations on gastric acidity before and after development of carcinoma of the stomach. *Am. J. Dig. Dis.*, 4:673–679.
27. Crespi, M. (1981): Patchy gastritis. *Hepato. Gastroenterol.*, 28:178.
28. Crespi, M., Bigotti, A., and Casale, V. (1977): High risk categories for gastric cancer and actual possibilities for a selection. In: *Gastric Precancerosis*, edited by I. A. Figus and L. Simon, pp. 211–216. Akademiai Kiado, Budapest.
29. Davenport, H. W. (1968): Destruction of the gastric mucosal barrier by detergents and urea. *Gastroenterology*, 53:175–181.
30. Davidson, W. M. B., and Markson, J. L. (1955): The gastric mucosa in iron deficiency anaemia. *Lancet*, 269:639–643.
31. De Boer, W. G. R. M., Forsyth, A., and Nairn, R. C. (1969): Gastric antigens in health and disease. Behaviour in early development, senescence, metaplasia and cancer. *Br. Med. J.*, iii:93–94.
32. Dodero, M., Celle, G., and Cheli, R. (1962): L'antrite ed i suoi rapporti con la frogosi del fundus. *Minerva Med.*, 53:1175–1180.
33. Doig, B. K., and Wood, J. J. (1952): Gastritis: study of 112 cases diagnosed by gastric biopsy. *Med. J. Aust.*, 39:593–599.
34. Elster, K., Carson, W., Wild, A., and Thomasko, A. (1979): Evaluation of histological classification in early gastric cancer. (An analysis of 300 cases). *Endoscopy*, 3:203–206.
35. Fieschi, A., and Cheli, R. (1956): *Le gastriti*, L. Pozzi, Rome.
36. Findley, J. W., Kirsner, J. B., and Palmer, W. L. (1950): Atrophic gastritis: a follow up study of 100 patients. *Gastroenterology*, 16:347–351.
37. Fischer, J. M., and Taylor, K. B. (1965): A comparison of autoimmune phenomena in pernicious anaemia and chronic atrophic gastritis. *N. Engl. J. Med.*, 722:499–503.
38. Fujimura, K. (1973): The gastric antibodies (intrinsic factor antibody and parietal cell antibody) and their clinical significance. Pernicious anaemia and atrophic gastritis. *Hiroshima J. Med. Sci.*, 22:221–227.
39. Giacosa, A., and Cheli, R. (1980): Smoke and chronic gastritis. *Abstracts IV Congress European Society of Digestive Diseases*, p. 14. Hamburg.
40. Giacosa, A., and Cheli, R. (1981): Gastrite chronique dans l'ulcere duodenal. *Gastroenterol. Clin. Biol.*, 5 (I bis):215 A.
41. Giacosa, A., Molinari, F., and Cheli, R. (1979): Analyse quantitative et qualitative des cellules inflammatoires dans les gastrites chroniques. *Acta Endosc.*, 9:105–110.
42. Giacosa, A., Turello, V., and Icardi, A. (1978): Sécrétion gastrique acide, gastrinémie et masse cellulaire pariétale dans les gastrites chroniques. *Gastroenterol. Clin. Biol.*, 2:133–137.
43. Guiss, L. W., and Stewart, F. W. (1943): Chronic atrophic gastritis and cancer of the stomach. *Arch. Surg.*, 46:823–828.
44. Heinkel, K., and Henning, N. (1964): Diagnose und klinisches Erkrankungsbild der chronischen Gastritis. *Radiologe*, 4:83–87.
45. Henning, N. (1959): Die chronische Gastritis im Lichte moderner Untersuchungsmethoden. *Gastroenterologia*, 92:307–313.
46. Hitchcock, C. R., McLean, L. D., and Sullivan, W. A. (1957): The secretory and clinical aspects of achlorhydria and gastric atrophy as precursors of gastric cancer. *J. Natl. Cancer Inst.*, 18:795–801.
47. Hurst, A. F. (1929): On the precursor of carcinoma of the stomach. *Lancet*, 217:1023–1027.
48. Jenner, A. W. F. (1939): Perniziose anämie und Magenkarzinom. *Acta Med. Scand.*, 102:529–534.
49. Johansen, A. (1981): *Early Gastric Cancer. A Contribution to the Pathology and to Gastric Cancer Histogenesis.* Poul Petri Bogtryk, Copenhagen.
50. Lambert, R. (1972): Chronic gastritis. A critical study of the progressive atrophy of the gastric mucosa. *Digestion*, 7:83–89.
51. Lambling, A. (1951): Role du reflux dans la pathologie digestive. *Presse Méd.*, 72:1496–1502.
52. Laurén, P. (1965): The two histological main types of gastric carcinoma: diffuse and so called intestinal-type carcinoma. *Acta Pathol. Microbiol. Scand.*, 64:31–49.
53. Magnus, H. A. (1958): A reassessment of gastric lesions in pernicious anaemia. *J. Clin. Pathol.*, II:289–294.
54. Magnus, H. A., and Ungley, C. C. (1938): The gastric lesions in pernicious anemia. *Lancet*, 1:420–423.
55. Markson, J. L., and Davidson, W. M. B. (1956): Gastric biopsy in megalobastic anemia. *Scott. Med. J.*, I:259.
56. Masala, C., Pala, A. M., Andreoli, F., De Philippis, C. V., and Ciardi-Dupré, G. F. (1970): Gastriti croniche atrofiche e anticorpi antimucosa gastrica. *Folia Allergol.*, 17:30–45.

57. Moll, A., and Petzel, H. (1964): Die Saugbiopsie ans dem Magenantrum und ihr Vergleich mit der Fundusbiopsie. *Gastroenterologia*, 101:41–45.
58. Morson, B. C. (1955): Intestinal metaplasia of the gastric mucosa. *Br. J. Cancer*, 9:365–376.
59. Morson, B. C., and Dawson, I. M. P. (1972): *Gastrointestinal Pathology*. Blackwell Scientific Publications, Oxford.
60. Moutier, F., and Cornet, A. (1955): *Les gastrites*. Masson, Paris.
61. Nagayo, T. (1980): Dysplastic changes of the digestive tract related to cancer. *Acta Endosc.*, 10:69–79.
62. Nieburgs, H. E., and Glass, G. B. J. (1963): Gastric cell maturation disorders in atrophic gastritis, pernicious anaemia and carcinoma. *Am. J. Dig. Dis.*, 8:135–141.
63. Rigler, R. G., and Kaplan, H. S. (1945): Pernicious anemia and the early diagnosis of tumors of the stomach. *JAMA*, 128:426–432.
64. Samloff, I. M., Kleinmann, M. S., and Turner, M. D. (1968): Blocking and binding antibodies to intrinsic factor and parietal cell antibody in pernicious anemia. *Gastroenterology*, 55:575–581.
65. Schindler, R. (1947): *Gastritis*. Grune and Stratton, New York, London.
66. Siurala, M., Isokoski, M., Varis, K., and Kekki, M. (1968): Prevalence of gastritis on a rural population. Bioptic study of subjects selected at random. *Scand. J. Gastroenterol.*, 3:211–223.
67. Varis, K., Pyovala, K., Krohn, K., Isokoski, M., and Siurala, M. (1970): Genetics of atrophic gastritis. In: *Abstracts of the 4th World Congress of Gastroenterology*. Copenhagen, edited by P. Riis et al., p. 154, Danish Gastroenterol. Assoc.
68. Siurala, M., and Seppala, K. (1960): Atrophic gastritis as a possible precursor of gastric carcinoma and pernicious anemia. *Acta Med. Scand.*, 166:455–461.
69. Siurala, M., Varis, K., and Wiljasalo, M. (1966): Studies of patients with atrophic gastritis: a 10-15 year follow up. *Scand. J. Gastroenterol.*, 1:40–46.
70. Stemmerman, G. N. (1967): Comparative study of histochemical patterns in non-neoplastic and neoplastic gastric epithelium. A study of Japanese in Hawaii. *J. Natl. Cancer Inst.*, 39:375–382.
71. Strickland, R. G., and McKay, I. R. (1973): A reappraisal of the nature and significance of chronic atrophic gastritis. *Am. J. Dig. Dis.*, 18:426–440.
72. Tarpila, S., Telkkä, A., and Siurala, M. (1969): Ultrastructure of various metaplasias of the stomach. *Acta Pathol. Microbiol. Scand.*, 77:187–195.
73. Varis, K. (1971): A family study of chronic gastritis: histological; immunological and functional aspects. *Scand. J. Gastroenterol (Suppl.)*, 6(13):1–56.
74. Varis, K., Ihamäki, T., Härkonën, M., Samloff, I. M., and Siurala, M. (1979): Gastric morphology, function, and immunology in first-degree relatives of probands with pernicious anemia and controls. *Scand. J. Gastroenterol.*, 14:129–139.
75. Villako, K., Tamm, A., Savisaar, E., and Ruttas, M. (1976): Prevalence of antral and fundic gastritis in a randomly selected group of an Estonian rural population. *Scand. J. Gastroenterol.*, 11:817–822.
76. Walker, I. R., Strickland, R. G., Ungar, B., and McKay, R. (1971): Simple atrophic gastritis and gastric carcinoma. *Gut*, 12:906–913.
77. Whitehead, R. (1979): *Mucosal Biopsy of the Gastrointestinal Tract*. W. B. Saunders Co., Philadelphia.
78. Wood, I. J., and Taft, L. I. (1958): *Diffuse Lesions of the Stomach*. Arnold, London.
79. Zeitoun, P., Potet, F., and Zyberberg, L. (1969): Histologie de la muqueuse antrale. In: *L'antre gastrique*. Masson, Paris.

Precancerous Lesions of the Gastrointestinal Tract, edited by P. Sherlock, B. C. Morson, L. Barbara, and U. Veronesi. Raven Press, New York © 1983.

Gastric Polyps: Pathology and Malignant Potential

Aage Johansen

Institute of Pathology, Bispebjerg Hospital, DK-2400 Copenhagen NV, Denmark

Polyps of the gastrointestinal tract are found at two major localisations: the stomach and the colon. Gastric polyps are relatively rare. They can be dealt with as self-contained units, but the advantages of comparing them with the much more intensively studied colonic polyps are numerous. Our knowledge about colonic polyps is better grounded, both regarding nomenclature and classification and in particular regarding malignant potential; when the different histology of the two organs is taken into consideration, transferring experience from the colonic polyps to the gastric polyps can be useful.

NOMENCLATURE AND CLASSIFICATION

A gastric polyp is a tumour that clearly projects from the mucosa into the lumen. The name is used for routine communication and will never disappear. It gives a certain impression of the macroscopic appearance of the tumour but is not well defined. The basis for a precise nomenclature must be the histologic type of the tissue forming the polyp, just as the histologic type and the genesis must be the basis for the classification of polyps.

Epithelial gastrointestinal polyps are usually divided into two main groups: the non-neoplastic and the neoplastic. The division is important, because only the neoplastic polyps have a malignant potential. The division implies a clear and unequivocal definition of neoplasia separating this growth disturbance from others. Autonomous growth owing to abnormal cellular metabolic processes, continuation of proliferation after cessation of the stimulus that has caused the growth, and abnormal delay of cell maturation are all factors usually entering into the definition of neoplasia. No gastrointestinal polyp fulfills such demands completely. The autonomy of the growth of all polyps is restricted; their growth seems to stop at a certain level, and some may even disappear, as it is seen for those polyps left behind in the rectal stump after colectomy in patients with familial adenomatosis of the colon (13).

Although it is not logical to call some gastrointestinal polyps neoplastic in the light of the definition of neoplasia, pathologists nevertheless work with such a concept and name these polyps adenomatous polyps or simply adenomas.

In all textbooks of pathology, adenoma is defined as a benign tumour originating from glandular epithelium. In the gastrointestinal tract, however, this definition has been changed or narrowed so that only benign tumours revealing dysplasia are adenomas (19).

It is tempting to discuss why the definition of an ordinary tumour type such as an adenoma in the gastrointestinal tract has been altered to such an extent that we now literally are talking about a dysplastic lump having the appearance of an adenoma (polyp) (17) instead of an adenoma (polyp) showing dysplasia; but first it is necessary to characterise dysplasia.

Epithelial dysplasia is a histologic more than a pure cytologic change. It comprises three main features: cellular atypia, abnormal differentiation, and disorganised mucosal architecture (20). Whether the simultaneous presence of all three features is mandatory for making the diagnosis dysplasia or whether one of the features may be lacking without rejecting the diagnosis has not been fully established, but it is possible to mention dysplastic lesions where for instance disorganised mucosal architecture is lacking. Recently microadenomas in the colon from patients not suffering familial adenomatosis have been described (28). They do not show a disturbed mucosal architecture. Similar lesions are also seen in the colonic mucosa in familial adenomatosis between the polyps (4). On the other hand, it can also be mentioned that all polyp-shaped adenomas automatically reveal a disturbed mucosal architecture, so that the significance of this feature is limited.

The incorporation and emphasis on dysplasia in the definition of gastrointestinal adenomas have several causes. The most important is that dysplastic changes are a constant finding in tumours usually considered adenomas irrespective of their macroscopic shape and histologic structure. It seems reasonable to include a constantly present characteristic of a lesion into its definition. Another cause is the expressed correlation between the degree of dysplasia and the presence of different parameters of the adenomas usually looked upon as reliable markers of cancer risk (18). A large, sessile, villous adenoma shows significantly more often severe degrees of dysplasia than a small, pedunculated, tubular adenoma. This also underlines the significance of dysplasia.

The above-mentioned considerations have primarily been used for colonic polyps but can be applied to gastric polyps as well.

GASTRIC POLYPS

Hyperplastic Polyps

The most common polyp of the stomach is usually looked upon as being nondysplastic because cellular atypia is lacking. On the other hand, abnormal differentiation and disorganised mucosal architecture are often present. These polyps are sometimes divided into two variants (6). The first is a smaller one that is built up of elongated foveolae covered with tall mucous secreting cells. Only preformed elements are seen in such polyps. The foveolae are cysticly dilated, but cysts without connection to the original foveolae are not seen, and if glands persist they are normal. The lamina propria between the changed foveolae does not differ from that of the neighbourhood. The genesis of the small polyps is uncertain. They may be caused by inflammation and regeneration, but since this is uncertain it seems most reasonable to call them hyperplastic polyps in accordance with their appearance. The cells of the polyp-forming elements are more numerous than those in the corresponding elements of the adjacent mucosa. They correspond to the type II polyps of Nakamura (25). Elster (6) has proposed the name focal foveolar hyperplasia, which is just as good, although it invites us to include lesions that are not real polyps in the strict sense of the word.

The other variant of this group of polyps is larger. It also shows hyperplastic foveolae, and groups of normal looking glands may be found, but besides this a varying number of more or less cysticly dilated glands localised between and below the foveolae are seen. The glands are covered with an epithelium of just the same type as the foveolae. Careful studies of serial sections (21) have revealed that some of the dilated glands correspond to the foveolae; others are new formations having no connection to the original structures. The stroma is proliferating, edematous, and contains many capillaries. Bundles of disorderly arranged smooth muscle fibres are common. The genesis of these glands is also uncertain. Usually they are looked upon as hyperplastic or reparative phenomena, but I think it is wise to agree with Muto and Oota (21), who stated that "the problem of whether or not the proliferated ducts are neoplastic remains obscure." To the best of my knowledge no cell kinetic studies, which might have given guidelines, have been carried out. The polyps were called regenerative by Ming and Goldman (16) in 1965, but in 1973 Ming (15) in the volume on Stomach Pathology of the Armed Forces Institute's *Atlas* designated them hyperplastic adenomatous polyps. In a previous volume of the same atlas, Stout (26) in 1953 had used the name adenomatous polyps like many other American pathologists at that time. In nearly every report, however, the benign nature of the polyps is underlined and the name has apparently been used only to indicate a lesion originating from glandular tissue.

From the literature it clearly appears that many who use the name do not consider the polyps as truly neoplastic. Elster (6), who has studied the polyp in detail uses the name hyperplasiogenous polyp (Greek: hyperplasi-o-genesis) and consequently stresses hyperplasia as the dominant factor for the development. Morson and Dawson (19) call the polyps generative polyps and Nagayo (23,24) uses the name hyperplastic for all polyps of non-neoplastic origin.

Adenomatous Polyps

A rather small group of gastric polyps shows varying degrees of dysplasia and they are thus, according to the general view, adenomas. Their macroscopic shape differs much from that of colonic adenomas, in fact it is extremely rare to see a gastric adenoma of classic polyp shape with stalk and head; also, the typical villous adenoma is rare in the stomach. Usually the tumours are sessile or the stalk is short and broad. A common variant is the small well-demarcated, wart-like lesion with small grooves on its surface, but principally similar lesions may cover a great part of the gastric mucosa. Adenomas appearing as a large fold have been described (10).

The degree of dysplasia of gastric polyps are graded into mild, moderate, and severe. Carcinoma *in situ*, the designation used elsewhere to indicate the most severe degree of epithelial, precancerous changes, is generally not used for lesions of the gastrointestinal tract. In the Japanese and German literature (8,22,27) the designation borderline lesion is often seen. The name is particularly applied to flat, sessile adenomas of a rather special type, with such a severe degree of dysplasia that the differential diagnosis towards early gastric cancer is very difficult or impossible to make. The diagnosis reflects an uncertainty that is well known from adenocarcinomas of other organs (7,10).

The adenomas are thought to originate from a neoplastic proliferation of the deeply situated foveolar cells. In his survey on gastric polyps Elster (6) mentioned an adenoma-like lesion of papillary appearance also originating from foveolar cells but not showing dysplasia. These tumours are most often localised in the cardiac region. Furthermore, Elster (6) described an adenoma-like lesion apparently arising from the *glands* of the pyloric and cardiac region. Neither of these lesions shows dysplasia and they are very rare. They are probably a hyperplastic phenomenon. When localised in the pyloric region they may correspond to what is generally called Brunner-gland adenomas of the duodenum.

All the polyps mentioned have an epithelial origin. Nearly every mesenchymal gastric tumour sometimes attains a polypoid appearance. Those tumours will not be mentioned in this paper. Neither will hamartomatous polyps, common to all parts of the gastrointestinal tract, nor will polyps based on heterotopia be discussed. Their malignant potential is negligible.

TABLE 1. *Number of epithelial polyps in 1,346 consecutively collected resection specimens*

No. specimens with	Polyps	
	Adenomatous	Hyperplastic
EGC, 73	3	12
AGC, 382	4	31
Carcinoma total, 455	7	43
Gastric ulcers, 613	4	58
Duodenal ulcers, 278	0	15
Ulcers total, 891	4	73
Specimens total, 1,346	11	116

RESEARCH RESULTS

Adenomas

My attitude to ordinary epithelial gastric polyps is that from a practical point of view they are best divided into two groups: those with and those without dysplasia. The first mentioned are adenomatous polyps, the last hyperplastic polyps. I do not distinguish between a small and a large variant of hyperplastic polyps because I find the transition too smooth. The following figures are based exclusively on polyps found in specimens resected for another localised lesion. The distribution of polyps according to the lesion that caused the resection is seen in Table 1. The adenomas were significantly most common in specimens resected for gastric cancer. Hyperplastic polyps were also most common in this group, but the difference was insignificant. There were no adenomatous polyps and only 15 hyperplastic polyps in specimens resected for duodenal ulcer.

Among the 455 resected carcinomas, 25 (5.6%) (Table 2) were judged to be malignantly transformed adenomas, as the greater part of these tumours showed an adenomatous structure. In 7 cases the structure was so marked that the differential diagnosis towards carcinoma was difficult to make when invasion through the lamina muscularis mucosae was absent (Fig. 1). In the other 18 cases parts of adenomatous tissue were still present at the margin of the carcinomas, but this was not a dominant feature (Fig. 2). For the sake of convenience, the 25 tumours are called malignant polyps.

The localisation of the adenomas including the malignant polyps is seen in Table 3. The most common position was the pyloric mucosa and only three polyps were found in the body mucosa. The size expressed by the largest diameter is given in Table 4. Two sessile adenomas measured more than 5 cm in proximal-distal extent.

TABLE 2. *Carcinomas originating in adenomas*

Type of carcinoma	Origin in an adenoma		Total
	Certain	Likely	
EGC, 73	5	6	11
AGC, 382	2	12	14
Total, 455	7	18	25

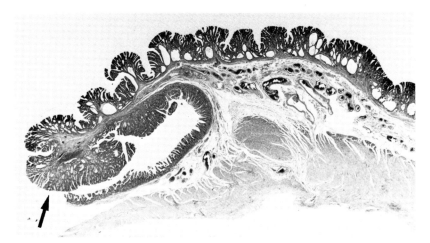

FIG. 1. Large, sessile adenoma with transition into intramucosal carcinoma at the top of the fold (*arrow*). H.-E., ×5.

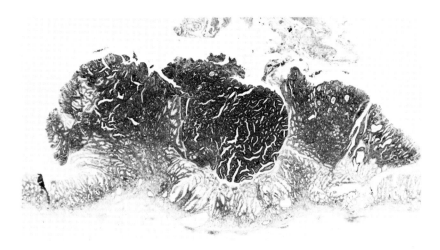

FIG. 2. Intramucosal carcinoma originating in a sessile adenoma. H.-E., ×5.

TABLE 3. *The localisation of the centres of adenomas, "malignant polyps," and hyperplastic polyps according to the type of gastric mucosa*

Type of polyp	Type of gastric mucosa		
	Pyloric	Transitional	Body
Adenomatous, 11	9	1	1
"Malignant", 25	16	7	2
Hyperplastic, 116	63	32	21

TABLE 4. Size of adenomas, "malignant polyps," and hyperplastic polyps (largest diameter)

Type of polyp	Largest diameter (mm)			
	<10	11–20	21–30	>30
Adenomatous, 11	2	5	1	3
"Malignant", 25	2	12	7	4
Hyperplastic, 116	88	17	10	1

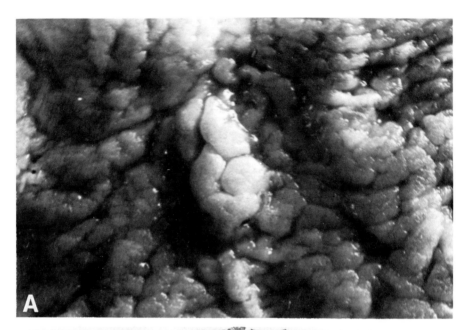

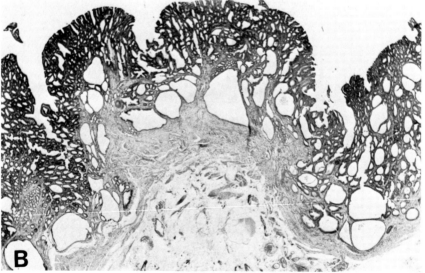

FIG. 3. A: Small, sessile, wart-like polyp 12 mm of proximal-distal extent. B: Section through the polyp. There is a moderate dysplasia and numerous cysts around the muscularis mucosae. H.-E., ×3.

The tumours showed very different shapes. Only two had the appearance of a classic, pedunculated, colonic adenoma. Most were nodular without any well-defined stalk. Some were rather sharply demarcated elevations with an irregular humpy surface. Among these there were very small tumours (Fig. 3), but also the largest tumours. Finally, some of them had the appearance of a giant mucosal fold projecting into the lumen (10).

The degree of dysplasia (Fig. 4) is given in Table 5. The adenomatous remains found in the malignant polyps showed in all cases severe dysplasia, and a similar grade was found in three pure adenomas.

Apart from this common feature the histological structure varied considerably. A villous pattern (Fig. 5) was extremely rare and a structure quite similar to what is known from tubular colonic adenomas was infrequent too. Yet, tubes were the most usual structure in the adenomas. Sometimes they appeared like the original foveolae covered with an atypical epithelium, sometimes the tubes were branched or dilated (Fig. 6). The degree of cellular atypia varied in the single adenoma and areas with normal foveolae were sometimes found. Owing to such areas and to the presence of brush border and goblet cell remains in foveolae covered with atypical epithelium, it was obvious that intestinal metaplastic epithelium was the basis for the dysplastic changes, but in some cases normal nonmetaplastic epithelium also had contributed.

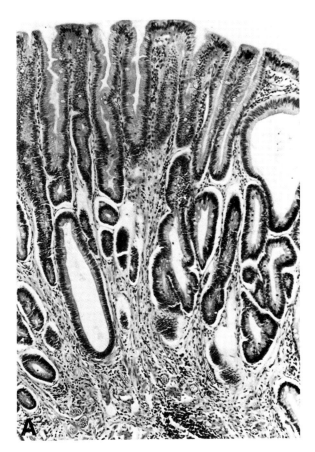

FIG. 4.A–D *(above and following pages)* Different degrees of dysplasia from four adenomas. **A:** Mild dysplasia. ×68.

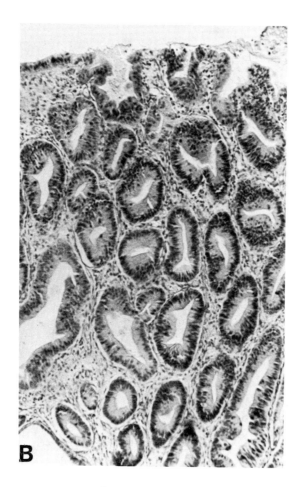

FIG. 4 *(continued)* **B:** Moderate dysplasia. ×68.

Quite as common as the tubes were cysts (Fig. 1), found in the mucosa below the level of the tubes in close connection with the muscularis mucosae, sometimes splitting up this layer (Fig. 6). The cysts were also covered with an atypical epithelium, but the degree of atypia was often milder and the epithelium of many cysts showed no atypia at all.

The original pyloric or body glands were very atrophic, in many cases they had even disappeared completely, but sometimes groups of normal pyloric glands were still present.

The stroma between the cysts and the tubes was usually sparse, probably due to compression. A slight increase in the number of chronic inflammatory cells was the rule, but some adenomas revealed a heavy inflammatory reaction with many Russell bodies. Erosion of the surface and acute inflammation were seldom. However, three cases were exceptions. In these cases the stroma was proliferating with considerable edema and there were erosions of the surface of the tumours.

Since the number of benign adenomas was 11 and the number of malignantly transformed adenomas 25, the rate of carcinomas developed in adenomas was 69.4%.

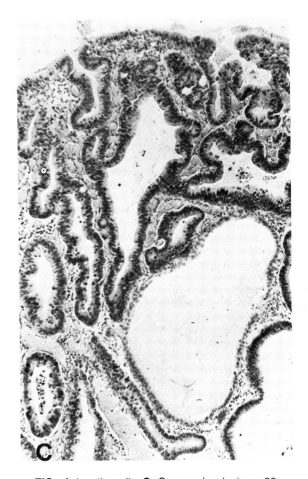

FIG. 4 *(continued)* **C:** Severe dysplasia. ×68.

Hyperplastic Polyps

As mentioned, all polyps without dysplasia made up a group called hyperplastic polyps. The localisation of these polyps is given in Table 3 and the size in Table 4. Their shape differed. The small ones were sessile and well marked (Fig. 7). The larger ones were often pedunculated (Fig. 8). Their surface was smooth or slightly lobulated. The smaller ones were sometimes localised on the rugal folds of the gastric mucosa.

The histological structure varied. The foveolae were elongated and branched. There were many cysts even in the smallest polyps, some of them without connection to the foveolae. The cysts often compressed and even split up the muscularis mucosae (Fig. 9). There was a proliferation of the original pyloric glands and body glands were replaced by pseudopyloric glands.

The epithelium covering the foveolae, cysts, and glands was usually of original gastric type, but both incomplete and complete intestinal metaplastic epithelium were seen. Usually an increased mucous secretion was found both in the original foveolar epithelium and in the metaplastic goblet cells which were enlarged.

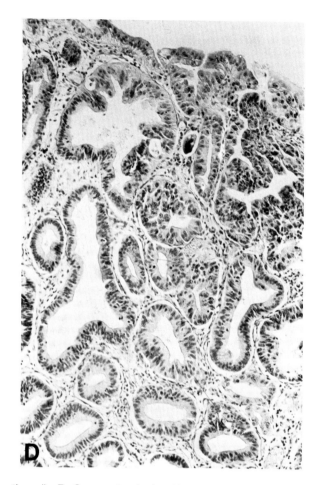

FIG. 4 *(continued)*   **D:** Severe dysplasia with transition into carcinoma. H.-E., ×68.

TABLE 5. *Degree of dysplasia of adenomas and of the adenomatous remnants of "malignant polyps"*

Type of polyp	Degree of dysplasia		
	Mild	Moderate	Severe
Adenomatous, 11	3	5	3
"Malignant", 25	—	—	25

FIG. 5.   A: Small, villous tumours localised on a mucosal fold. H.-E. ×5. **B:** Section from **A** (*arrow*). There is only a mild degree of dysplasia. H.-E. ×68.

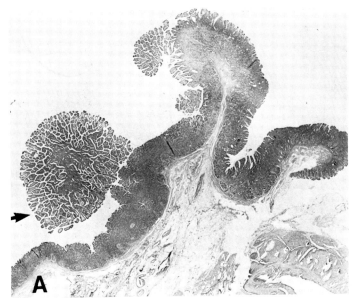

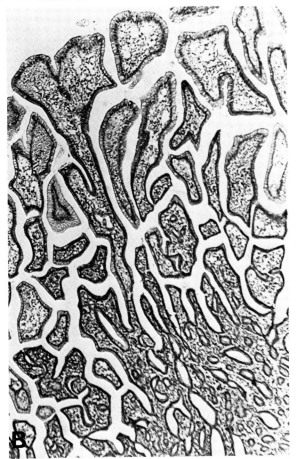

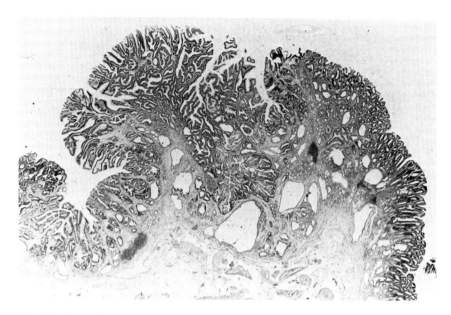

FIG. 6. Papillary adenoma with many cysts. There is only a mild degree of dysplasia. Fig. 4A is from this tumour. H.-E. ×100.

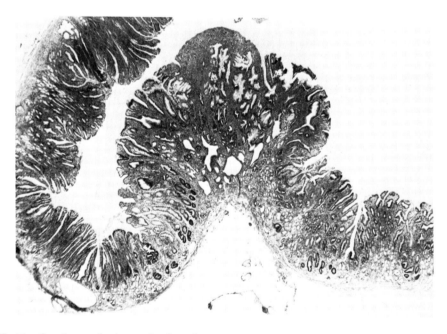

FIG. 7. Small, sessile, hyperplastic polyp measuring twice the height of the mucosa. A few cysts are present. H.-E. ×10.

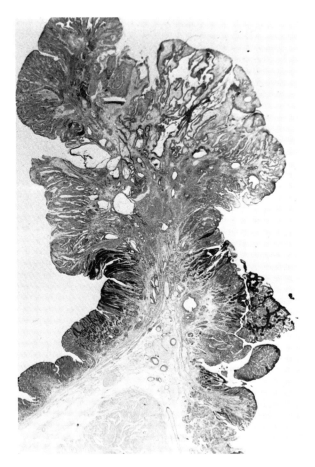

FIG. 8. Large, pedunculated, hyperplastic (hyperplasiogenous) polyp with many cysts. Alcian blue. ×7.

The stroma of the polyps was rather characteristic. It was abundant and edematous. It was provided with many capillaries and there were bundles of muscle fibres in it, most of which could be traced back to a splitting of the muscularis mucosae. The number of inflammatory cells differed and there were not so many Russell bodies as in the adenomatous polyps.

None of the singly situated hyperplastic polyps showed signs of malignant transformation, and none of the carcinomas showed remains of a hyperplastic polyp. In one specimen a large number of densely situated polyps was found. They had an appearance compatible with hyperplastic polyps, and not the slightest degree of cellular atypia was found, but a great part of the epithelium was metaplastic. This tumour, which I have depicted elsewhere (10), resulted in metastases to the skin and the liver.

The above-mentioned specimen was one of six with polyps in large numbers examined in this institute during the last 20 years. Two others were resection specimens with more

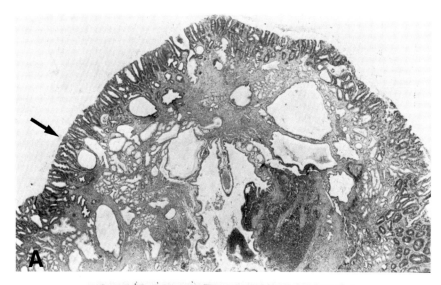

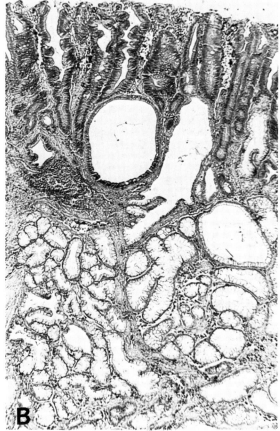

FIG. 9. **A:** A dome-shaped adenoma from an 85-year-old man. H.-E. ×6. **B:** Section from the tumour *(arrow)*. Note the group of nearly normal or slightly dilated pyloric glands. The foveolar zone shows mild dysplasia only. H.-E. ×40.

anemia or type A gastritis may be advisable particularly when upper abdominal symptoms are present or if there is a family history of gastric cancer. Although there are convenient and reliable screening methods available for type A gastritis (29,30), screening of type A gastritis from a general population for detection of gastric cancer is questionable from the cost-benefit point of view. Over all, ethical aspects and also technical restrictions caused by the limited endoscopy capacity in most countries may be decisive when the performance of endoscopic examinations are considered at an individual level.

REFERENCES

1. Cheli, R., Santi, L., Ciancamerla, G., and Canciani, G. (1973): A clinical and statistical follow-up study of atrophic gastritis. *Dig. Dis.*, 18:1061–1066.
2. Cheli, R., Simon, L., Aste, H., Figus, I. A., Nicoló, G., Bajtai, A., and Puntoni, R. (1980): Atrophic gastritis and intestinal metaplasia in asymptomatic Hungarian and Italian populations. *Endoscopy*, 12:105–108.
3. Correa, P. (1980): The epidemiology and pathogenesis of chronic gastritis: Three etiological entities. *Front. Gastrointest. Res.*, 6:98–108.
4. Correa, P., Cuello, C., and Duque, E. (1970): Carcinoma and intestinal metaplasia of the stomach in Colombian migrants. *J. Natl. Cancer Inst.*, 44:297–306.
5. Dutz, W., Kohout, E., and Vessal, K. (1979): Epidemiologic studies of gastric carcinoma: comparison between Iranians and two racial groups of the USA. *Israel J. Med. Sci.*, 15:410–413.
6. Elsborg, L., Andersen, D., Myhre-Jensen, O., and Bastrup-Madsen, P. (1977): Gastric mucosal polyps in pernicious anaemia. *Scand. J. Gastroenterol.*, 12:49–52.
7. Elsborg, L., and Mosbech, J. (1979): Pernicious anaemia as a risk factor in gastric cancer. *Acta Med. Scand.*, 206:315–318.
7a. Finnish Cancer Registry—The Institute for Statistical and Epidemidological Cancer Research (1981): Cancer incidence in Finland. Cancer Society of Finland, publ. no. 28, pp. 16–19, Helsinki.
8. Gregor, O., Blaha, J., Mertl, L., Svoboda, M., Cholt, M., Bednar, B., and Reisenaur, R. (1977): Gastric cancer detection among risk groups and their longitudinal follow-up. In: *Current Views in Gastroenterology*, edited by V. Varró and G. A. Bálint, pp. 541–545. Hungarian Society of Gastroenterology, Hungary.
9. Hakulinen, T., Pukkala, E., Hakama, M., Lehtonen, M., Saxén, E., and Teppo, L. (1981): Survival of cancer patients in Finland in 1953–1974. *Ann. Clin. Res. (Suppl.)*, 13(31):27–30.
10. Hitchcock, C. R., Sullivan, W. A., and Wangensteen, O. H. (1955): The value of achlorhydria as a screening test for gastric cancer. *Gastroenterology*, 29:621–632.
11. Hoffman, N. R. (1970): The relationship between pernicious anemia and cancer of the stomach. *Geriatrics*, 25:90–95.
11a. Ihamäki, T. et al. (1979): Morphological, functional, and immunological state of the gastric mucosa in gastric carcinoma families. Comparison with a computer-matched family sample. *Scand. J. Gastroenterol.*, 14:801–812.
12. Irvine, W. J., Cullen, D. R., and Mawhinney, H. (1974): Natural history of autoimmune achlorhydric atrophic gastritis. *Lancet*, 2:482–485.
13. Jørgensen, J. (1951): The mortality among patients with pernicious anemia in Denmark and the incidence of gastric carcinoma among the same. *Acta Med. Scand.*, 139:472–481.
14. Kaplan, H. S., and Rigler, L. G. (1945): Pernicious anemia and carcinoma of the stomach—autopsy studies concerning their interrelationship. *Am. J. Med. Sci.*, 209:339–348.
15. Kobler, E., Nüesch, H. J., Rhyner, K., and Deyhle, P. (1977): Perniziosa und Magenkarzinom. *Schweiz. Rundschau Med.*, 66:659–660.
16. Kuster, G. G. R., ReMine, W. H., and Dockerty, M. B. (1972): Gastric cancer in pernicious anemia and in patients with and without achlorhydria. *Ann. Surg.*, 175:783–789.
17. Lauren, P. (1965): The two histological main types of gastric carcinoma, diffuse and so-called intestinal type carcinoma. *Acta Pathol. Microbiol. Scand.*, 64:31–49.
18. Morson, B. C., Sobin, L. H., Grundmann, E., Johansen, A., Nagayo, T., and Serck-Hanssen, A. (1980): Precancerous conditions and epithelial dysplasia in the stomach. *J. Clin. Pathol.*, 33:711–721.
19. Mosbech, J., and Videbaek, A. (1950): Mortality from and risk of gastric carcinoma among patients with pernicious anaemia. *Br. Med. J.*, 2:390–394.
20. Munoz, N., and Asvall, J. (1971): Time trends of intestinal and diffuse types of gastric cancer in Norway. *Int. J. Cancer*, 8:144–157.
21. Munoz, N., and Connelly, R. (1971): Time trends of intestinal and diffuse types of gastric cancer in the United States. *Int. J. Cancer*, 8:158–164.
22. Nomura, A. M. Y., Stemmermann, G. N., and Samloff, I. M. (1980): Serum pepsinogen I as a predictor of stomach cancer. *Ann. Intern. Med.*, 93:537–540.

23. Pedersen, A. B., and Mosbech, J. (1969): Morbidity of pernicious anaemia. *Acta Med. Scand.*, 185:449–452.
24. Ruddell, W. S. J., Bone, E. S., Hill, M. J., and Walters, C. L. (1978): Pathogenesis of gastric cancer in pernicious anaemia. *Lancet*, 1:521–523.
25. Siurala, M., Varis, K., and Wiljasalo, M. (1966): Studies of patients with atrophic gastritis; a 10–15 years follow-up. *Scand. J. Gastroenterol.*, 1:40–48.
26. Strickland, R. G., and MacKay, I. R. (1973): A reappraisal of the nature and significance of chronic atrophic gastritis. *Am. J. Dig. Dis.*, 18:426–440.
27. Varis, K. (1971): A family study of chronic gastritis; histological, immunological, and functional aspects. *Scand. J. Gastroenterol. (Suppl.)*, 6(13):36–41.
28. Varis, K., Ihamäki, T., Härkönen, M., Samloff, I. M., and Siurala, M. (1979): Gastric morphology, function and immunology in first-degree relatives of probands with pernicious anemia and controls. *Scand. J. Gastroenterol.*, 14:129–139.
29. Varis, K., and Isokoski, M. (1981): Screening of type A gastritis. *Ann. Clin. Res.*, 13:133–138.
30. Varis, K., Samloff, I. M., Ihamäki, T., and Siurala, M. (1979): An appraisal of tests for severe atrophic gastritis in relatives of patients with pernicious anemia. *Am. J. Dig. Dis.*, 23:187–191.
31. Varis, K., Samloff, I. M., Tiilikainen, A., Ihamäki, T., Kekki, M., Sipponen, P., and Siurala, M. (1980): Gastritis in first-degree relatives of pernicious anemia, gastric cancer patients and controls. In: *The Genetics and Heterogeneity of Common Gastrointestinal Diseases*, edited by J. I. Rotter, I. M. Samloff, and D. L. Rimoin, pp. 171–191. Academic Press, New York.
32. Varis, K., and Siurala, M. (1981): Genetics of gastric diseases. In: *Stomach in Health and Disease*, edited by W. Domschke, and K. Wormsley, pp. 94–102. Thieme Publishers, Stuttgart.
33. Varis, K., Stenman, U.-H., Lehtola, J., and Siurala, M. (1978): Gastric lesion and pernicious anaemia: a family study. *Acta Hepatogastroenterol.*, 25:62–67.
34. Zamcheck, N., Grable, E., Ley, A., and Norman, L. (1955): Occurrence of gastric cancer among patients with pernicious anemia at the Boston City Hospital. *N. Engl. J. Med.*, 252:1103–1110.

Precancerous Lesions of the Gastrointestinal Tract, edited by P. Sherlock, B. C. Morson, L. Barbara, and U. Veronesi. Raven Press, New York © 1983.

Markers of Cancer Risk and Surveillance of the Gastric Stump

J. Myren

Department of Gastroenterology, Department of Medicine 9, Ullevål Hospital, Oslo 1, Norway

In 1922 Balfour (2) directed attention to factors that may influence the life expectancy of patients operated on for benign gastric ulcers. He observed that out of 130 patients with partial gastrectomies, 3% died subsequently from gastric cancer. Since then numerous reports have dealt with the following problems: *What are the risk and markers of cancer of the gastric stump? How shall patients with gastric stumps be followed in order to detect the markers or premalignancies?*

Most authors have tried to give answers to these problems by retrospective studies of series of patients operated on with partial gastrectomy for mortality from gastric stump carcinoma, or by analysing patients with stump carcinomas following a primary operation for a benign gastric disease. To avoid errors in diagnosis of the primary benign lesion, only malignancies occurring later than 5 years post-operatively have been considered as primary cancer of the gastric stump (1,10,12,14,16,19,20,21,22,27,28,35,37,41,47,48).

In these studies (Table 1) great variations (1.9–17%) have been observed in the frequency of carcinomas of the gastric stump. In some studies the observed occurrence has been

TABLE 1. *Occurrence of gastric stump carcinoma*

Ref.	No. of pat.	No. of carcinoma	%	In relation to expected
16; mortality tracing	222	11	5.0	3.38[a]
22; mortality	361	25	7.7	11.3
27; mortality	616	9	9.6	
45; autopsy, matched	630	55	8.7	3.0[a]
7; clinical + endoscopy with biopsy	214	6	2.8	
43; gastroscopy + biopsies	108	4	3.7	
10; endoscopy + biopsies	111	2	0.8	
39; endoscopy + biopsy	117	1	0.9	
5; mortality	517	16	3.1	1.9[a]
17; autopsy	371	30	8.2	5.4[a]
3; selected	250	35	17	
1; uncertain	234	5	1.9	

[a] = $p < 0.01$.

TABLE 2. *Clinical symptoms in patients with gastric stump carcinoma*

Ref.	No. of pat.	Years after operation	Abdom. pain	Anorexia, weight loss	Bleeding, anemia
16	11	19	dyspepsia last year in all cases		
24	23	14	symptoms in all cases		
40	18	19		79	37
8	310	20	24	75	16
30	18	25	22	39	56
12	26	?	76	92	4
36	46		62	86	17
47	36	28	56	78	25
49	35	21	90	80	

compared to that expected for the same sex and age group estimated from official death certificates. Most authors conclude with a higher risk for cancer in the gastric remnant than in the not-operated stomach. The majority are found in the stoma, with some being observed in the proximal part of the gastric remnant (31). The authors further agree that the malignancies are detected at an average of about 20 years after the primary operation (Table 2), rarely before 10 years have elapsed (1,3,5–7,10,12,14–17,22,23,27,39,43,45,47,48). According to the studies performed before the introduction of fiberoptic endoscopy, a majority of the patients with stump carcinoma got symptoms of dyspepsia (Table 2), anorexia with loss in body weight, anemia, and blood in stool after a period of well-being following the gastric surgery (6–8,16,23,36).

The conclusion from these retrospective studies based on mortality and autopsy statistics was that patients subjected to partial gastric resection, particularly when a Billroth II anastomosis had been performed, should be reexamined at regular intervals for detection of new symptoms, occult bleeding, anemia, and changes demonstrable by roentgenological tech-

TABLE 3. *Results of surgical treatment in patients with carcinoma of the gastric stump*

Ref.	No. of cases	Gastrectomy	Survival (years)				No. of early carcinoma
			−1	−2	−3	−5 more	
35	18	6	2	2			
24	23	2	0				
23	29	14	primary mortality			10	
18	102	42	6	8		2	
40	18	14	1	1	1	3	
30	18	12	4	2	1	1	
33	28	11		1		1 (died)	
12	27	11				5	
47	31	17				1	
29	39	18	7	2		1	
42	35	10	3			1	
42	36	17	9	living, time not given			4
46	7	5		1	4		4

TABLE 4. *The occurrence of gastritis in the gastric stump*

Ref.	% Cases with		No. of cases
	A.G.	+ I.M.	
21; gastroscopy + biopsy			
Gastric resection	44	28	25
Gastric ulcer	35	21	109
Duodenal ulcer	32	8	37
Controls	22	28	249
26			
BII	57	41	70
BI	92	3	35
Duodenal ulcer	3	1	100
7; gastroscopy + biopsy	84	33	188
6; gastroscopy 1976	96	40	74
10	51	54	106

A.G., atrophic gastritis; I.M., intestinal metaplasia.

niques. It seemed rational to start such a follow-up after about 10 years after the primary surgery. However, the result of treatment by surgical intervention for these mostly advanced carcinomas was poor because of a low resectability and rather high primary mortality among the advanced age of the patients. The 5-year survival varied between 5% and 10% of those treated radically (Table 3) (12,18,23,24,29,30,33,35,37,40,42,46).

During recent years the reliability of the reports based on retrospective studies of mortality statistics, autopsy, and clinical observations in selected series, has been doubted. More controlled studies have been performed, the aims of which were to show the "true" occurrence of malignancies in the gastric stumps, and a better way to detect the early stages providing an improvement of the surgical therapy. Some of these studies will be dealt with here and the opinions on surveillance discussed.

In a study performed by Stahlsberg and Taksdal (45), 630 cases with carcinoma of the gastric stump were examined post-mortem, and the results were compared to those of matched controls. It was found that patients with a previous gastric operation for benign ulcer had three times higher mortality from carcinoma than matched controls, both with respect to gastric and duodenal ulcer (Table 1). The average time lapse since operation was 26.4 years. The data indicated that until 15 years after operation, the risk of developing stomach cancer may be lower than in the general population. Thereafter, a steadily increased cancer risk appeared. The authors admit that a necropsy material may be biased by the patients selected for autopsy. However, on the basis of official statistics it is estimated that more than 80% of the cases were subjected to necropsy examination. The authors believe that the establishment of a gastrojejunostomy with resulting gastritis, increase in bacterial growth (9), and reflux of bile, and intestinal and pancreatic juices into the stomach, is the main contributing factor to the malignancies which were overrepresented in cases with gastroenterostomy and in those with gastroenterostomy plus partial gastrectomies.

According to the suggestions of this study, operative procedures for the treatment of peptic ulcer not using gastroenterostomy with or without partial gastrectomy should be preferred, as for example parietal cell vagotomy. Another possibility would be to improve the diagnostic abilities for detection of the earliest stages of malignancies. Such an approach has been performed by Domellöf et al. (6,7), who made a follow-up of 459 patients operated on for benign peptic ulcers between 1952 and 1956. Out of these cases 140 were dead at the follow-up in 1976, 60 of whom had an autopsy performed. In the other cases the official death certificates were registrated. An endoscopic follow-up was performed in 214 patients with histology on multiple biopsies.

Among the patients who had died, 3 carcinomas were detected, and among those subjected to endoscopy plus biopsy, 6 carcinomas were found, of which 2 were classified as early ones. One case with precancerous changes, 2 with tubular adenomas, and 20 with regenerative polyps were also found. The macroscopic and microscopic changes were most pronounced at the stoma, which showed the preferential site of the malignancies. The histological changes of atrophic gastritis, intestinal metaplasia, and cystic dilatations of the gastric glands were, however, similar in cases with and without the malignant changes, indicating that these alterations were poor markers on cancer developments. The authors stressed that all malignancies were found in men. Possible explanations might be differences in diet, abuse of tobacco and alcohol, and a sex-linked factor. They discussed also the role of biliary reflux as a cause of gastritis (Table 4), which has been suggested by several others to provide a disposition for malignant change (15,22,26,27,36,38,44).

A similar approach was followed by Schrumpf et al. (43), who reported on a follow-up of 421 patients operated on during the years 1950 to 1955 with a Billroth II partial gastrectomy for duodenal ulcer. Out of these cases 220 patients were still alive at the time of follow-up in 1976, but only 191 were living in the Oslo area, and were asked for a clinical reexamination with gastroscopy with at least 20 biopsies from the gastric remnant. A satisfying examination was performed in 108 cases.

The results of this study showed that one case (0.9%) had advanced carcinoma, 3 cases had early carcinoma (2.3%), and 3 had severe dysplasia or carcinoma in situ (2.3%). In the remaining 101 cases a nearly normal mucosa was observed histologically in 1, atrophic gastritis in 12, and intestinal metaplasia in 24. In addition atrophic gastritis without or with intestinal metaplasia in combination with mild dysplasia were found in 52 cases and with moderate dysplasia in 12.

It was pointed out by the authors that there was no correlation between the endoscopic findings and histological changes of dysplasia or malignancies. The patients had no symptoms that might indicate the early alterations of malignancy. The importance of obtaining at least 20 biopsies from each remnant of the stomach was stressed by the observation that only 10% of the biopsies from those with a malignancy showed a positive result. In the present series cytology did not add to the results obtained, but it is rational to obtain snare resections from suspicious lesions if biopsies do not show a positive result (34).

The present study showed, as did Domellöf et al.'s, a higher incidence of malignancies in the gastric stump than expected. In addition, the present series of cases had a higher incidence of dysplasia amounting to 62%, mostly of mild and moderate degrees. The significance of this finding is unknown. The occurrence of chronic gastritis was similar to that reported by several others (Table 4) (7,21,26). As observed by Gjeruldsen et al. (11,13), chronic gastritis is frequently found as early as 3 months after operation when compared to preoperative histology on biopsy specimens. This study observed a higher incidence of gastritis in patients subjected to a two-thirds partial gastrectomy compared to a one-third, suggesting that the degree of gastric resection may play a role.

The findings of Schrumpf et al. (43) indicated that the occurrence of dysplasia in the gastric remnant might be a marker for cancer development, thus being a guide to the frequency of follow-up. They also stressed the inability of clinical symptoms and observations as well as endoscopy to detect these premalignant markers and the early stages of malignancies. A similar view was also held by Ewert (10), who performed a follow-up of 569 patients operated on during the period 1950 to 1953 in the Stockholm area. Endoscopy with biopsy was performed in 111 cases. Chronic gastritis was observed in the majority of cases. Dysplasia was found in 6 patients (5.7%) of which one was considered severe. No case of carcinoma was found in the living patients, whereas in 130 of the 230 dead patients 3 cases of carcinoma were recorded.

An association between dysplasia and malignancies was strongly suggested by Hammar (15), who analysed the localization of precancerous changes and carcinoma after a previous gastric operation for a benign condition. In 65 cases reoperated 20 years after the first surgical intervention, he found that 9 had precancerous changes of atypia, probably representing moderate dysplasia, 22 had carcinoma *in situ*, or severe dysplasia, and 34 had infiltrating carcinoma. In 35 of these cases the preoperative specimens could be traced and did not show any changes suggesting premalignancies or malignancies.

The answer to the first question about the occurrence of carcinoma of the gastric stump and the markers thus may be the following: Malignancies of the gastric stump are more frequent than in unoperated stomachs. The reason for this statement may be changes connected with surgical intervention in function and histopathology. However, the preoperative changes of the gastric mucosa has to be considered to evaluate the follow-up of such patients, particularly those of dysplasia, which seems to be the most prominent histologically detectable marker. Thus, the development of carcinoma from epithelial dysplasia seems to be most important to know in order to establish a rational follow-up of patients.

In order to explore the significance of these histological markers further, Stokkeland et al. (46) performed a second follow-up study 3 years after the first one by Schrumpf et al. (43).

The reexamination was performed as reported in the previous study. Since then 7 patients had died, but none from carcinoma of the gastric stump. A satisfactory endoscopy with at least 20 biopsies was obtained in 58 cases. In addition, the outcome of the 7 patients with malignant lesions detected at the first follow-up was recorded. At the second follow-up the authors could not demonstrate any malignancy or severe dysplasia. It was also encouraging that 4 of the 7 patients with malignancies or severe dysplasia were still alive at the second follow-up. Three of these had been operated on for early carcinoma, and the fourth for severe dysplasia. One of the patients who had advanced carcinoma died 1 year after gastrectomy. Out of 2 with severe dysplasia but not operated on, 1 died with metastases.

The authors conclude that no progression of dysplasia had occurred during the observation time of 3 years in the present cases. Although the reproducibility of the bioptical method used may vary considerably, the findings suggested that a follow-up of patients with mild or moderate dysplasia should be performed every 3 to 5 years, including gastroscopy with at least 20 biopsies from the gastric remnant. However, prospective studies of follow-up of dysplasia are needed before the final conclusion of the follow-up procedures can be decided correctly.

The answer to the question of dysplasia in the not–operated stomach before surgical intervention for a benign lesion seems to be little known. Meister et al. (28) examined surgical specimens from patients operated on for peptic ulcer ($n = 18$) and early and advanced carcinoma ($n = 31$). In patients with benign peptic ulcers mild dysplasia was observed in about 60% of the cases compared with 95% in patients with malignancies. Moderate dysplasia was detected in 40% and 93% and severe dysplasia in 10% and 60%, respectively. The unexpected high incidence of severe dysplasia in benign peptic ulcer disease needs further exploration.

The occurrence of dysplasia in patients with chronic gastritis was studied by Myren and Serck-Hanssen (32) in a retrospective series of 108 patients (36 women) at Ullevål Hospital. The examinations were performed consecutively in patients subjected to gastroscopy with multiple biopsies. At the same time they were asked for clinical symptoms and previous occurrence of peptic ulcer. The results showed that 14 of the patients had dysplasia of the glands, 11 mild and 3 moderate (13%). The age and symptomatology did not differ from that of patients with gastritis. The occurrence of dysplasia was slightly less in patients with previous peptic ulcer history and slightly higher in the canalis than in the body of the stomach. A larger series of patients should be studied prospectively in order to obtain conclusive results (Tables 5–8).

TABLE 5. *Epithelial dysplasia and gastritis in the not-operated stomach*

Histological diagnosis[a]	No. of patients	Age (years)	Sympt. (years)
A.G.			
(M)	20	54	6
(F)	18	63	7
A.G. + I.M.			
(M)	21	67	7
(F)	35	70	6
Dysplasia			
(M)	11	62	6
(F)	3		
Total	108	68	6.2

[a]M, male; F, female; A.G., atrophic gastritis; I.M., intestinal metaplasia.

TABLE 6. *Epithelial dysplasia and gastritis in the not-operated stomach—clinical observations*

Histological diagnosis	% with dyspepsia	Previous ulcer
A.G.	81	21
A.G. + I.M.	66	32
Dysplasia	64	43

A.G., atrophic gastritis; I.M., intestinal metaplasia.

TABLE 7. *Epithelial dysplasia and gastritis in the not-operated stomach—gastroscopical observations*

Histological diagnosis	N	Sg	A.G. antrum	Body	Other
A.G.	10	5	29	42	14
A.G. + I.M.		5	27	48	20
Dysplasia	7	7	28	36	22

N, normal; Sg, superficial gastritis; A.G., atrophic gastritis; I.M., intestinal metaplasia.

TABLE 8. *Epithelial dysplasia and gastritis in the not-operated stomach*

Histological diagnosis	% Changes in Antrum	Body
A.G.	61	39
A.G. + I.M.	36	64
Dysplasia	64	36

A.G., atrophic gastritis; I.M., intestinal metaplasia.

CONCLUSIONS

The conclusions from the present review may be summarized:

1. Patients operated on for benign gastric lesions (gastric stumps) represent a high-risk group for cancer of the gastric remnant.
2. The most promising premalignant marker seems to be glandular dysplasia, particularly that of severe grade.
3. Patients with severe dysplasia need close supervision for a malignant disease.
4. Patients with mild to moderate dysplasia should be reexamined every 3 to 5 years with gastroscopy and at least 20 biopsies. Future research must determine the exact routine for follow-up.
5. Patients without symptoms or dysplasia but with chronic gastritis should be followed with clinical examination, including gastroscopy with multiple biopsies, every 5 years.
6. Reoperation should be considered in relation to operative risk and stage of malignancy.

REFERENCES

1. Bähr, R., Röhrle-Lehmann, S., and Geisbe, H. (1980): Statische Untersuchungen zur Ätiologie des Magenstumpfkarzinoms. *Med. Welt.*, 31:123–127.
2. Balfour, D. C. (1922): Factors influencing the life expectancy of patients operated on for gastric ulcer. *Ann. Surg.*, 76:405–408.

3. Bosseckert, von H., and Kreibich, U. (1980): Magenstumpfkarzinom bei Routinegastroskopien. *Dtsch. Z. Verdau. Stoffwechselkr.*, 40:63–70.
4. Cardenas, F., and Coffey, R. J. (1964): Clinical features of first carcinoma of the gastric stump following gastric resection for benign peptic ulcer. *Am. J. Gastroenterol.*, 42:77–83.
5. Cheli, R., Molinary, F., Santi, L., Ciancamerla, G., and Puntoni, R. (1978): Gastric stump cancer: Statistical evaluation. *Rendic. Gastroenterol.*, 9:169–172.
6. Domellöf, L., Eriksson, S., and Janunger, K.-G. (1976): Late precancerous changes and carcinoma of the gastric stump after Billroth I resection. *Ann. J. Surg.*, 132:26–31.
7. Domellöf, L., Eriksson, S., and Janunger, K.-G. (1977): Carcinoma and possible precancerous changes of the gastric stump after Billroth II resection. *Gastroenterology*, 73:462–468.
8. Dony, A., Witte, Cl. de, Serste, J.-P., and Deschreyer, M. (1973): Le cancer du moignon gastrique aprés gastrectomie pour ulcere. *Acta Gastroenterol. Belgica*, 36:544–560.
9. Enander, L. K., Nilsson, F., Rydén, A.-C., and Schwan, A. (1979): Bacteriology of the gastric remnant. *Acta Chir. Scand. (Suppl.)*, 493:15.
10. Ewerth, S. (1978): The incidence of carcinoma in the gastric remnant after resection for benign ulcer disease. *Acta Chir. Scand. (Suppl.)*, 482:2–5.
11. Fretheim, B., Myren, J., and Gjeruldsen, S. T. (1966): Clinical findings before and after a graded gastrectomy for duodenal ulcer. *Scand. J. Gastroenterol.*, 1:188–198.
12. Gazzola, L. M., and Saegesser, F. (1975): Cancer of the gastric stump following operations for benign gastric or duodenal ulcers. *J. Surg. Oncol.*, 7:293–298.
13. Gjeruldsen, S., Myren, J., and Fretheim, B. (1968): Alterations of gastric mucosa following a graded partial gastrectomy for duodenal ulcer. *Scand. J. Gastroenterol.*, 3:465–470.
14. Griesser, G., and Schmidt, H. (1964): Statische Erhebungen über die Häufigkeit des Karzinoms nach Magenoperation wegen eines Geschwürsleidens. *Med. Welt.*, 35:1836–1840.
15. Hammar, E. (1976): The localization of precancerous changes and carcinoma after previous gastric operation for benign condition. *Acta Pathol. Microbiol. Scand.*, 84:495–507.
16. Helsingen, N., and Hillestad, L. (1956): Cancer development in the gastric stump after partial gastrectomy for ulcer. *Ann. Surg.*, 143:173 179.
17. Hilbe, G., Salzer, G. M., Hussl, H., and Kutschera, H. (1968): Die Carcinomgefährdung des Resektionsmagens. *Langenbecks Arch. Klin. Chir.*, 323:142–153.
18. Huber, P., Hilbe, G., and Bösmüller-Linz, H. (1969): Die Prognose des Magenstumpfcarcinoms. *Langenbecks Arch. Klin. Chir.*, 325:461–466.
19. Ito, S., Murakami, T., Tanaka, M., Kishi, S., and Akagi, G. (1976): Early cancer of the type IIa developed in the remnant stomach. *Stomach and Intestine*, 11:449–453.
20. Klarfeld, J., and Resnick, G. (1979): Gastric remnant carcinoma. *Cancer*, 44:1129–1133.
21. Kobayashi, S., Prolla, J. C., and Kirsner, J. B. (1970): Late gastric carcinoma developing after surgery for benign conditions. *Am. J. Dig. Dis.*, 15:905–912.
22. Krause, U. (1958): Late prognosis after partial gastrectomy for ulcer. *Acta Chir. Scand.*, 114:341–354.
23. Kronberger, L., and Hafner, H. (1968): Über das "primäre Stumpfcarcinom" nach Ulcusresektion. *Chirurg*, 39:118–122.
24. Kuss, A. B., and Bartsch, W. M. (1964): Das Karzinom im Restmagen. *Med. Klinik*, 59:1413–1417.
25. Langhans, P., Heger, R. A., Hohenstein, J., and Bünte, H. (1981): Gastric stump carcinoma—New aspects deduced from experimental results. *Scand. J. Gastroenterol. (Suppl.)*, 16(67):161–164.
26. Lazzlo, S., Figus, A. I., and Bajtai, A. (1973): Chronic gastritis following resection of the stomach. *Am. J. Gastroenterol.*, 60:477–487.
27. Liavaag, K. (1962): Cancer development in gastric stump after partial gastrectomy for peptic ulcer. *Ann. Surg.*, 155:103–106.
28. Meister, H., Holubarsch, Ch., Haferkamp, O., Schlag, P., and Herfarth, Ch. (1979): Gastritis, intestinal metaplasia and dysplasia versus benign ulcer in stomach and duodenum and gastric carcinoma. A histotopographical study. *Path. Res. Pract.*, 164:259–269.
29. Meyer, H.-J., Ziegler, H., and Pichlmayr, R. (1979): Problems associated with the surgical treatment of cancer of the gastric stump. Gastr. cancer. Herforth, C. H., and Schlag, P. Springer-Verlag, Berlin.
30. Morgenstern, L., Yamakawa, T., and Seltzer, D. (1973): Carcinoma of the gastric stump. *Am. J. Surg.*, 125:29–38.
31. Morson, B. C., Sobin, L. H., Grundman, E., Johansen, A., Nagayo, T., and Serck-Hanssen, A. (1980): Precancerous conditions and epithelial dysplasia in the stomach. *J. Clin. Pathol.*, 33:711–721.
32. Myren, J., and Serck-Hanssen, A. (1981): Gastritis and epithelial dysplasia seen from a clinical point of view. In: *Diseases of the Upper Gastrointestinal Tract*, Hässle Symposium, edited by B. Arnesjö and A. Skarstein.
33. Nichols, J. C. (1974): Carcinoma of the stomach following partial gastrectomy for benign gastroduodenal lesions. *Br. J. Surg.*, 61:244–249.
34. Osnes, M., Løtveit, T., Myren, J., and Serck-Hanssen, A. (1977): Early gastric cancer in patients with a Billroth II partial resection. *Endoscopy*, 9:45–49.

35. Pack, G. T., and Banner, R. L. (1958): The late development of gastric cancer after gastroenterostomy and gastrectomy for peptic ulcer and benign pyloric stenosis. *Surgery*, 44:1024–1033.

36. Peitsch, W., and Burkhardt, K. (1976): Zur Pathogenese und Klinik des Magenstumpfcarcinoms. *Lagenbecks Arch. Chir.*, 341:195–203.

37. Rehner, M., Soehendra, N., Eichfuzz, H. P., Dahm, K., Eckert, P., and Mitschke, H. (1974): Frühcarzinome im (Billroth-II-) Resektionsmagen. *Dtsch. med. Wschr.*, 99:533–534.

38. Reynolds, K. W., Johnson, A. G., and Fox, B. (1975): Is intestinal metaplasia of the gastric mucosa a premalignant lesion? *Clin. Oncol.*, I:101–109.

39. Rösch, W., and Prütling, E. (1978): Das Karzinom im operierten Magen. *Klinik Art.*, 7:386–390.

40. Saegesser, F., and Jämes, D. (1972): Cancer of the gastric stump after partial gastrectomy (Billroth II principle) for ulcer. *Cancer*, 29:1150–1159.

41. Schmid, von E. (1979): Magenstumpfkarzinom. *Krebsgeschehen*, 11:110–112.

42. Schönleben, K., Langhans, P., Schlake, W., Kautz, G., and Bünte, H. (1979): Gastric stump carcinoma —Carcinogenic factors and possible preventive measures. *Acta Hepatogastroenterol.*, 26:239–247.

43. Schrumpf, E., Serck-Hanssen, A., Stadaas, J., Aune, S., Myren, J., and Osnes, M. (1977): Mucosal changes in the gastric stump 20-25 years after partial gastrectomy. *Lancet*, II:467–469.

44. Siurala, M., Varis, K., and Wiljasalo, M. (1966): Studies of patients with atrophic gastritis: a 10–15 years follow-up. *Scand. J. Gastroenterol.*, 1:40–48.

45. Stalsberg, H., and Taksdal, S. (1971): Stomach cancer following gastric surgery for benign conditions. *Lancet*, II:1175–1177.

46. Stokkeland, M., Schrumpf, E., Serck-Hanssen, A., Myren, J., Osnes, M., and Stadaas, J. (1981): Incidence of malignancies of the Billroth II operated stomach. *Scand. J. Gastroenterol. (Suppl.)*, 16(67):169–171.

47. Terjesen, T., and Erichsen, H. G. (1976): Carcinoma of the gastric stump after operation for benign gastroduodenal ulcer. *Acta Chir. Scand.*, 142:256–260.

48. Wanzjan, von E. N., Astrozhnikov, Y. V., and Tschernousov, A. F. (1977): Stumpfkarzinom nach Magenresektion wegen Ulkuskrankheit und adenomatöser Polypen. *Zbl. Chirurgie*, 102:1358–1364.

49. Wolf, O., Pannenborg, G., and Voigtsberger, P. (1977): Über das primäre Magenstumpfkarzinom. *Zbl. Chirurgie*, 102:1183–1187.

Precancerous Lesions of the Gastrointestinal Tract, edited by P. Sherlock, B.C. Morson, L. Barbara, and U. Veronesi. Raven Press, New York © 1983.

Precancerous Conditions of the Small Intestine

Henry Thompson

University of Birmingham, General Hospital Birmingham, Birmingham B4 6NH, United Kingdom

Precancerous and prelymphomatous conditions of the small intestine have been recognised in recent years following clinical and pathological research into specific disease entities. The conditions are listed in Table 1.

Precancerous lesions of the small intestine are fewer in number and are listed in Table 2. These will be discussed in relation to each disease entity.

ADULT COELIAC DISEASE

This is a disease of chronic ill health that is associated with the malabsorption syndrome and steatorrhoea. Iron deficiency anaemia or folic acid deficiency anaemia may be the first indication of this disorder. A proportion of patients develop osteomalacia or neuropathy.

The diagnosis is established by jejunal biopsy procedure, dissecting microscopy and histology (30). The mucosa in untreated adult coeliac disease is flat (Fig. 1) or convoluted with or without a mosaic pattern. The biopsy also shows total, subtotal (Fig. 2), or partial villous atrophy. Additional histological features include cuboidal surface epithelium (Figs. 3 and 4), increased numbers of lymphocytes in the surface epithelium, crypt hyperplasia, increased numbers of lymphocytes and plasma cells in the lamina propria, and, in approximately one-third of the cases, a narrow zone of subepithelial hyalin that stains as collagen. Morphometric studies (9,10,15,20,33), such as cell counts and determination of crypt villous ratio, confirm the diagnosis.

Patients with coeliac disease are sensitive to gluten, which in some peculiar way damages the mucosa of the jejunum with cell loss leading to a more rapid turnover of cells in the enterocyte escalator system, that is, crypt hyperplasia. Treatment with a gluten-free diet leads to marked improvement in their clinical state and to a gradual restoration of normal villous architecture. It is essential that there should be strict adherence to a rigid gluten-free

TABLE 1. *Small intestine precancerous conditions*
Adult coeliac disease
Alpha chain disease
Crohn's disease
Polyps papillomata
Clinical syndromes

TABLE 2. *Small intestine premalignant lesions*
Dysplasia
Adenoma
Malignant histiocytosis
Ulceration?
Lymphomatous polyposis

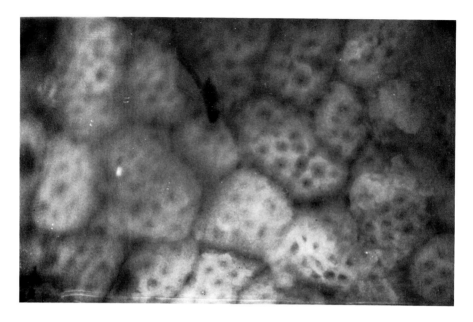

FIG. 1.   Flat mosaic jejunal biopsy from patient with adult coeliac disease. Dissecting microscopy.

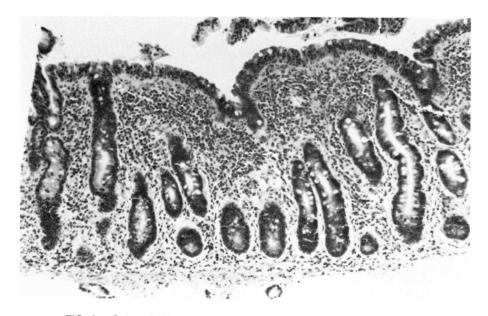

FIG. 2.   Subtotal villous atrophy in untreated adult coeliac disease.

diet for the rest of the patient's life if the malabsorption syndrome is to be cured. Failure to do so will lead to relapse or to chronic ill health. Occasionally a patient will fail to respond to the gluten-free diet and will require treatment with steroids or milk-free diet. Some patients

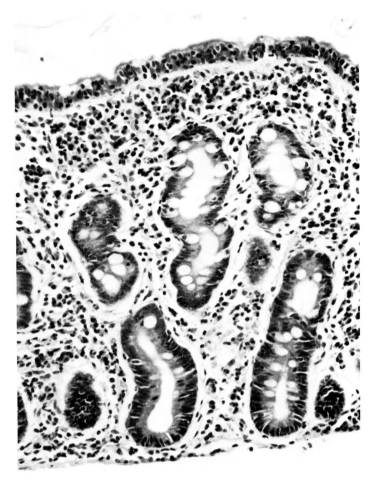

FIG. 3. Crypt hyperplasia in untreated adult coeliac disease. Surface epithelium is abnormal and there is an excess of plasma cells in the lamina propria.

will only respond after treatment of complications. Clinical and villous response to a gluten-free diet is a desirable aspect of our concept of adult coeliac disease, but it is not essential, since resistant cases are occasionally encountered.

In 1962 Gough et al. (12) described 3 cases of lymphoma complicating the course of adult coeliac disease. These cases were originally identified as reticulosarcoma and then (1967) as Hodgkin's disease (2). Harris et al. (17), in a larger statistical study of 202 patients with adult coeliac disease and idiopathic steatorrhoea, encountered 31 cases of malignancy representing an incidence of 15%. There were 14 cases (7%) of malignant lymphoma and of these 10 were classified as reticulum cell sarcoma and 4 as Hodgkin's disease. The incidence of carcinoma principally of the gastrointestinal tract was 6.4%. In my 1976 paper on the extended Birmingham series, I classified the lymphoma as reticulum cell sarcoma, rejecting Hodgkin's disease except for 1 case, and found the necropsy incidence to be 42%. The total incidence of malignancy in the necropsy series including cancer was 58%. Isaacson and Wright (23) described the lymphoma complicating coeliac disease as malignant histio-

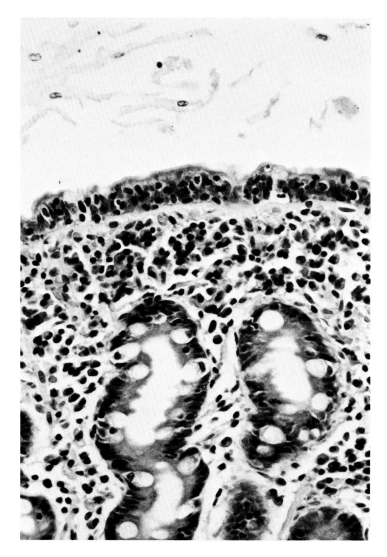

FIG. 4. Cellular cuboidal surface epithelium showing lymphocytic infiltration. Excess plasma cells are noted in the lamina propria.

cytosis, since the cells contained polyclonal immunoglobulin. Issacson and co-workers have since identified the cells as histiocytic on the basis of enzyme markers, namely, alpha 1 antitrypsin (22), acid phosphatase, nonspecific esterase, etc. (P. Isaacson, *personal communication*, 1981). The tumour cells may also show erythrophagocytosis. Immunoglobulin accumulation may be associated with a prominent plasmacytoid appearance of the tumour cells. Multinucleated cells resembling Reed-Sternberg cells are frequently present. Infiltration with eosinophils and fibrosis are occasional features. Reexamination of the Birmingham series confirms that the majority of cases represent malignant histiocytosis (Fig. 5) with a small incidence of other lymphomas.

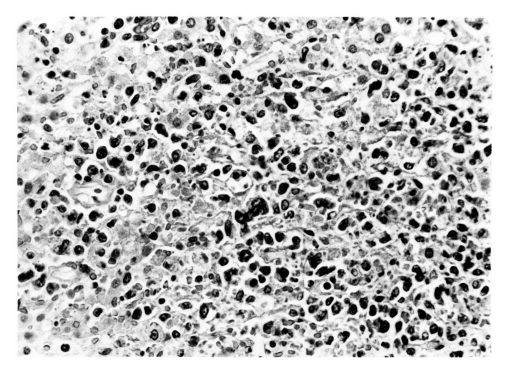

FIG. 5. Malignant histiocytosis complicating adult coeliac disease. The tumour cells gave positive α-1-antitrypsin result with the immunoperoxidase technique.

The Northwick Park M.R.C. study (34) has confirmed the Birmingham observations, showing an equal incidence of malignant lymphoma and carcinoma complicating coeliac disease. A few patients developed both lymphoma and carcinoma. Occasionally patients with dermatitis herpetiformis and coeliac disease succumbed to malignancy.

The majority of patients with malignant lymphoma deteriorated rapidly and died within 6 months to 2 years, despite surgical resection or chemotherapy. We have 2 long-term survivals. One patient with coeliac disease and Hashimoto's disease developed malignant lymphoma of the thyroid gland, which was treated by thyroidectomy and chemotherapy. He has survived 6 years. Another coeliac patient with Hodgkin's disease stage 1 localised to the neck was treated by excision biopsy and radiotherapy. He survived 26 years. A few months before his death, haemolytic anaemia appeared and at necropsy he was found to be harbouring foci of malignant lymphoma in lumbar vertebrae, although there was no evidence of tumour elsewhere in the body. The cytology of the vertebral lymphoma was totally different from the previous Hodgkin's disease and showed no Reed-Sternberg cells, although these had been a prominent feature in the original cervical lymph node biopsy.

Perforation of ulcerated lesions in the small intestine may be a presenting or complicating feature leading to generalised peritonitis or localised abscess. Careful examination of the perforated lesion reveals malignant lymphoma, but the correct diagnosis can be overlooked by the pathologist inexperienced in the study of gastrointestinal disease, who may erroneously attribute it to nonspecific ulceration.

Malignant histiocytosis, however, can exist as a precursor state with foci of neoplastic cells in intestine, liver, spleen, and bone marrow. These microscopic foci may ultimately develop into macroscopic tumour tissue and eventually progress rapidly as florid lymphoma. In this respect, there is some resemblance to mycosis fungoides in the premycotic stage.

It is probable that the cases of steatorrhoea lymphadenopathy described by Whitehead (38) correspond to malignant histiocytosis. Lymphoid hyperplasia or reticuloendothelial hyperplasia in itself is not a precursor of malignancy.

Liver biopsy may provide evidence of occult malignant histiocytosis in a coeliac patient and the disorder may remain clinically silent for a number of years. Nonspecific ulceration of the small intestine may be a feature of malignant histiocytosis and may precede lymphoma. We have studied 1 patient who had a resection for nonspecific ulceration of the small intestine followed by dramatic improvement in his clinical state. There was no clinical or histological evidence of malignant histiocytosis at this stage, even on later review by a panel of pathologists. He succumbed to malignant lymphoma 7 years later. A mortality rate of 75% from nonspecific ulceration of the small intestine is documented in the literature, but some of these cases probably represented unrecognised or undiagnosed malignant histiocytosis. There are certainly other causes of nonspecific ulceration, such as polyarteritis nodosa, enteric coated potassium tablets. We have a number of patients under observation who have had a resection for ulceration, but they still show no evidence of lymphoma.

Other types of lymphoma are occasionally encountered (e.g., Hodgkin's disease, histiocytic lymphoma, and unclassified lymphoma). One of our cases of lymphoma presented as mycosis fungoides d'emblee and another developed Raynaud's phenomenon and digital gangrene (fingers). It would be surprising if occasional cases of other types of lymphoma (e.g., B cell lymphoma) did not occur. We have also seen 1 case of myeloid leukaemia.

Carcinoma of the small intestine in coeliac disease was described by Brzechwa-Ajdukiewicz et al. (5) and there have also been 4 cases reported from Birmingham (21). Squamous carcinoma of the oesophagus was reported by Harris et al. (17) and others (39); cases have also appeared in our series. We have also encountered carcinoma of the stomach, second part of the duodenum, jejunum, colon, rectum, pharynx, palate, and tongue. Carcinoma outside the gastrointestinal system has been documented in the Birmingham and Northwick Park series.

The cause of malignancy in coeliac disease is still unknown, but loss of immune surveillance and viral oncogenesis are possible explanations. Lymphoreticular atrophy is fairly common in coeliac disease, but it is not always associated with malignancy.

ALPHA CHAIN DISEASE

This fascinating entity is a malabsorption disease in which plasma cell or lymphoplasmacytic proliferation (26,29,31,32,35,37) in the lamina propria proceeds to malignant lymphoma. It differs from coeliac disease in that the enterocyte population and villi appear normal in the early stages, although the mucosa may be relatively flat in the later stages of the disease. The plasma cells contain alpha heavy chain immunoglobulin, which can be identified in serum, urine, jejunal fluid, and saliva. Immunofluorescent and immunoperoxidase techniques demonstrate alpha chain immunoglobulin within the plasma cells, although not all cells give a positive reaction. The proliferation of plasma cells extends to involve the colon, rectum, stomach, nasopharyngeal tissues, lymph nodes, and bone marrow. Malignant lymphoma develops with extensive thickening of the bowel wall, ulceration, or multiple tumour masses. The mesenteric lymph nodes enlarge with tumour. The fully developed picture is comparable to that of Mediterranean lymphoma. The tumour is a B cell

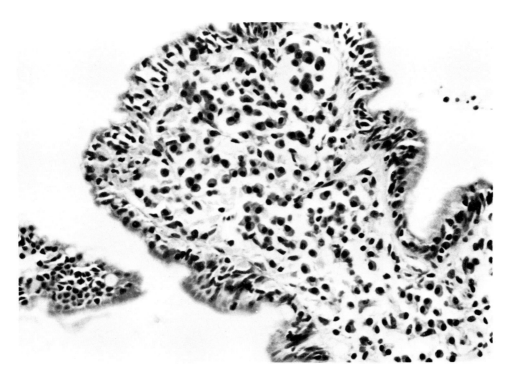

FIG. 6. Alpha chain disease confirmed by serum immunoglobulin studies.

lymphoma (19) or immunoblastic sarcoma (27), although it has originally been described as reticulum cell sarcoma or histiocytic lymphoma. Enzyme markers for histiocytic origin are absent.

The gastrointestinal phase of the disease that corresponds to immunocytic enteropathy without tumours may respond to antibiotic therapy. The later tumour phase requires chemotherapy to achieve a temporary remission. The aetiology of alpha chain disease has been related to parasitic disease and possible enteric infection. The diagnosis rests on identification of heavy chain alpha immunoglobulin in the serum by immunoselection technique (8) and confirmatory jejunal biopsy (Fig. 6).

The relationship between Mediterranean lymphoma and alpha chain disease is still controversial (7,11,25,28) and denied by some authors but accepted by others. The syndrome of chronic diarrhoea, abdominal pain, clubbing, and diffuse lymphoplasmacytic lymphoma (Fig. 7) of the upper small intestine may or may not be associated with alpha heavy chain production. This immunoglobulin can also be produced by North American intestinal polypoid lymphomas (6) and in a respiratory form. Gamma heavy chain disease (3) can also simulate alpha chain disease in its gastrointestinal phase.

Alpha chain production was demonstrated in two-thirds of a series of 145 malignant lymphomas of the small intestine in Iraq by Al-Saleem (1). In this series, patients with lymphoma were almost 8 years older than those with immunocytic enteropathy. Intracytoplasmic as well as intranuclear PAS positive inclusions have also been described in the proliferating cells.

The highest incidence of alpha chain disease is in the Middle East, Mediterranean littoral, Iraq, and Iran, but it has also been reported in South Africa, Pakistan, South America, the

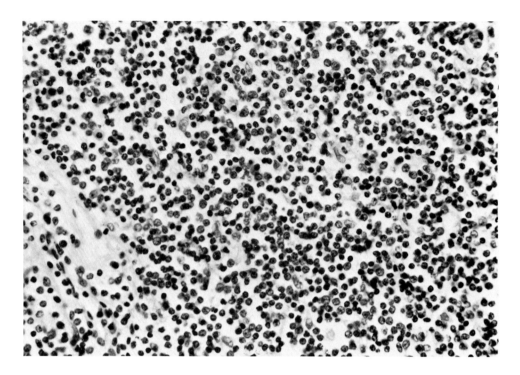

FIG. 7. Lymphocytic plasmacytic lymphoma complicating alpha chain disease.

Far East, and Nigeria. Occasionally cases occur in Britain, predominantly among the immigrant population.

CROHN'S DISEASE

Statistical studies (16) reveal a fourfold increased incidence of colorectal carcinoma (Fig. 8) in patients with Crohn's disease and a slightly increased incidence of carcinoma in the upper gastrointestinal tract. In this statistical study there was only 1 case of carcinoma of the small intestine.

During an 18-year period in the General Hospital, Birmingham, we have encountered 3 cases of carcinoma of the small intestine complicating Crohn's disease (18). Two were located in the ileum and 1 involved the jejunum. I have also encountered 2 further cases in other hospitals, making a total of 5 cases in one pathologist's experience of examining specimens of Crohn's disease. One of these other cases proved to be a small argentaffin carcinoma.

The carcinomas complicating Crohn's disease were diffusely infiltrating lesions (Figs. 9a,9b,10) and could not be seen by naked eye, with the exception of the youngest patient, age 24, who had obvious peritoneal seedlings and neoplastic enlargement of the mesenteric lymph nodes confirmed by frozen section. All patients had longstanding Crohn's disease and there was no clinical or pathological evidence of a primary tumour in any other organ. These tumours are easily overlooked and can only be detected by examining multiple blocks.

A total of 61 cases have been described in the literature, but it is difficult to carry out a proper statistical study, since carcinoma of the small intestine is a relatively rare tumour

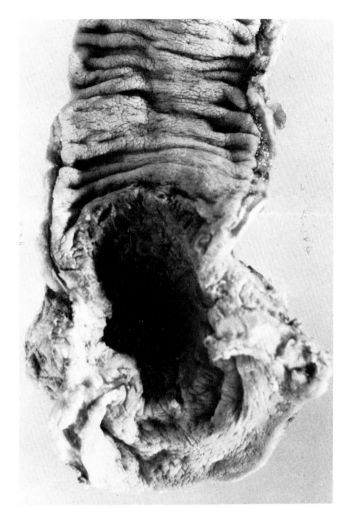

FIG. 8. Carcinoma of the rectum complicating Crohn's disease.

and the policy of surgical resection in the treatment of regional ileitis reduces the incidence of malignancy by removing the grossly diseased tissues. Greenstein et al. (13,14) reported a series of cases of carcinoma developing in the bypassed loop. We have not encountered this in Birmingham, since bypass surgery has long since been abandoned. Our experience of 3 cases in a single hospital, however, indicates that it is a genuine complication of Crohn's disease. An endometriosis-like pattern has been described in the literature and this was a feature in 3 of the 5 cases. Dysplasia has been observed in 12 cases in the literature and this was well developed in 1 of our cases and present as foci in the other 2. Dysplasia is occasionally encountered in regional ileitis with no evidence of carcinoma.

The histological features of dysplasia included nuclear pleomorphism hyperchromatism, mitoses, disorderly architecture, cytoplasmic basophilia, and loss of polarity of the cells.

We have also observed 3 cases of carcinoma developing in fistulae associated with Crohn's disease. The first was a rectovaginal fistula, the second a cystic remnant from a previous caecostomy, and the third arose from remnants of a fistula involving small intestine, rectum,

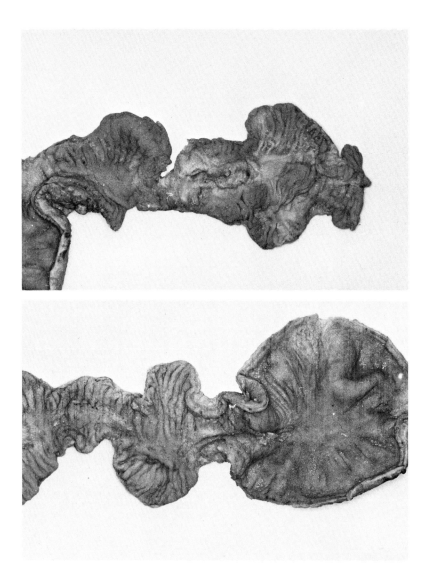

FIG. 9. Carcinoma of the small intestine *(top)* complicating regional ileitis *(bottom)*.

and vagina. These were all longstanding fistulae and it is probable that dysplastic epithelium extended into the fistula leading eventually to carcinoma.

Lymphoma of the small intestine has been reported as a rare association by Lee et al. (24). We have not encountered lymphoma in the small intestine, but there have been 2 cases involving the colon. There is, however, no statistical evidence of an increased incidence of malignant lymphoma in Crohn's disease or indeed in ulcerative colitis.

POLYPS AND PAPILLOMAS

Tubular Adenoma

Tubular adenoma, tubulo-villous, and villous adenoma are rare in the small intestine but are occasionally encountered in random autopsies. Dypslasia and carcinoma can supervene in the same way as colorectal and gastric polyps can become malignant.

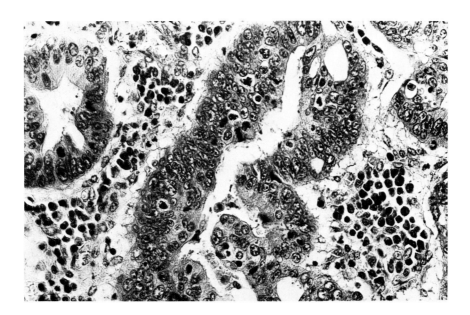

FIG. 10. Adenocarcinoma of small intestine complicating Crohn's disease.

The lesions can also occur in the periampullary second part of the duodenum, where progression to carcinoma is a likely consequence. The polyps frequently show argentaffin and Paneth cells and have to be differentiated from Peutz-Jeghers polyps.

Islet Cell Tumours of the Duodenum

These polypoid tumours, whether functioning or nonfunctioning, have a malignant potential. The argyrophil reaction is usually positive. These lesions are capable of producing various endocrine syndromes, for example, V.I.P. syndrome, and the cells belong to the amine precursor uptake and decarboxylisation (APUD) system.

Carcinoid Tumour

All carcinoid tumours of the small intestine behave as low-grade argentaffin carcinomas (Fig. 11). The cells give the argentaffin or argyrophil reaction (Fig. 12) and fine subnuclear eosinophiliac granules are often visible in hematoxylin-eosin (H.-E.) preparations. The tumours secrete 5-hydroxytryptamine, which can be detected in the urine. The carcinoid syndrome is associated with metastatic deposits in the liver. A scirrhous reaction is frequently present and this can lead to fibrous contracture of mesentery and fibroelastosis of the mesenteric vessels. Ischaemic lesion of the intestine can occur as a complication. Multiple carcinoid tumours can also occur in the small intestine.

Brookes et al. (4) reported a 41.9% 5-year survival figure and, for those treated with radical surgery, a 56.3% 5-year survival rate. Carcinoid tumours can also occur in Meckel's diverticulum and the clinical behaviour is comparable to that in the small intestine.

CLINICAL SYNDROMES

Carcinoma of the small intestine rarely develops in polyposis coli, multiple gastrointestinal cancer cases, Peutz-Jeghers syndrome, and juvenile polyposis coli. Malignant lymphoma rarely complicates multiple lymphomatous polyposis and immune deficiency syndromes.

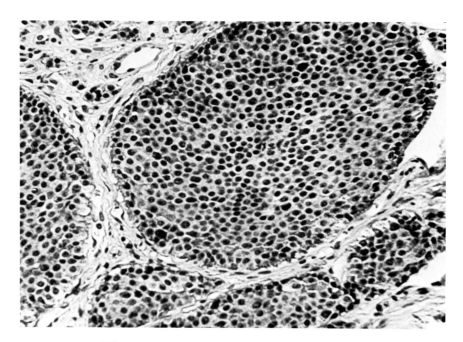

FIG. 11. Argentaffin carcinoma of small intestine.

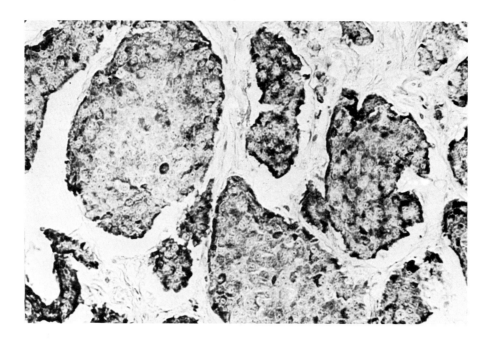

FIG. 12. Positive subnuclear argentaffin granules in argentaffin carcinoma stained by the Masson Fontana method.

One of our patients with multiple gastrointestinal cancers had a right hemicolectomy for carcinoma of the caecum and tubular adenomatous polyps in 1966, partial gastrectomy for ulcer cancer of the stomach in 1972, and at necropsy in 1973 was found to have carcinoma of the jejunum and polyps in the small intestine. The morphology of the cancers in each site was different and the carcinoma of the jejunum showed evidence of Paneth cell differentiation in some areas. Dysplasia was noted in the polyps and also in the mucosa adjacent to the carcinoma of the jejunum. The aetiology of such cases is not clear, but search for chromosomal break abnormalities should be considered.

Malignant tumours in the small intestine should always raise a strong suspicion of a precursor state, but it may be difficult to obtain sufficient evidence in individual cases.

CONCLUSIONS

1. Adult coeliac disease, alpha chain disease, and Crohn's disease represent precancerous conditions of the small intestine.
2. Precancerous lesions include dysplasia, adenoma, and malignant histiocytosis.
3. Carcinoma and lymphoma may also complicate rare clinical syndromes.

REFERENCES

1. Al-Saleem, T., and Zardani, I. M. (1979): Primary lymphomas of the small intestine in Iraq: a pathological study of 145 cases. *Histopathology*, 3:89–106.
2. Austad, W. I., Cornes, J. C., Gough, K. R., McCarthy, C. F., and Read, A. E. (1967): Steatorrhoea and malignant lymphoma. The relationship of malignant tumours of lymphoid tissue and coeliac disease. *Am. J. Dig. Dis.*, 12:475–490.
3. Bender, S. W., Danon, F., Preudhomme, J. L., Posselt, H. G., Roettger, P., and Seligman, M. (1978): Gamma heavy chain disease simulating alpha chain disease. *Gut*, 19:1148–1152.
4. Brookes, V. S., Waterhouse, J. A. H., and Powell, D. J. (1968): Malignant lesions of the small intestine. *Br. J. Surg.*, 55:405.
5. Brzechwa-Ajdukiewicz, A., McCarthy, C. F., Austad, N. I., Cornes, J. C., Harrison, N. J., and Read, A. (1966): Carcinoma, villous atrophy and steatorrhoea. *Gut*, 7:572–577.
6. Cohen, J. H., Gonzalvo, A., Krook, J., Thompson, T. T., and Kremer, W. B. (1978): New presentation of alpha chain disease: North American polypoid gastro-intestinal lymphoma. *Cancer*, 41:1161–1169.
7. Doe, W. F. (1975): Alpha chain disease—clinicopathological features and relationship to so-called Mediterranean lymphoma. *Br. J. Cancer (Suppl.)*, 31(11):350–355.
8. Doe, W. F., Henry, K., Hobbs, J. R., Jones, F. A., Dent C. E., and Booth, C. C. (1972): Five cases of alpha chain disease. *Gut*, 13:947.
9. Dunhill, M. S., and Whitehead, R. (1972): A method for the quantitation of small intestinal biopsy specimens. *J. Clin. Pathol.*, 25:243–246.
10. Ferguson, A., and Murray, D. (1971): Quantitation of intraepithelial lymphocytes in human jejunum. *Gut*, 12:988–994.
11. Gallian, A., Lecestre, M. J., Scotto, J., Bognel, C., Matuchansky, C., and Rambaud, J. C. (1976): Pathological study of alpha chain disease with special emphasis on evolution. *Cancer*, 39:201–210.
12. Gough, K. R., Read, A. E., and Naish, J. M. (1962): Intestinal reticulosis as a complication of idiopathic steatorrhoea. *Gut*, 3:232–239.
13. Greenstein, A. J., Sachar, D., and Pucillo, A. (1978): Cancer in Crohn's disease after diversionary surgery. *Am. J. Surg.*, 135:86–90.
14. Greenstein, A. J., Sachar, D. B., and Smith, H. (1980): Patterns of neoplasia in Crohn's disease and ulcerative colitis. *Cancer*, 46:403–407.
15. Guix, M., Skinner, J. M., and Whitehead, R. (1979): Measuring intraepithelial lymphocytes, surface area and volume of lamina propria in the jejunal mucosa of coeliac patients. *Gut*, 20:275–278.
16. Gyde, S. N., Prior, P., Macartney, J. C., Thompson, H., Waterhouse, J. A. H., and Allan, R. N. (1980): Malignant in Crohn's disease. *Gut*, 21:1024–1029.
17. Harris, O. D., Cooke, W. T., Thompson, H., and Waterhouse, J. A. H. (1967): Malignancy in adult coeliac disease and idiopathic steatorrhoea. *Am. J. Med.*, 42:899–912.

18. Hawker, P., Gyde, S. N., Thompson, H., and Allan, R. N. (1982): Carcinoma of the small intestine complicating Crohn's disease. *Gut*, 23:188–193.
19. Henry, K., and Farrer-Brown, G. (1977): Primary lymphomas of the gastrointestinal tract. 1. Plasma cell tumours. *Histopathology*, 1:53–76.
20. Holmes, G. K. T., Asquith, P., Stockes, P. J., and Cooke, W. T. (1973): Cellular infiltrate of jejunal biopsies in adult coeliac disease (A.C.D.) in relation to gluten withdrawal. *Gut*, 14:429.
21. Holmes, G. K. T., Dunn, G. I., Cockel R., and Brookes, V. S. (1980): Adenocarcinoma of the upper small bowel complicating Coeliac disease. *Gut*, 21:1010–1016.
22. Isaacson, P., Jones, D. B., Millward-Sadler, G. H., Judd, M. A., and Payne, S. (1981): Alpha-1-antitrypsin in human macrophages. *J. Clin. Pathol.*, 34:982–990.
23. Isaacson, P., and Wright, D. H. (1978): Intestinal lymphoma associated with malabsorption. *Lancet*, 1:67–70.
24. Lee, G. B., Smith, P. M., and Seal, R. M. E. (1977): Lymphosarcoma in Crohn's disease. *Dis. Colon Rectum*, 20:351–354.
25. Lewin, K. J., Kahn, L. B., and Novis, B. H. (1976): Primary intestinal lymphoma of "Western" and "Mediterranean" type alpha chain disease and massive plasma cell infiltration. *Cancer*, 38:2511–2528.
26. Morson, B. C., and Dawson, I. M. P. (1979): *Gastro-intestinal Pathology*, p. 414. Blackwell Scientific Publications. Oxford, London.
27. Nassar, V. H., Salem, P. A., Shahid, M. J., Alami, S. Y., Balikian, J. B., Salem, A. A., and Nasrallah, S. M. (1978): Mediterranean abdominal lymphoma or immunoproliferative small intestinal disease. *Cancer*, 41:1346–1354.
28. Rambaud, J. C., and Matuchansky, C. (1973): Alpha chain disease; pathogenesis and relation to Mediterranean lymphoma. *Lancet*, 1:1430–1432.
29. Rappaport, H., Ramot, B., Hulu, N., and Park, J. K. (1972): The pathology of so-called Mediterranean abdominal lymphoma with malabsorption. *Cancer*, 29:1509.
30. Rubin, C. E., Brandborg, L. L., Phelps, P. C., and Taylor, Jr., H. C. (1960): Studies of coeliac disease. 1. The apparent identical and specific nature of the duodenal and proximal jejunal lesion in coeliac disease and idiopathic steatorrhoea. *Gastroenterology*, 38:28–49.
31. Seligman, M. (1975): Alpha chain disease—immunoglobulin abnormalities, pathogenesis and current concepts. *Br. J. Cancer (Suppl.)*, 31(11):356.
32. Shahid, M. J., Alami, S. Y., Nasser, V. H., Balikian, J. B., and Salem, A. A. (1975): Primary intestinal lymphoma with paraproteinaema. *Cancer*, 35:848.
33. Shiner, M., and Doniach, I. (1960): Histopathologic studies in steatorrhoea. *Gastroenterology*, 38:419–440.
34. Swinson, C. M., Slavin, G., Coles, E. C., and Booth, C. C. (1981): Coeliac disease and malignancy. *Gut*, 22:A872.
35. Tabbane, S., Tabbane, F., Cammoun, M., and Mourali N. (1976): Mediterranean lymphoma with alpha heavy chain monoclonal gammopathy. *Cancer*, 38:1989–1996.
36. Thompson, H. (1976): Pathology of coeliac disease. In: *Current Topics in Pathology, Vol. 63: Pathology of the Gastrointestinal Tract*, edited by B. C. Morson, pp. 49–75. Springer Verlag, Berlin.
37. Whicker, J. T., Ajdukiewicz, A., and Davies, J. D. (1977): Two cases of alpha chain disease from Nigeria. *J. Clin. Pathol.*, 30:678.
38. Whitehead, R. (1968): Primary lymphadenopathy complicating idiopathic steatorrhea. *Gut*, 9:569–575.
39. Wright, J. T., and Richardson, P. C. (1967): Squamous carcinoma of the thoracic oesophagus in malabsorption syndrome. *Br. J. Med.*, 1:540–542.

Precancerous Lesions of the Gastrointestinal Tract, edited by P. Sherlock, B.C. Morson, L. Barbara, and U. Veronesi. Raven Press, New York © 1983.

The Influence of Dietary Cholic Acid and Beta-Sitosterol on MNU-Induced Colon Carcinogenesis

Eleanor E. Deschner

Memorial Sloan-Kettering Cancer Center, New York, New York 10021

A diet rich in saturated fats derived from animal and diary products is commonly consumed in the United States and Western Europe, areas of the world with a high incidence of colon cancer. In contrast, the Japanese and the American Seventh Day Adventists who rely principally on a vegetarian type diet show a relatively low colorectal cancer incidence. High saturated fat consumption has as one of its consequences an increase in bile acid output and ultimately high excretion levels of its bacterial metabolites. Measurements of fecal bile acids and cholesterol metabolites in various colonic disease states have suggested a possible relationship between them and colon cancer incidence.

Experimentally, intrarectal instillation of secondary bile acids induced a significantly increased incidence of colonic neoplasia among N-methyl-N'-nitro-N-nitrosoguanidine treated rats (5). Likewise, chronic ingestion of cholic acid at a 0.2% level increased the frequency of neoplasms induced by the carcinogen N-methyl-N-nitrosourea (MNU) from 54% (1.1 tumor/animal) to 62% (1.8 tumor/animal) ($p < 0.05$) (1). Apparently, augmentation of bile acid levels via either route effected an increase in tumor formation among carcinogen-treated rodents, leading to the premise that bile acids act as tumor promotors.

The main components of a vegetarian diet are the plant sterols of which beta-sitosterol is one. Since beta-sitosterol is not absorbed in the colon, fecal analysis of this component serves as a measure of dietary plant intake. Fecal samples from strict vegetarians demonstrate significantly higher beta-sitosterol excretion levels than those of the general population (4).

Experimentally, dietary supplementation with beta-sitosterol has been shown to protect against MNU-induced colonic neoplasia. A significantly reduced tumor incidence was demonstrated in rats fed beta-sitosterol concurrently with intrarectal instillation of the carcinogen (6).

Examination of the acute and chronic effect of these agents on epithelial cell proliferation was undertaken to shed light on their mechanism of action against chemically induced colonic tumor formation (2,3).

MATERIALS AND METHODS

Male Fischer rats were employed in both studies and were allowed free access to food and water. For chronic ingestion purposes, cholic acid was added to rat chow at a level of 0.2% of diet. Acute studies used a 1.0% concentration. The bile acid was mixed in ground Purina rat chow and repelleted.

Beta-sitosterol fed at a level of 0.2% of diet was also assessed following acute and chronic administration. One batch of food was prepared by adding the plant sterol to ground meal and repelleting. All food was stored in a cool dry environment and used as needed.

The colon carcinogen MNU was administered intrarectally as a 2-mg dose in 0.5 ml sterile 0.9% saline solution. It was provided at four separate intervals (days 1,4,7, and 10), giving a total dose of 8 mg/rat, a dose that induces a 50% incidence of colonic tumors.

CHOLIC ACID

Consumption of 1.0% cholic acid in the diet for 3 days caused an increase in the number of colonic epithelial cells per crypt column accompanied by an increased population of DNA synthesizing cells per column compared with control or 0.2%-cholic-acid-fed rats. These additional cells were recruited from the middle third of the crypt. The leading edge of labeled epithelial cells was further up the cryptal wall of cholic-acid-fed rats and migration to the luminal surface of crypts was faster in these animals than was seen in the control or 0.2%-cholic-acid-treated rats.

The 0.2% concentration of cholic acid created a detectable proliferative effect after ingestion for 1 week. The number of DNA synthesizing cells per column was increased from 3.0 for control to 4.0 for cholic-acid-treated rats.

Chronic feeding for 12 and 28 weeks demonstrated the continued extension of the proliferative compartment beyond that seen in the control chow-fed rats with a higher frequency of labeled cells per column in bile-acid-fed rodents. Similar to the acute feeding study, additional DNA synthesizing cells were supplied from the middle third of the gland encompassing cell positions 9 to 27.

BETA-SITOSTEROL

Three days dietary exposure to the plant sterol reduced the total number of epithelial cells per crypt column. Moreover, the labeling index (L.I.), or ratio of labeled cells to total cells scored, was reduced from the control group (13.2% $\pm$ 2.3) to 11.9% $\pm$ 1.9. This translated to 3.9 labeled cells per crypt column in the beta-sitosterol group compared with 4.7 for the controls. The decrease in labeled cells was brought about by the suppression of DNA synthesis in the middle third of the crypt or upper region of the proliferative compartment.

Long-term feeding with 0.2% beta-sitosterol revealed continued reduced levels of cell proliferation and slower rate of migration of labeled cells when compared with control rats. As was seen in the acute study, suppression of DNA synthesis occurred in the middle third of the crypts from plant-sterol-treated rats and L.I. in the basal regions were enhanced.

MNU-treated rats ingesting 0.2% beta-sitosterol had 3.3 labeled cells per crypt column, whereas MNU-treated rats on control chow had 5.4, indicating the suppression of DNA synthesis by the plant sterol. In addition, beta-sitosterol effectively compressed the proliferative compartment so that the leading edge of MNU-labeled cells reached position 30 in contrast to position 24 in MNU- and beta-sitosterol-treated rats.

CONTRASTED RESPONSE

Cholic acid and beta-sitosterol serve as a study in contrasts. The plant sterol diet reduces epithelial cell proliferation and migration and brings about a decrease in the size of the proliferative compartment. On the other hand, cholic acid supplementation enhances cell proliferation, expands the proliferative compartment, and speeds up migration of epithelial cells along the cryptal wall.

Each of these agents in contact with a carcinogen-treated colon influences proliferation in the same manner as occurred in the untreated, control large bowel mucosa. Cholic acid stimulates epithelial cells in the already active MNU-treated tissue to express an even more heightened degree of DNA synthesis, whereas beta-sitosterol acts to suppress the proliferative activity induced by MNU. The response in both instances is one that successfully alters the incidence of colonic neoplasia. The plant sterol acts as a protective substance by restraining the expression of malignant transformation within certain members of the stem cell compartment. Cholic acid on the other hand, by increasing the number of proliferating epithelial cells, provides a greater opportunity for the malignant genotype to be uncovered and allowed to form a dysplastic site.

ACKNOWLEDGMENTS

The author gratefully acknowledges the technical assistance of Ms. Florence Long, Susan Herrmann, and Mary Hakissian. This work was supported in part by NCI Grants CA-08748, CA-14991, and CA-18651, the latter as part of the National Large Bowel Cancer Project.

REFERENCES

1. Cohen, B. I., Raicht, R. F., Deschner, E. E., Takahashi, M., Sarwal, A. N., and Fazzini, E. (1980): Effect of cholic acid feeding on N-methyl-N-nitrosourea-induced colon tumors and cell kinetics in rats. *J. Natl. Cancer Inst.*, 62:573–578.
2. Deschner, E. E., Cohen, B. I., and Raicht, R. F. (1981): The acute and chronic effect of dietary cholic acid on colonic epithelial cell proliferation. *Digestion*, 21:290–296.
3. Deschner, E. E., Cohen, B. I., and Raicht, R. F. (1982): The kinetics of the protective effect of beta-sitosterol against MNU induced colonic neoplasia. *J. Cancer Res. Clin. Oncol.*, 103:49–54.
4. Miettinen, T. A., and Tarpila, S. (1978): Fecal beta-sitosterol in patients with diverticular disease of the colon and in vegetarians. *Scand. J. Gastroenterol.*, 13:573–576.
5. Narisawa, T., Magadia, N. E., Weisburger, J. H., and Wynder, E. L. (1974): Promoting effect of bile acids on colon carcinogenesis after intrarectal instillation of N-methyl-N′-nitro-N-nitrosoguanidine. *J. Natl. Cancer Inst.*, 55:1093–1097.
6. Raicht, R. F., Cohen, B. I., Fazzini, E. P., Sarwal, A. N., and Takahashi, M. (1980): Protective effect of plant sterols against chemically-induced colon tumors in rats. *Cancer Res.*, 40:403–405.

Precancerous Lesions of the Gastrointestinal Tract, edited by P. Sherlock, B.C. Morson, L. Barbara, and U. Veronesi. Raven Press, New York © 1983.

Mechanisms of Colorectal Carcinogenesis in Animal Models: Possible Implications in Cancer Prevention

Alain P. Maskens

Avenue Lambeau 62, B-1200 Brussels, Belgium

THE MULTISTEP NATURE OF CARCINOGENESIS IN GENERAL

Studies of the biological side of carcinogenesis are of three main types, all of which point to the conclusion that malignant transformation occurs stepwise, that is, that it involves a succession of discrete changes in the affected cells.

The first approach is based on the classical observations of Berenblum and Shubick (7,8) and Mottram (74). These authors showed that mouse skin cancer can be induced by a biphasic procedure. If a single application of a carcinogenic hydrocarbon, at a dose too small to cause tumors alone ("initiator"), is followed by multiple applications of a material such as croton oil, which, alone, would never induce tumors at any dose ("promoter"), multiple tumors will rapidly develop. Whereas the prevalent view is that initiation is probably a mutational event, the essence of promotion remains a debated matter [see the review by Slaga et al. (99)]. The main interest of these studies, in our opinion, is that they represent the first experimental demonstration of the multistep nature of chemical carcinogenesis. In addition, they have clearly shown that several compounds, some of which can be found in our natural environment (38,92), can in fact greatly facilitate or accelerate the development of cancer, even if they have no carcinogenic properties when tested alone. The relevance of this model in our understanding of the specific steps involved in carcinogenesis is limited, however, by the fact that the tumor most frequently obtained is a benign papilloma, often reversible.

The second main approach to this problem is based on the more recent development of experimental liver carcinogenesis (26,99). Several models have in fact extended to the liver the initiation/promotion procedure for cancer induction (80,82). Characteristic here is the observation that a series of successive stages can be recognized on histological, histochemical, or even biochemical (15) bases. One drawback again is that the specificity of these intermediary benign growths to the malignant transformation is not clearly established.

The third approach attempts to determine the mathematical consequences of the multistep concept. This has been mainly applied in human situations, based on the analysis of age distribution of the most frequent cancers (1,2,13,32,67,78,105). It was shown that, provided transformation rates from a given stage to the next one remain constant throughout life, tumor prevalence will increase with the nth power of age if n steps are involved in the carcinogenesis process (1,81). In the case of colorectal cancers, for instance, epidemiologic observations indicate that prevalence varies with the 5.0th to the 6.3rd power of age (1,3,67,108), and it has been concluded that this indeed could represent the number of steps that separate a normal enterocyte from a carcinomatous cell (1,3,108). It should be noted that the terms *change* and *step* apply here only in situations where

1. the modification is unequivocal, that is, involves an all-or-nothing type of qualitative change; and
2. the modification has a relatively low probability of occurring, that is, only an occasional cell within a tissue will be affected (81).

Thus, when a cell or group of cells undergo a rather automatic succession of progressive changes, these are not regarded as separate steps in the present context.

In recent years, several analyses have been published that conclude that most observations are in fact consistent with a mechanism requiring no more than two essential steps, although the analyses confirm the multistep essence of carcinogenesis at large. We have shown, for instance, that a two-step model can produce 5th- or 6th-power functions of prevalence versus age, provided the rates of each of the two steps vary with age, a phenomenon likely to occur (64). Similarly, Moolgavkar and co-workers (71,72) have indicated that, when the possibility of growth and differentiation of the normal and intermediate cells is taken into account, most human incidence data can be accounted for by the two-step hypothesis. Perhaps one of the most convincing evidences in support of this hypothesis has been provided by Knudson's analyses of incidence data from hereditary and nonhereditary retinoblastoma. These data were indeed perfectly fitted by a model in which the disease resulted from precisely two consecutive cellular events, the first being a recessive mutation, germinal in the hereditary form and somatic in the nonhereditary variant (40,47,48).

DEMONSTRATION OF TWO-STEP CARCINOGENESIS IN AN EXPERIMENTAL COLON CANCER MODEL

At the experimental level, it is in the field of colorectal carcinogenesis that one of the best opportunities was recently provided to confirm the two-step model. Tumors obtained in various rodent species treated with symmetrical 1,2-dimethylhydrazine (DMH) or other related hydrazine derivatives happened indeed to share several properties highly desirable for such a purpose. Unlike the liver and skin systems, carcinomas can be obtained in DMH-treated rats without preliminary benign tumor stages (57,59,66,86). In addition, this carcinogen is potent enough to cause colon cancers after one single dose (56,62,95,104); repeated injections will result in large numbers of tumors, up to 20 or more per colon. In such a system, it is thus possible both to follow histologically the entire development of the carcinomatous lesions and to test the mathematical predictions of multistep models. Again, it was found in two detailed analyses that precisely two specific changes were necessary and sufficient to induce the malignant growth (59,62).

We will illustrate this conclusion using the tumor prevalence data observed after a short exposure to three different doses of DHM (Fig. 1). More complete data and discussion are given elsewhere (62,66). The carcinogen was given subcutaneously (S.C.) once weekly, at a dose of 20 mg/kg of the hydrochloride form. The number of injections was 1, 4, and 8, respectively, for series I, II, and III. The animals were sacrificed per groups of 6 at various intervals after the first injection. All tumors in the colon and rectum were submitted to histological analysis; 95% were glandular neoplasms, of which 92% were invading through the muscularis mucosae and classified as adenocarcinomas. Analysis of microscopic lesions revealed no benign adenoma stage preceding the carcinomatous change. Two findings need

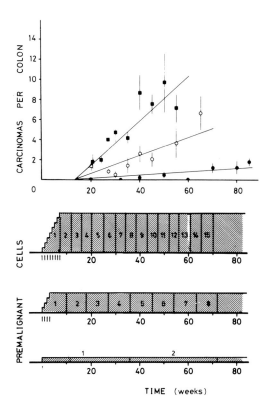

FIG. 1. Top: Mean number of macroscopically visible adenocarcinomas observed in the large intestine of rats sacrificed per groups of 3–6 at various intervals after 1 (*closed circles*), 4 (*open circles*), and 8 (*closed squares*) weekly injections of symmetrical 1,2-dimethylhydrazine (DMH). The lines represent the best-fitting linear regression curves of tumor prevalence versus (t-w), where t is the time from first injection, and w the time needed for tumors to grow from a volume of one cell to a visible nodule (93 days). **Bottom**: The two-step carcinogenesis concept is illustrated. It is proposed that each injection of the carcinogen (*arrows*) induces an equal mean number of intermediate or premalignant cells, which accumulate with successive treatments. These cells have no phenotypic expression in terms of proliferative advantage, but they are at risk for a second transformation capable of initiating tumor growth. The surface areas delineated by columns in the shaded areas of the diagram are all equal and each represent the probability of one such definitive transformation. Tumor incidence is thus expected to be proportional to the total dose of DMH, as actually observed.

to be emphasized. First, there was in all series a positive correlation between tumor prevalence and time, no plateau phase being reached after as long as 85 weeks. Thus, new tumors continued to originate in the colon long after cessation of the immediate biologic effects of DMH. This indicates that at least two steps were required for tumor induction; the first one was obviously caused by DMH, its effects being transmitted within the mucosa for prolonged periods. Second, the incidence rate was constant in each of the three groups, and directly proportional to the total dose of DMH, with an average of 1.0 carcinoma per colon per dose of DMH per year. These observations are consistent with a two-step model in which a number of normal cells will undergo a first step toward malignancy as a consequence of DMH treatments. The number of these intermediate or "precancer" cells will thus be proportional to the dose of DMH. The risk that one of these intermediate cells becomes fully malignant is on the average constant; tumor incidence will thus be proportional to their total number or to the total dose of DMH.

THE FIRST STEP IN DMH-INDUCED CARCINOGENESIS: A SOMATIC MUTATION

What are the speculative possibilities about the nature of each of the two steps? For the first one, the most logical assumption is that it represents a somatic mutation. Several facts strongly support this view:

1. DMH is a potent alkylator of DNA in the target organs (14,37,52,85,94,106). Among others, production of 06-methylguanine has been demonstrated. Several experiments have supported the hypothesis that 06-methylguanine is a promutagenic DNA lesion that may play a signficant role in the induction of cancer by monofunctional alkylating agents (33,46,55,77,79).

2. DMH carcinogenicity necessitates not only DNA alkylation but also cell proliferation to be effective (60). Indeed, although DNA alkylation is more severe in hepatocytes compared to enterocytes (37,52,85,106), DMH-induced tumors in the liver are exceedingly rare (24,86,110), unless cell proliferative stimulus is provided shortly after administration of the carcinogen (12,121,122). This observation is consistent with the hypothesis that DNA replication in the presence of alkylated bases—mainly 06-methylguanine—can produce mutations as a result of base mispairing (50,55,88,93,113).

3. DMH and its metabolites do indeed exhibit potent mutagenic effects. The mutagenic properties of methylazoxymethanol were documented as early as 1966 (100,107). DMH was not detected as a mutagen in the Salmonella/microsome test (69), but it exhibited potent mutagenicity in the host-mediated assay (73); this property was inhibited by pretreatment of the host with disulfiram, a chemical that blocks the metabolism of DMH.

4. There exists a clear correlation between the alkylating, mutagenic, and carcinogenic activities of DMH. The link between the alkylation of nucleic acids in the intestinal epithelium, as observed after DMH treatments, and carcinogenicity can be deduced from the observation that those alkylhydrazines that are not carcinogenic to the gut (e.g., monomethylhydrazine, diethylhydrazine) do not alkylate nucleic acids in that organ (37,85). Furthermore, it was recently shown that after a DMH injection higher concentrations of 7-methylguanine and 06-methylguanine were obtained in the enterocytes of those mouse strains most susceptible to DMH tumorigenesis (14). Similarly, when mouse strains of different sensitivity to DMH carcinogenesis (27) were used in the host-mediated mutagenesis assay, mutagenicity was well correlated with carcinogenicity (73). Disulfiram, which protects animals from DMH carcinogenesis (114–116), prevents both the alkylation of nucleic acids (106) and the mutagenic activity caused by this agent (73).

5. The appearance of new colon carcinomas more than one year after one single injection of DMH clearly indicates that the changes induced by the carcinogen in the mucosa are stable and transmissible upon cell renewal.

Thus, each DMH injection is probably capable of inducing, on a random basis, a first specific mutation in a given proportion of colon cells. Those precancer, or intermediate, cells will thereafter be at risk for the second change, which will allow expression of the cancer phenotype.

CHEMICALLY INDUCED SOMATIC MUTATIONS: A COMMON PHENOMENON IN COLORECTAL CARCINOGENESIS

Chemical carcinogens initiating the process of malignant transformation via a somatic mutation now appears to be a quite general phenomenon (70). We should then ask, Does chemical carcinogenesis play any significant role in colon cancers or is the DMH model a rather artificial system? A large body of evidence favors the first alternative.

First, the list of chemicals reported to induce colon tumors in animals is by no means limited to the hydrazine derivatives (Table 1); most such compounds have proven mutagenic properties (69,73). Second, recent studies have shown that hydrazine derivatives can theoretically arise during the metabolism of endogenous aliphatic amines such as methylamine (30). Furthermore, methylazoxymethanol has been reported to induce tumors, including colon adenomas, in nonhuman primates (98). Third, mutagenic and/or co-mutagenic activity has been detected by several investigators in the stools of individuals at risk for colon cancer (11,89,90); possible dietary factors capable of producing mutagenic chemicals have been proposed by Weisburger et al. (118).

TABLE 1. *Colon carcinogens in experimental animals*

Category	Compound	Ref.
Cholanthrenes	1,2,5,6-dibenzanthracene	54
	20-methylcholanthrene	43,54
Aromatic amines	4–aminodiphenyl	109
	3:2'-dimethyl-4-aminodiphenyl	101,109
	N,N'-2,7-fluorenylenebisacetamide	120
Hydrazine derivatives	1,2-dimethylhydrazine	25,66
	methylazoxymethanol	68,123
	azoxymethane	24,112
	1-methyl-2-butyl-hydrazine	24
	methyl-azoxybutane	24
Alkylnitrosamides	N-methyl-N'-nitroso-N-nitrosoguanidine	75
	N-methyl-N-nitrosourea	51,111
	N-nitrosobis(2-oxopropyl)amine	83
Miscellaneous agents	extracts of bracken or fiddlehead fern	28,42
	substituted carbamates	36
	aflatoxin b1	76

CHARACTERISTICS OF THE SECOND STEP IN DMH CARCINOGENESIS: A THEORETICAL MODEL OF MALIGNANT TRANSFORMATION

How far can we speculate on the nature of the second event in malignant transformation? The experimental setting of the DMH studies referred to above allows its main characteristics to be specified, thus narrowing the range of possible interpretations.

As the number of successful occurrences of this event equals the number of observed carcinomas [assuming a clonal origin of tumor (31)], its frequency reaches no more than once per year per dose of DMH, for a population of intermediate cells probably on the order of 10^4 (64). The number of tumors per colon is compatible with a Poisson distribution (59); their location in the colon is variable. Thus, the second step is a rare event randomly affecting the population of intermediate cells. Also important is the observation that this second step does not require the presence of the carcinogen, and that its average frequency appears to be quite constant in a given tissue. Finally, the effect of the second change is transmissible upon cell renewal, as it will allow for the development of a neoplastic clone.

We thus have to think of the second step as a rare cellular event occurring spontaneously at a given rate in a given tissue, which will be capable of expressing the first DMH-induced mutation so as to induce the proliferation of a tumoral cell line. Not many cellular phenomena share all these specific properties, and we have suggested that somatic recombination of homologous genes, or other mitotic accidents capable of rendering a cell homozygous for a recessive gene, might do the job quite well (62,63). This hypothesis has been proposed as a possible mechanism in several human cancer conditions as well (48).

One can thus theorize that one of the ways in which a colorectal cancer can be caused is based on the following two essential steps (Fig. 2):

1. A mutagen will cause, in a number of normal cells, a specific mutation. The affected cells (intermediate cells) will not express this mutation (recessive mutants), at least in terms of proliferative advantage.
2. Expression of the cancer phenotype will result from a second event capable of rendering

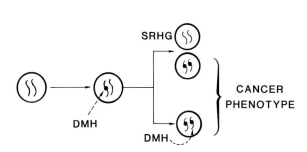

FIG. 2. Suggested mechanisms by which a cell heterozygous for a 1,2-dimethylhydrazine (DMH)-induced recessive cancer mutation can express the cancer phenotype. One first possibility, which can occur independently from further carcinogenic treatments, is a mitotic error resulting in a recombination of the homologous genes. Continued exposure to the carcinogen can also independently affect the homologous gene in one of the intermediate cells. SRHG, somatic recombination of homologous genes.

some of the intermediate cells homozygous for the recessive mutation. Spontaneous mitotic errors can be one such event. In addition, continued exposure to the carcinogen can also independently affect the homologous gene in one of the intermediate cells.

USE OF THE MODEL IN UNDERSTANDING CARCINOGENIC AND COCARCINOGENIC FACTORS

The risk of cancer in a given tissue will thus essentially depend on (a) the number of intermediate cells and (b) the rate at which the second step occurs. The number of intermediate cells will in turn result from two main factors. The first is the amount of active carcinogen ultimately reaching the target cells. It will obviously depend on (a) the amount of carcinogen to which the individual is being exposed and (b) the metabolic pathways that will be available to the carcinogenic chemical.

In the particular case of experimental colon cancer, dose/response effects have been clearly documented (21,62,111). Agents such as disulfiram, which interfere with DMH metabolism, have been shown to protect against its carcinogenic effects (114–116). Specific tissue enzymes capable of enhancing the metabolism of DMH derivatives in the organs more susceptible to harbor tumors have been detected by Zedeck et al. (34,124).

The second factor interfering with the first step is the efficiency with which mutations can be fixed in the genetic material. Of central importance here is the replicative activity of the target cells (12,60,88,121,122). The chemical structure of the carcinogen as well as repair and other properties of DNA also play a prominent role in this respect (45,46,70).

As for the second event, the risk that a mitotic error, leading to expression of a recessive mutant, occurs ought to be essentially dependent on the mitotic rate. It is therefore to be expected that factors that enhance cell proliferation will promote cancer formation. Beyond that, it is reasonable to hypothesize that some tissues or species can be more susceptible to this type of mitotic error than others. It is in fact known that a human genetic disease, Bloom's syndrome, where homologous chromosome exchange is known to occur, is highly susceptible to various kinds of cancers (29).

PROLIFERATIVE AND CLONOGENIC PROPERTIES OF TISSUES: TWO KEY ELEMENTS IN EVALUATING THE CANCER RISK

Among the tissue properties that significantly affect the carcinogenic risk in given conditions of exposure to mutagens, the two most important are probably cell proliferation and clonogenicity.

The two-step carcinogenesis model presented above clearly underlines the importance of cell proliferation, as this element is central in each of the two steps. The importance of DNA replication for the fixation of chemically induced mutations has already been alluded to. Its importance for the ultimate step(s) of malignant transformation has also been clearly established in experimental systems other than the colon (4,5,87,96). In DMH colon carcinogenesis, it is significant that several factors known as activators of cell proliferation do in fact promote tumors. These include bile derivatives (23,91,92), nonspecific injury (84), and transmissible murine colonic hyperplasia (6). Along the same line, one of the ways in which dietary fat might promote carcinogenesis is via an increase in bile excretion in the intestinal lumen. Also relevant is the recent suggestion that dietary selenium, which markedly decreases the incidence of DMH-induced tumors (44), is in fact also responsible for a selective decrease in DNA synthesis in the colon (35).

Clonogenicity is another, probably less well understood, tissue factor that can greatly multiply the cancer risk in tissues exposed to chemical carcinogens. It is the normal fate of adult renewing tissues to be organized into small structural units, such as the crypts of Lieberkühn. In this frame, any recessive mutant cell will be forced to remain unique or, at most, to form small groups not exceeding the size of the tissue unit where it was born. On the other hand, germinal mutations, and mutations occurring early during development or growth of a tissue, or in a benign tumor, will be multiplied by factors of thousands, millions, or even billions. If this mutation is carcinogenic, what will happen is thus a multiplication of the number of intermediate cells, with a corresponding rise in the risk that the second step will occur. The mathematical consequences of this phenomenon have been incorporated in the two-step model recently published by Moolgavkar and Knudson (72). Of note is the fact that although cell proliferation can occur in the absence of clonal expansion, the reverse is not true. Clonogenic tissues are by definition always proliferative and thus twice at risk.

DYSPLASIA AND BENIGN GROWTHS OF THE COLORECTAL MUCOSA: THEIR SIGNIFICANCE IN RELATION TO THE CARCINOGENESIS MODEL

What is the relevance of the two-step model in understanding the biological significance of the precursor lesions in the human colon and rectum? Under the pathologist's microscope, the commonest lesion seen to precede carcinomas is the dysplasia (B. C. Morson, *this volume*). It is usually associated—with varying degrees of severity—with lesions such as tubular adenomas, villous tumors, or long-standing ulcerative colitis. Although the exact etiology and biological meaning of dysplasia is not known, one certain fact is that all these situations are characterized by an increased proliferative activity (18–20,22,58,61,119). Dysplasia also appears to be more severe and associated with a greater cancer risk in larger adenomas (B. C. Morson, *this volume*), that is, in lesions with greater clonogenic properties. The implications of the two-step carcinogenesis model are thus in good agreement with current views on the cancer risk associated with various forms of dysplasia, as summarized in Table 2. Furthermore, they provide a biological basis for the hypothesis, proposed by Hill et al. (41), that "the major factor in determining the incidence of carcinoma is the one which causes adenomas to grow to a large size rather than the one which actually causes the carcinomatous change."

One important theoretical question then remains to be addressed: does the adenomatous or dysplastic tissue represent a clone of cells having already undergone the first specific step towards cancer? If this were the case, they would represent a mandatory prerequisite before the occurrence of a cancer. Several observations seem to indicate that this is not the case. In experimental carcinogenesis, it is now well documented that most carcinomas arise *de*

TABLE 2. *Proliferative activity, clonogenicity, and cancer risk associated with various conditions of the colorectal mucosa*

Condition	Proliferation	Clonogenicity	Cancer risk
Normal crypt	+	0	Minimal
Hyperplastic polyp	+	0	Minimal
Dysplasia in flat mucosa	+ + +	0 (?)	+
Small tubular adenoma	+ +	+	+
Large tubular adenoma	+ + +	+ + +	+ + +
Villous tumor	+ + +	+ + +	+ + +

novo in flat mucosa, in the absence of preexisting benign neoplasms (66); it was recently shown that in rats given a low dose of DMH, carcinomas continue to be produced in the absence or after subsidence of a temporary hyperplastic and/or dysplastic reaction resulting from the acute effects of the carcinogen (62). That adenomas and carcinomas constitute in fact genetically distinct entities was strongly suggested by the observation that this same carcinogen will in some animal strains, mainly mice, induce adenomas exclusively or predominantly, whereas in most rat strains, carcinomas will be largely preponderant (66). In the human situation, carcinomas arising in flat mucosa have also been reported (39,97,102,103,117). We would therefore favor the opinion that the specific genetic alterations leading to cancer of the colon and rectum are distinct from those leading to the precursor lesions. Dysplastic or adenomatous changes are thus not obligatory stages before cancer; however, they greatly contribute to the risk that the cancer changes will be acquired and expressed. This implies that the risk that cancer develops in a histologically normal crypt, although extremely low, is not zero; considering that the number of normal crypts in a human colon is on the order of tens of billions, the "chance" that carcinomas arise in some of them must be significant.

CONCLUSIONS

In conclusion, several features of the two-step model of carcinogenesis as demonstrated in the rat DMH system appear to have relevance for human colorectal cancer as well. They can help in better understanding the type of measures most likely to be effective in preventing and detecting this disease.

Preventive measures should be of two main types:

1. recognition and elimination of substances that can have a mutagenic effect on the colon epithelium, or factors that can enhance the metabolism of their precursors;
2. recognition and elimination of factors or conditions that can enhance the proliferative or clonogenic activity of the epithelial cells.

As for early detection, it will be directed toward recognition of clinical or histological evidence of increased proliferative or clonogenic activity of the epithelial cells. Dysplasia, with or without neoplastic changes, is probably the main such signal. In this context, thymidine incorporation studies, which are capable of tracing even earlier proliferative modifications, represent a major investigative as well as clinical tool (9,10,16–20,22,53,65).

REFERENCES

1. Armitage, P., and Doll, R. (1954): The age distribution of cancer and a multi-stage theory of carcinogenesis. *Br. J. Cancer*, 8:1–12.
2. Ashley, D. J. B. (1969): The two "hit" and multiple "hit" theories of carcinogenesis. *Br. J. Cancer*, 23:313–328.
3. Ashley, D. J. B. (1969): Colonic cancer arising in polyposis coli. *J. Med. Gen.*, 6:376–378.
4. Barbason, H., and Betz, E. H. (1982): Proliferation of preneoplastic lesions after discontinuation of chronic DENA feeding in the development of hepatomas in rats. *Br. J. Cancer*, 44:561–566.
5. Barbason, H., Smoliar, V., Fridman-Manduzio, A., and Betz, E. H. (1979): Effect of discontinuation of chronic feeding of diethylnitrosamine on the development of hepatomas in adult rats. *Br. J. Cancer*, 40:260–267.
6. Barthold, S. W., and Jonas, A. M. (1977): Morphogenesis of 1,2-dimethylhydrazine-induced lesions and latent period reduction of colon carcinogenesis in mice by a variant of citrobacter freundii. *Cancer Res.*, 37:4352–4360.
7. Berenblum, I. (1941): The mechanism of cocarcinogenesis: a study of significance of cocarcinogenic action and related phenomena. *Cancer Res.*, 1:807–814.
8. Berenblum, I., and Shubick, P. (1949): An experimental study of the initiating stage of carcinogenesis, and a re-examination of the somatic cell mutation theory of cancer. *Br. J. Cancer*, 3:109–118.
9. Bleiberg, H., Mainguet, P., and Galand, P. (1972): Cell renewal in familial polyposis: comparison between polyps and healthy mucosa. *Gastroenterology*, 63:240–245.
10. Bleiberg, H., Mainguet, P., Galand, P., Chretien, J., and Dupont-Mairesse, N. (1970): Cell renewal in the human rectum. "In vitro" autoradiographic study on active ulcerative colitis. *Gastroenterology*, 58:851–855.
11. Bruce, W. R., Varghese, A. J., Furrer, R., and Land, P. C. (1977): A mutagen in the feces of normal humans. In: *Origins of Human Cancer*, edited by H. H. Hiatt, J. D. Watson, and J. A. Winsten, pp. 1641–1646. Cold Spring Harbor Laboratory, Cold Spring Harbor, New York.
12. Columbano, A., Rajalakshmi, S., and Sarma, D. S. R. (1980): Requirement of cell proliferation for the induction of presumptive preneoplastic lesions in rat liver by a single dose of 1,2-dimethylhydrazine. *Chem. Biol. Interact.*, 32:347–351.
13. Cook, P. J., Doll, R., and Fellingham, S. A. (1969): A mathematical model for the age distribution of cancer in man. *Int. J. Cancer*, 4:93–112.
14. Cooper, H. K., Buecheler, J., and Kleihues, P. (1978): DNA alkylation in mice with genetically different susceptibility to 1,2-dimethylhydrazine-induced colon carcinogenesis. *Cancer Res.*, 38:3063–3065.
15. de Gerlache, J., Lans, M., Mercier, M., and Roberfroid, M. (1980): Comparison of biochemical and histochemical analyses of liver hyperplastic nodules. *Toxicol. Lett. (Suppl)*, 1:241.
16. Deschner, E. E. (1979): Colorectal biopsy and lavage for the evaluation of high risk groups. *Acta Endosc.*, 9:181–185.
17. Deschner, E. E. (1980): Aspects of normal and altered epithelial cell proliferation in the human intestine. In: *Cell Proliferation in the Gastrointestinal Tract*, edited by D. R. Appleton, J. P. Sunter, and A. J. Watson, pp. 370–381. Pitman Medical, Tunbridge Wells (U.K.).
18. Deschner, E. E., Lewis, C. M., and Lipkin, M. (1962): In vitro H3-thymidine incorporation into human rectal mucosa. *Clin. Res.*, 10:189.
19. Deschner, E. E., Lewis, C. M., and Lipkin, M. (1963): In vitro study of human rectal epithelial cells. I. Atypical zone of H3 thymidine incorporation in mucosa of multiple polyposis. *J. Clin. Invest.*, 42:1922–1928.
20. Deschner, E. E., Lipkin, M., and Solomon, C. (1966): Study of human rectal epithelial cells in vitro. II. H3-Thymidine incorporation into polyps and adjacent mucosa. *J. Natl. Cancer Inst.*, 36:849–857.
21. Deschner, E. E., Long, F. C., and Maskens, A. P. (1979): Relationship between dose, time, and tumor yield in mouse dimethylhydrazine-induced colon tumorigenesis. *Cancer Lett.*, 8:23–28.
22. Deschner, E. E., and Maskens, A. P. (1982): Significance of the labelling index and labelling distribution as kinetic parameters in colo-rectal mucosa of cancer patients and DMH treated animals. *Cancer*, 50:1136–1141.
23. Deschner, E. E., and Raicht, R. F. (1979): Influence of bile on kinetic behavior of colonic epithelial cells of the rat. *Digestion*, 19:322–327.
24. Druckrey, H. (1970): Production of colonic carcinomas by 1,2-dialkylhydrazines and azoxyalkanes. In: *Carcinoma of the Colon and Antecedent Epithelium*, edited by W. J. Burdette, pp. 267–279. Charles C Thomas, Springfield.
25. Druckrey, H., Preussmann, R., Matzkies, F., and Ivankovic, S. (1967): Selektieve Erzeugung von Darmkrebs bei Ratten durch 1,2-Dimethylhydrazin. *Naturwissenschaften*, 54:285–286.
26. Emmelot, P., and Scherer, E. (1980): The first relevant cell stage in rat liver carcinogenesis. A quantitative approach. *Biochem. Biophys. Acta*, 605:247–304.
27. Evans, J. T., Hauschka, T. S., and Mittelman, A. (1974): Differential susceptibility of four mouse strains to induction of multiple large-bowel neoplasms by 1,2-dimethylhydrazine. *J. Natl. Cancer Inst.*, 52:999–1000.
28. Evans, I. A., and Mason, J. (1965): Carcinogenic activity of Bracken. *Nature*, 208:913–914.

29. Festa, R. S., Meadows, A. T., and Boshes, R. A. (1977): Leukemia in a black child with Bloom's syndrome: somatic recombination as a possible mechanism for neoplasia. *Cancer*, 44:1507–1510.
30. Fiala, E. S. (1980): The formation of azoxymethane, a colon carcinogen, during the chemical oxydation of methylamine. *Carcinogenesis*, 1:57–60.
31. Fialkow, P. J. (1979): Clonal origin of human tumors. *Ann. Rev. Med.*, 30:135–143.
32. Fisher, J. C. (1958): Multiple-mutation theory of carcinogenesis. *Nature*, 181:651–652.
33. Goth, R., and Rajewsky, M. G. (1974): Persistence of 06-ethylguanine in rat brain DNA: correlation with nervous system-specific carcinogenesis by ethylnitrosourea. *Proc. Natl. Acad. Sci.*, 71:639–643.
34. Grab, D. J., and Zedeck, M. S. (1977): Organ-specific effects of the carcinogen methylazoxymethanol related to metabolism by nicotinamide adenine dinucleotide-dependent dehydrogenase. *Cancer Res.*, 37:4182–4189.
35. Harbach, P. R., Denlinge, R. H., Ficsor, G., Beuving, L., and Swenberg, J. A. (1980): Effect of selenium on 1,2-dimethylhydrazine (DMH) metabolism and DNA alkylation. *Proc. Am. Assoc. Cancer Res.*, 21:64.
36. Harris, P. N., Gibson, W. R., and Dillard, R. D. (1970): The oncogenicity of two 1,1-diaryl-2-propynyl N-cycloalkylcarbamates. *Cancer Res.*, 30:2952–2954.
37. Hawks, A., and Magee, P. N. (1974): The alkylation of nucleic acids of rat and mouse in vivo by the carcinogen 1,2-dimethylhydrazine. *Br. J. Cancer*, 30:440–447.
38. Hecker, E. (1978): Structure-activity relationships in diterpene esters irritant and cocarcinogenic to mouse skin. In: *Carcinogenesis, Vol. 2: Mechanisms of Tumor Promotion and Cocarcinogenesis*, edited by T. J. Slaga, A. Sivak, and R. K. Boutwell, pp. 11–48. Raven Press, New York.
39. Hellwig, E. B. (1947): The evolution of adenomas of the large intestine and their relation to carcinoma. *Surg. Gynecol. Obstet.*, 84:36–49.
40. Hethcote, H. W., and Knudson, A. G. (1978): A model for the incidence of embryonal cancers: application to retinoblastoma. *Proc. Natl. Acad. Sci.*, 75:2453–2457.
41. Hill, M. J., Morson, B. C., and Bussey, H. J. R. (1978): Aetiology of adenoma-carcinoma sequence in large bowel. *Lancet*, i:245–247.
42. Hirono, I., Shibuya, C., Fushimi, K., and Haga, M. (1970): Studies on carcinogenic properties of bracken, Pteridium aquilinum. *J. Natl. Cancer Inst.*, 45:179–188.
43. Homburger, F., Hsuek, S. S., Kerr, C. S., and Russfield, A. B. (1972): Inherited susceptibility of inbred strains of syrian hamsters to induction of subcutaneous sarcomas and mammary and gastrointestinal carcinomas by subcutaneous and gastric administration of polynuclear hydrocarbons. *Cancer Res.*, 32:360–366.
44. Jacobs, M. M., Jansson, B., and Griffin, A. C. (1977): Inhibitory effects of selenium on 1,2-dimethylhydrazine and methylazoxymethanol acetate induction of colon tumors. *Cancer Lett.*, 2:133–138.
45. Kanagalingam, K., and Balis, A. E. (1975): In vivo repair of rat intestinal damage by alkylating agents. *Cancer*, 36:2364–2372.
46. Kleihues, P., and Margison, G. P. (1974): Carcinogenicity of N-methyl-N-nitrosourea: possible role of excision repair of 06-methylguanine from DNA. *J. Natl. Cancer Inst.*, 53:1839–1841.
47. Knudson, A. G. (1971): Mutation and cancer: statistical study of retinoblastoma. *Proc. Natl. Acad. Sci.*, 68:820–823.
48. Knudson, A. G. (1981): Human cancer genes. In: *Genes, Chromosomes, and Neoplasia*, edited by F. E. Arrighi, P. N. Rao, and E. Stubblefield, pp. 453–462. Raven Press, New York.
49. Knudson, A. G., Hethcote, H. W., and Brown, B. W. (1975): Mutation and childhood cancer: A probabilistic model for the incidence of retinoblastoma. *Proc. Natl. Acad. Sci.*, 72:5116–5120.
50. Lawley, P. D. (1974): Some chemical aspects of dose-response relationships in alkylation mutagenesis. *Mutat. Res.*, 23:283–295.
51. Lev, R., and Herp, A. (1978): Pathogenesis of rat colon carcinomas induced by N-methyl-N-nitrosourea. *J. Natl. Cancer Inst.*, 61:779–786.
52. Likhachev, A. J., Margison, G. P., and Montesano, R. (1977): Alkylated purines in the DNA of various rat tissues after administration of 1,2-dimethylhydrazine. *Chem. Biol. Interact.*, 18:235–240.
53. Lipkin, M. (1974): Phase I and phase II proliferative lesions of colonic epithelial cells in diseases leading to colonic cancer. *Cancer*, 34:878–888.
54. Lorenz, E., and Stewart, H. L. (1941-42): Intestinal carcinoma and other lesions in mice following oral administration of 1,2,5,6-dibenzanthracene and 20-methylcholanthrene. *J. Natl. Cancer Inst.*, 1:17–40.
55. Loveless, A. (1969): Possible relevance of 06-alkylation of deoxyguanosine to the mutagenicity and carcinogenicity of nitrosamines and nitrosamides. *Nature*, 223:206–207.
56. Martin, M.-S., Martin, F., Justrabo, E., Knopf, J. F., Bastien, H., and Knobel, S. (1974): Induction de cancers coliques chez le rat par injection unique de 1,2-dimethylhydrazine. *Biol. Gastroenterol.*, 7:37–42.
57. Maskens, A. P. (1976): Histogenesis and growth pattern of 1,2-dimethylhydrazine-induced rat colon adenocarcinoma. *Cancer Res.*, 36:1585–1592.
58. Maskens, A. P. (1978): Distribution du compartiment proliferatif dans la muqueuse recto-colique normale, preneoplasique et neoplasique. *Acta Gastroenterol. Belg.*, 41:226–240.
59. Maskens, A. P. (1978): Mathematical models of carcinogenesis and tumor growth in an experimental colon adenocarcinoma. In: *Gastrointestinal Tract Cancer*, edited by M. Lipkin and R. Good, pp. 361–384. Plenum Press, New York.
60. Maskens, A. P. (1979): Significance of the karyorrhectic index in 1,2-dimethylhydrazine carcinogenesis. *Cancer Lett.*, 8:77–86.

61. Maskens, A. P. (1979): Histogenesis of adenomatous polyps in the human large intestine. *Gastroenterology*, 77:1245–1251.
62. Maskens, A. P. (1981): Confirmation of the two-step nature of chemical carcinogenesis in the rat colon adenocarcinoma model. *Cancer Res.*, 41:1240–1245.
63. Maskens, A. P. (1981): Quantitative analysis of the "somatic recombination of homologous genes" (SRHG) hypothesis in the dimethylhydrazine (DMH)-induced rat colon carcinoma model. *Proc. Am. Assoc. Cancer Res.*, 22:72.
64. Maskens, A. P. (1982): Multistep models of colorectal carcinogenesis. In: *Falk Symposium 31: Colonic Carcinogenesis*, edited by R. A. Malt and R. C. N. Williamson, pp. 211–219. MTP Press Limited, Lancaster (U.K.).
65. Maskens, A. P., and Deschner, E. E. (1977): Tritiated thymidine incorporation into epithelial cells of normal-appearing colorectal mucosa of cancer patients. *J. Natl. Cancer Inst.*, 58:1221–1224.
66. Maskens, A. P., and Dujardin-Loits, R. M. (1981): Experimental adenomas and carcinomas of the large intestine behave as distinct entities: most carcinomas arise de novo in flat mucosa. *Cancer*, 47:81–89.
67. Maskens, A. P., and Vandenberghe, A. (1979): Epidemiologie du cancer du gros intestin en Belgique. *Acta Endosc.*, 9:155–160.
68. Matsubara, N., Mori, H., and Hirono, I. (1978): Effect of colostomy on intestinal carcinogenesis by methylazoxymethanol acetate in rats. *J. Natl. Cancer Inst.*, 61:1161–1163.
69. Mc Cann, J., Choi, E., Yamasaki, E., and Ames, B. N. (1975): Detection of carcinogens as mutagens in the Salmonella/microsome test: assay of 300 chemicals. *Proc. Natl. Acad. Sci.*, 72:5135–5139.
70. Miller, E. C., and Miller, J. A. (1981): Mechanisms of chemical carcinogenesis. *Cancer*, 47:1055–1064.
71. Moolgavkar, S. H., Day, N. E., and Stevens, R. G. (1980): Two-stage model for carcinogenesis: epidemiology of breast cancer in females. *J. Natl. Cancer Inst.*, 65:559–569.
72. Moolgavkar, S. H., and Knudson, A. G. (1981): Mutation and cancer: a model for human carcinogenesis. *J. Natl. Cancer Inst.*, 66:1037–1052.
73. Moriya, M., Kato, K., Watanabe, K., Watanabe, Y., and Shirasu, Y. (1978): Detection of mutagenicity of the colon carcinogen 1,2-dimethylhydrazine by the host-mediated assay and its correlation to carcinogenicity. *J. Natl. Cancer Inst.*, 61:457–460.
74. Mottram, J. C. A. (1944): Developing factors in epidermal blastogenesis. *J. Pathol. Bacteriol.*, 6:439–484.
75. Narisawa, T., Sato, T., Hayakawa, M., Sakuma, A., and Nakano, H. (1971): Carcinoma of the colon and rectum of rats by rectal infusion of N-methyl-N'-nitro-N-nitrosoguanidine. *Gan*, 62:231–234.
76. Newberne, P. M., and Rogers, A. (1973): Rat colon carcinomas associated with aflatoxin and marginal vitamin A. *J. Natl. Cancer Inst.*, 50:439–448.
77. Nicoll, J. W., Swann, P. F., and Pegg, A. E. (1975): Effect of dimethylnitrosamine on persistence of methylated guanines in rat liver and kidney DNA. *Nature*, 254:261–262.
78. Nordling, C. D. (1953): A new theory on the cancer inducing mechanism. *Br. J. Cancer*, 7:68–72.
79. Pegg, A. E. (1977): Formation and metabolism of alkylated nucleosides: possible role in carcinogenesis by nitroso compounds and alkylating agents. *Adv. Cancer Res.*, 25:195–269.
80. Peraino, C., Fry, R. J. M., Staffeldt, E., and Kisielski, W. E. (1973): Effects of varying the exposure to phenobarbital on its enhancement of 2-acetylaminofluorene-induced hepatic tumorigenesis in the rat. *Cancer Res.*, 33:2701–2705.
81. Peto, R. (1977): Epidemiology, multistage models, and short-term mutagenicity tests. In: *Origins of Human Cancer*, edited by H. H. Hiatt, J. D. Watson, and J. A. Winsten, pp. 1403–1428. Cold Spring Harbor Laboratory, Cold Spring Harbor, New York.
82. Pitot, H. C. (1977): The natural history of neoplasia. *Am. J. Pathol.*, 89:401–412.
83. Pour, P. (1978): A new and advantageous model for colorectal cancer: its comparison with previous models for a common human disease. *Cancer Lett.*, 4:293–298.
84. Pozharisski, K. M. (1975): The significance of nonspecific injury for colon carcinogenesis in rats. *Cancer Res.*, 35:3824–3830.
85. Pozharisski, K. M., Kapustin, Y., Likhachev, A., and Shaposhnikov, J. (1975): The mechanism of carcinogenic action of 1,2-dimethylhydrazine (SDMH) in rats. *Int. J. Cancer*, 15:673–683.
86. Pozharisski, K. M., Likhachev, A. J., Klimashevski, V. F., and Shaposhnikov, J. D. (1979): Experimental intestinal cancer research with special reference to human pathology. *Adv. Cancer Res.*, 30:165–237.
87. Rabes, H., and Hartenstein, R. (1970): Specific stages of cellular response to homeostatic control during diethylnitrosamine induced liver carcinogenesis. *Experientia, 26:1356–1359.*
88. Rajewsky, M. F. (1972): Proliferative parameters of mammalian cell systems and their role in tumor growth and carcinogenesis. *Z. Krebsforsch.*, 78:12–30.
89. Rao, B. G., Mac Donald, I. A., and Hutchison, D. M. (1981): Nitrite-induced volatile mutagens from normal human feces. *Cancer*, 47:889–894.
90. Reddy, B. S., Sharma, C., and Wynder, E. (1980): Fecal factors which modify the formation of fecal co-mutagens in high- and low-risk population for colon cancer. *Cancer Lett.*, 10:123–132.
91. Reddy, B. S., and Watanabe, K. (1979): Effect of cholesterol metabolites and promoting effect of lithocholic acid in colon carcinogenesis in germ-free and conventional F344 rats. *Cancer Res.*, 39:1521–1524.
92. Reddy, B. S., Weisburger, J. H., and Wynder, E. L. (1978): Colon cancer: bile salts as tumor promoters.

In: *Carcinogenesis, Vol. 2; Mechanisms of Tumor Promotion and Cocarcinogenesis*, edited by T. J. Slaga, A. Sivak, and R. K. Boutwell, pp. 453–464. Raven Press, New York.

93. Roberts, J. J., Sturrock, J. E., and Ward, K. N. (1974): Enhancement by caffeine of alkylation-induced cell death, mutations and chromosomal aberrations in chinese hamster cells, as result of inhibition of post-replication repair. *Mutat. Res.*, 26:129.

94. Rogers, K. J., and Pegg, A. E. (1977): Formation of 06-methylguanine by alkylation of rat liver, colon and kidney DNA following administration of 1,2-dimethylhydrazine. *Cancer Res.*, 37:4082–4088.

95. Schiller, C. M., Curley, W. H., and McConnell, E. E. (1980): Induction of colon tumors by a single oral dose of 1,2-dimethylhydrazine. *Cancer Lett.*, 11:75–79.

96. Schulte-Hermann, R., Ohde, G., Schuppler, J., and Timmermann-Trosiener, I. (1981): Enhanced proliferation of putative preneoplastic cells in rat liver following treatment with the tumor promoters phenobarbital, hexachlorocyclohexane, steroid compounds, and nafenopin. *Cancer Res.*, 41:2556–2562.

97. Shamsuddin, A. K. M., Bell, H. G., Petrucci, J. V., and Trump, B. F. (1980): Carcinoma in-situ and "micro-invasive" adenocarcinoma of colon. *Pathol. Res. Pract.*, 167:374–379.

98. Sieber, S. M., Correa, P., Dalgard, D. W., McIntire, K. R., and Adamson, R. H. (1980): Carcinogenicity and hepatotoxicity of cycasin and its aglycone methylazoxymethanol acetate in nonhuman primates. *J. Natl. Cancer Inst.*, 65:177–189.

99. Slaga, T. J., Sivak, A., and Boutwell, R. K., editors (1978): *Carcinogenesis, Vol. 2: Mechanisms of Tumor Promotion and Cocarcinogenesis*. Raven Press, New York.

100. Smith, D. W. (1966): Mutagenicity of cycasin aglycone (methylazoxymethanol), a naturally occurring carcinogen. *Science*, 152:1273–1274.

101. Spjut, H. J., and Spratt, J. S. (1965): Endemic and morphologic similarities existing between spontaneous colonic neoplasms in man and 3:2'-dimethyl-4-aminobiphenyl induced colonic neoplasms in rats. *Ann. Surg.*, 161:309–324.

102. Spjut, H. J., Frankel, N. B., and Appel, M. F. (1979): The small carcinoma of the large bowel. *Am. J. Surg. Pathol.*, 3:39–46.

103. Spratt, J. S., Ackermann, L. V., and Moyer, C. A. (1958): Relationship of polyps of the colon to colonic cancer. *Ann. Surg.*, 148:682–696.

104. Springer, P., Springer, J., and Oehlert, W. (1970): Die Vorstufen des 1,2-Dimethylhydrazin-induzierten Dick- und Dundarmcarcinoms des Ratte. *Z. Krebsforsch.*, 74:236–240.

105. Stocks, P. (1953): A study of the age curve for cancer of the stomach in connection with a theory of the cancer producing mechanism. *Br. J. Cancer*, 7:407–417.

106. Swenberg, J. A., Cooper H. K., Buecheler, J., and Kleihues, P. (1979): 1,2-dimethylhydrazine-induced methylation of DNA bases in various rat organs and the effect of pretreatment with disulfiram. *Cancer Res.*, 39:465–467.

107. Teas, J., and Dyson, J. G. (1967): Mutation in Drosophila by methylazoxymethanol, the aglycone of cycasin. *Proc. Soc. Exp. Biol. Med.*, 125:988–990.

108. Utsunomiya, J., Murata, M., and Tanimura, M. (1980): An analysis of the age distribution of colon cancer in adenomatosis coli. *Cancer*, 45:198–205.

109. Walpole, A. L., Williams, M., and Roberts, D. C. (1952): The carcinogenic action of 4-aminodiphenyl and 3:2'-dimethyl-4-aminodiphenyl. *Br. J. Ind. Med.*, 9:255–263.

110. Ward, J. M. (1974): Morphogenesis of chemically induced neoplasms of the colon and small intestine in rats. *Lab. Invest.*, 30:505–513.

111. Ward, J. M., Sporn, M. B., Wenk, M. L., Smith, J. M., Feeser, D., and Dean, R. J. (1978): Dose response to intrarectal administration of N-methyl-N-nitrosourea and histopathological evaluation of the effect of two retinoids on colon lesions induced in rats. *J. Natl. Cancer Inst.*, 60:1489–1492.

112. Ward, J. M., Yamamoto, R. S., and Brown, C. A. (1973): Pathology of intestinal neoplasms and other lesions in rats exposed to azoxymethane. *J. Natl. Cancer Inst.*, 51:1029–1039.

113. Warwick, G. P. (1971): Effect of the cell cycle on carcinogenesis. *Fed. Proc.*, 30:1760–1765.

114. Wattenberg, L. W. (1975): Inhibition of dimethylhydrazine-induced neoplasia of the large intestine by disulfiram. *J. Natl. Cancer Inst.*, 54:1005–1006.

115. Wattenberg, L. W., and Fiala, E. S. (1978): Inhibition of 1,2-dimethylhydrazine-induced neoplasia of the large intestine in female CF1 mice by carbon disulfide. *J. Natl. Cancer Inst.*, 60:1515–1517.

116. Wattenberg, L. W., Lam, L. K. T., Fladmoe, A. V., and Borchert, P. (1977): Inhibitors of colon carcinogenesis. *Cancer*, 40:2432–2435.

117. Weingarten, M., and Turell, R. (1952): Carcinomatous mucosal excrescence of the rectum. *JAMA*, 179:1467–1469.

118. Weisburger, J. H., Reddy, B. S., Spingarn, N. E., and Wynder, E. J. (1980): Current views on the mechanisms involved in the etiology of colorectal cancer. In: *Colorectal Cancer: Prevention, Epidemiology, and Screening*, edited by S. J. Winawer, D. Schottenfield, and P. Sherlock. pp. 19–41. Raven Press, New York.

119. Wiebecke, B., Brandts, A., and Eder, M. (1974): Epithelial proliferation and morphogenesis of hyperplastic, adenomatous and villous polyps of the human colon. *Virchows Arch. [Pathol. Anat.]*, 364:35–49.

120. Yamada, S., Ito, M., and Nagayo, T. (1971): Histological and autoradiographical studies on intestinal tumors of rat induced by oral administration of N,N'-2,7-fluorenylenebisacetamide. *Gan.*, 62:471–478.
121. Ying, T. S., Sarma, D. S. R., and Farber, E. (1979): Induction of presumptive preneoplastic lesions in rat liver by a single dose of 1,2-dimethylhyudrazine. *Chem. Biol. Interact.*, 28:363–367.
122. Ying, T. S., Sarma, D. S. R., and Farber, E. (1981): Role of acute hepatic necrosis in the induction of early steps in liver carcinogenesis by diethylnitrosamine. *Cancer Res.*, 41:2096–2102.
123. Zedeck, M. S., Sternberg, S. S., McGowan, J., and Poynter, R. W. (1972): Methylazoxymethanol acetate: induction of tumors and early effects on RNA synthesis. *Fed. Proc.*, 31:1485–1492.
124. Zedeck, M. S., Grab, D. J., and Sternberg, S. S. (1977): Differences in the acute response of the various segments of rat intestine to treatment with the intestinal carcinogen methylazoxymethanol acetate. *Cancer Res.*, 37:32–36.

Precancerous Lesions of the Gastrointestinal Tract, edited by P. Sherlock, B.C. Morson, L. Barbara, and U. Veronesi. Raven Press, New York © 1983.

Role of Host-Tumor Interaction in the Growth Control of Chemically Induced Colon Cancer

F. Martin, A. Caignard, J. F. Jeannin, O. Olsson, and M. S. Martin

Research Group on Immunology of Digestive Tumors, CNRS-ERA 628 and INSERM U-45, Laboratory of Immunology, Faculté de Médecine, 21033 Dijon, France

Among other carcinogens, 1-2 dimethylhydrazine may induce in laboratory rodents colorectal carcinomas that are morphologically very close to human intestinal cancer (1,11). These carcinomas are invasive, kill the animals in a few months, and metastasize to lymph nodes and distant organs. If these tumors are induced in inbred, syngeneic animals, they can be grafted from animal to animal, keeping the histological and histochemical patterns and the metastatic potential of the original tumor (10). These tumors may also be established as cell culture lines, which are still able to produce carcinoma when they are injected in the syngeneic host (10). Chemically induced colorectal cancers, serially transplantable tumor grafts, and established cell cultures are suitable models for studying the interactions between host and intestinal cancer.

Several observations made on this experimental model suggest that host factors are able to control the growth of these tumors. First, even well-established colon cancer, transplanted to a syngeneic host, may sometimes regress. Second, there is a large difference in the doubling time of colon cancer growing *in vivo* as a tumor transplant (8–20 days) and *in vitro* as a cell culture (24–36 hr). Third, it is experimentally possible to enhance the growth of tumor graft, which suggests the suppression of natural inhibitory mechanisms (10). These control mechanisms may involve hormones, vasoactive mediators, or specific or nonspecific immunologic effectors.

HORMONAL CONTROL OF COLON CANCER GROWTH

Svet-Moldavski (15) demonstrated that repeated injections of gastrin significantly increased the mean tumor weight of colon carcinoma transplanted in syngeneic mice. This effect is probably specific, since gastrin does not change the growth of a hepatoma, a sarcoma or a duodenal carcinoma. This suggests that gastrointestinal hormones could play a role in the control of colon cancer growth. We have shown that two digestive hormonal peptides, glucagon and gastrin-related tetrapeptide, were able to enhance *in vitro* the growth rate of cancer cells obtained from a colonic tumor chemically induced in the rat (1a).

EFFECT OF VASOACTIVE MEDIATORS

Tutton and Barkla (17) found that the mitotic rate of rat colon carcinoma was increased by histamine and severely decreased by cimetidine, a potent histamine-2 receptor antagonist.

However, we observed no change in colon cancer cell cultures incubated in histamine or cimetidine (*unpublished data*). Therefore, the effect of histamine and cimetidine could be indirect, perhaps through histamine-dependent suppressor T lymphocytes (16).

EFFECT OF SPECIFIC IMMUNITY

Steele and Sjögren (13) and our experimental data (2) demonstrated that several antigenic modifications of cell surface were associated with chemically induced rat colon cancer. Some of these antigens were able to evoke a specific immune response (circulating antibodies or T lymphocytes) in the tumor-bearing host (6). These antigens are shared by rat intestinal cancer cells from different origin and also by fetal intestinal cells. Whether or not the immune response evoked by these antigens plays a role in the natural control of colon cancer growth is still controversial. Specific immunotherapy, using colon cancer cells or grafts to immunize animals, gave variable results. Although some degree of protection was obtained in some experiments (14), a patent enhancement of tumor growth and metastases was observed in others (8). For instance, an experiment challenging syngeneic rats with 10^6 colon cancer cells resulted in small tumors (mean weight: 0.4g) in only 10 of 17 control animals, and in large tumors (mean weight: 3.1g) in all the rats immunized by both transplantation of irradiated colon cancer grafts and injection of mitomycin-treated colon cancer cells. This experiment reminds us of the potential hazards of enhancement in the immunotherapy of animal or human tumors. It also means that natural control of colon cancer growth does exist, since it may be abrogated by immunologic manipulation of the host.

IMMUNOLOGIC NONSPECIFIC MECHANISMS: ROLE OF THE MACROPHAGE

Macrophages infiltrating the tumor may also play a role in the modulation of colon cancer growth. We observed that rabbits immunized with saline extracts of colorectal carcinomas chemically induced in the rat raised antibodies directed against an antigen common to a large variety of digestive tumors but absent in the normal intestine (3). At first we thought it was a tumor-associated antigen, but we later found that it was also present in saline extracts of spleen or lung, using Ouchterlony's technique. Using immunofluorescence, we discovered that the antigen was not present in the cancer cells but was present in large, mononuclear cells infiltrating the tumor. Similar cells were found in the spleen, surrounding lymphocytic nodules, and in the alveolar wall of the lung. Though peripheric polymorphs were also labeled, we assumed on morphologic and topographic data that antigen-containing cells found in the colorectal cancers were chiefly macrophages, except in the necrotic areas where labeled cells were chiefly polymorphs. When fluorescence studies were performed on the intestine of rats killed at different intervals after the beginning of carcinogen administration, mononuclear, fluorescent cells were found, from the very early stages of the tumor, surrounding small foci of mucous dysplasia, whereas they were absent from the mucosa of untreated animals.

The next step was to determine if colon cancer cells could be killed by macrophages. As intratumoral macrophages are very difficult to isolate, we have used peritoneal macrophages from syngenic rats. Peritoneal macrophages from untreated rats were not cytotoxic to colon cancer cells even after 3 days of mixed culture. On the contrary, peritoneal macrophages were strongly cytotoxic to colon cancer cells, when they came from rats treated by two intraperitoneal injections of bacillus Calmette-Guerrin (BCG) (5). As in other tumor models, tumor cell destruction by BCG-activated macrophages requires a direct contact between effector and target cells. Cinemicrographic studies demonstrated that tumor cells were not phagocytozed by macrophages but autolyzed a few hours after their contact with the macrophage.

At this stage, it was important to find out if BCG-activated macrophages could also be efficient on colon cancer cells growing *in vivo*. BCG was administered to rats in a large variety of experimental schedules: subcutaneously before or after challenge with colon cancer cells, intratumorally in transplanted colon cancer, as an adjuvant of surgical resection of these grafts, in association with specific immunotherapy, and orally and rectally during chemically induced colon carcinogenesis (7–9). In most of the experiments, BCG did not change the course of the tumor. When BCG was associated with specific immunotherapy with mitomycin-treated tumor cells, a major enhancement of tumor growth and metastases was observed.

Therefore, BCG, which was very efficient in inducing tumoricidal activity in macrophages, was unable to control tumor growth *in vivo*. Why tumor macrophages are not cytotoxic after BCG administration *in vivo* is not yet understood. The best explanation could be the production by tumor cells of factors(s) inhibiting macrophage-mediated cytotoxicity. Recently, Pollard and Luckert (12) published results demonstrating an inhibition of chemically induced colon cancer growth in rats receiving indomethacin, an inhibitor of prostaglandin synthesis. Prostaglandins are recognized inhibitors of macrophage-mediated tumor cell lysis and could therefore be involved in the resistance of cancer to macrophage toxicity.

ROLE OF BACTERIAL ENDOTOXINS

Endotoxins are lipopolysaccharidic components of the outer wall of gram-negative bacteria. They are very potent activators of macrophage for tumor cell killing. *In vitro* endotoxins are effectively able to induce peritoneal macrophages to kill intestinal tumor cells (4). Large amounts of endotoxins are produced by the bulk of gram-negative bacteria present in the intestinal lumen where they can directly interact with colorectal cancer. Experiments were performed to find out if bacterial endotoxins could interfere with the growth of a colorectal carcinoma transplanted in the syngenic animal. As a matter of fact, systemic treatment with endotoxin 1 or 6 days before a challenge with intestinal tumor cells shortened the median time for tumor appearance in comparison with untreated controls (20 days instead of 37 days, $p < 0.001$).

CONCLUSIONS

Manipulations of the host are able to modify the growth of experimental colorectal cancer. This suggests the existence of a natural resistance towards these tumors, even if the precise mechanisms of this resistance are incompletely known. Unfortunately, with the notable exception of indomethacin, it is still easier to weaken this resistance than to strengthen it.

ACKNOWLEDGMENTS

The work described in this chapter was supported by grant CRL 79-5-472-7 from the Institut National de la Santé et de la Recherche Médicale (INSERM).

REFERENCES

1. Druckrey, H., Preussmann, R., Matzkies, F., and Ivankovic, S. (1967): Selektive Erzeugung von Darmkrebs bei Ratten durch 1.2 Dimethylhydrazin. *Naturwissensch.*, 54:285–286.

1a. Kobori, O., Voillot, M. T., Martin, F. (1982): Growth response of rat stomach cancer cells to gastro-entero-pancreatic hormones. *Int. J. Cancer*, 30:65–67.

2. Martin, F., Knobel, S., Martin, M. S., and Bordes, M. (1975): A carcinofetal antigen located on the membrane of cells from rat intestinal carcinoma in culture. *Cancer Res.*, 35:333–336.

3. Martin, F., Martin, M. S., Bordes, M., and Knobel, S. (1975): Antigens associated with intestinal carcinomas chemically induced in rats. *Int. J. Cancer*, 15:144–151.

4. Martin, F., Martin, M. S., Jeannin, J. F., and Lagneau, A. (1978): Rat macrophage-mediated toxicity to cancer cells: effect of endotoxins and endotoxin inhibitors contained in culture media. *Eur. J. Immunol.*, 8:607–611.

5. Martin, F., Martin, M. S., Lagneau, A. (1978): Role of the macrophage in control of colon cancer growth. An in vitro study. *Eur. J. Cancer (Suppl. 1)*, 14:139–144.

6. Martin, F., Martin, M. S., Lagneau, A., Bordes, M., and Knobel, S. (1976): Circulating antibodies in rats bearing grafted colon carcinoma. *Cancer Res.*, 36:3039–3042.

7. Martin, M. S., Justrabo, E., Lagneau, A., Michel, M. F., and Martin, F. (1977): Effects of oral and rectal BCG administration on chemically-induced rat intestinal carcinoma. *Digestion*, 16:189–193.

8. Martin, M. S., Martin, F., Justrabo, E., Michel, M. F., and Lagneau, A. (1977): Immunoprophylaxis and therapy of grafted rat colonic carcinoma. *Gut*, 18:232–235.

9. Martin, M. S., Martin, F., Justrabo, E., Michel, M. F., and Lagneau, A. (1978): BCG-therapy as an adjuvant of surgery in treatment of 5 transplantable lines of rat colon cancer. *Eur. J. Cancer (Suppl. 1)*, 14:123–126.

10. Martin, M. S., Martin, F., Justrabo, E., Turc, C., and Lagneau, A. (1976): Lignées transplantables et cultures cellulaires obtenues à partir de carcinomes intestinaux chimio-induits chez le rat. *Biol. Gastroenterol.*, 9:186–192.

11. Martin, M. S., Martin, F., Michiels, R., Bastien, H., Justrabo, E., Bordes, M., and Viry, B. (1973): An experimental model for cancer of the colon and rectum. Intestinal carcinoma induced in the rat by 1,2 dimethylhydrazine. *Digestion*, 8:22–34.

12. Pollard, M., and Luckert, P. H. (1980): Indomethacin treatment of rats with dimethylhydrazine-induced intestinal tumors. *Cancer Treat. Rep.*, 64:1323–1327.

13. Steele, G., and Sjögren, H. O. (1974): Cross-reacting tumor-associated antigen(s) among chemically-induced rat colon carcinomas. *Cancer Res.*, 34:1801–1807.

14. Steele, G., and Sjögren, H. O. (1977): Cell surface antigen in a rat colon cancer model: correlation with inhibition of tumor growth. *Surgery*, 82:164–169.

15. Svet-Moldavsky, G. J. (1980): Dependence of gastrointestinal tumors on gastrointestinal hormones. Pentagastrin stimulates growth of transplanted colon adenocarcinoma in mice. *Biomedicine*, 33:259–261.

16. Thomas, Y., Huchet, R., and Granjon, D. (1981): Histamine-induced suppressor cells of lymphocyte mitogenic response. *Cell. Immunol.*, 59:268–275.

17. Tutton, P. J. M., and Barkla, D. H. (1976): A comparison of cell proliferation in normal and neoplastic intestinal epithelium following either biogenic amine depletion or monoamine oxidase inhibition. *Virchows Arch. (Zell Pathol)*, 21:161–168.

Precancerous Lesions of the Gastrointestinal Tract, edited by P. Sherlock, B.C. Morson, L. Barbara, and U. Veronesi. Raven Press, New York © 1983.

Tritiated Thymidine (ϕ_p,ϕ_h) Labeling Distributions and Associated Measurements in the Early Identification of Populations at High Risk for Cancer of the Large Intestine

Martin Lipkin

Memorial Sloan-Kettering Cancer Center, New York, New York 10021

Colorectal cancer poses a major health problem in the United States and many other countries. Recent figures in the U.S. indicate over 100,000 new cases annually and a high mortality rate. The likelihood of patients successfully surviving the disease varies with its extent at the time of diagnosis and initial therapy; detection of disease at an early stage is of primary importance for improved survival.

In recent years, new approaches to early detection and control of large bowel neoplasia have been explored. They include the identification of population groups at increased risk for colorectal cancer and a further search for environmental and physiologic factors that might contribute to the pathogenesis of colorectal neoplasms. In addition, therapeutic intervention in high-risk populations is being considered and attempts to prevent the progression of colorectal neoplasms have been initiated.

In this article new findings in each of the above-mentioned areas were reviewed. Emphasis was given to the early identification of risk factors in population groups having increased susceptibility to colorectal neoplasia, and proposed methods for the early detection and prevention of lesion development and progression. The various risk factors studied are associated with predisposition to familial cancer, and abnormalities that have been observed in the development of colonic and other cells have been studied.

MEMORIAL SLOAN-KETTERING REGISTRY OF POPULATION GROUPS AT HIGH RISK FOR CANCER OF THE LARGE INTESTINE

To facilitate this work, we have developed a comprehensive registry of individuals and familial groups at this Institution who are at high risk for cancer of the large intestine (30).

Hereditary Polyposis Syndromes (Familial Polyposis and Gardner's Syndrome)

At present, 31 families with familial polyposis are listed in our registry. They include 71 symptomatic subjects and 325 asymptomatic subjects who are at risk for the disease; 71 spouse family members also are available for measurement of risk parameters. Descriptions of the familial polyposis syndromes have previously been given (6,19,20,31,34). The pattern of inheritance of a familial aggregate having familial polyposis is shown in Fig. 1. Figure 2 illustrates the early age of appearance that characterizes the onset of cancer in familial polyposis, which helps to distinguish it from the onset of cancer in the general population.

Familial Colon Cancer Without Polyposis

Our population registry of familial groups having high frequencies of colon cancer without familial polyposis includes 15 families with mainly site-specific colon cancer, including 41 affected, and 178 asymptomatic at-risk subjects, available for this activity. In addition, 12 families with high frequencies of colonic and other cancers with 30 affected and 209 asymptomatic individuals are available. The pedigree of a typical familial aggregate is shown in Fig. 3. These individuals do not have the extensive colonic polyposis that characterizes familial polyposis (18,33) and are believed to have a hereditary form of colon cancer with an autosomal dominant mode of inheritance (2,33). The early age of onset of cancer of the large intestine is also shown in Fig. 2.

Multiple Cancers Including Colorectal

We now have a population registry of subjects available for call-up at Memorial Hospital of 324 individuals who have had colorectal plus other primary malignancies. In these individuals, the primary malignancies include breast (21% of individuals), gynecological (16% of individuals), genitourinary (11% of individuals), and other regions of the gastrointestinal tract (9% of individuals). The early age of onset of colorectal cancer in these individuals with colorectal plus other primary malignancies is shown in Fig. 4.

Single and Multiple Colorectal Adenomas

The presence of one or more adenomas occurs in 5% to 10% of the general population and is associated with the development of adenocarcinomas. Humans have also been reported showing an association of single and multiple adenomas with adenocarcinoma with an apparent genetic susceptibility (43). It has been estimated that 5% of all of these adenomas become malignant, and the development of villous characteristics in the adenomas is associated with increased frequency of malignancy. Colonic adenomas also appear with a peak incidence 5 to 10 years earlier than colon cancer in the general population. These adenomatous polyps have a similar epidemiologic distribution to colon cancer (9,34). Our registry of single and multiple adenomas recently included 634 individuals, and we now are developing age-incidence data for the appearance of multiple adenomas in these individuals.

Primary Colorectal Cancer in the General Population

Individuals in this category who have had colorectal cancer without other malignancy also are available for comparison with the aforementioned population groups (Fig. 5).

The age-incidence distribution in this group is closer to the age incidence of colon cancer in the general population of the U.S. and Japan. Our population registry recently consisted of 374 individuals having primary colorectal cancer; 59 individuals have a family history of colorectal cancer, 123 individuals have a family history of cancer other than colorectal, and 192 have no family history of cancer. In several studies, it has been shown that familial associations of colorectal cancer among index cases of colorectal cancer in the general population are higher than in control groups. Environmental, as well as inherited factors, could be associated with the development of neoplasms in these groups.

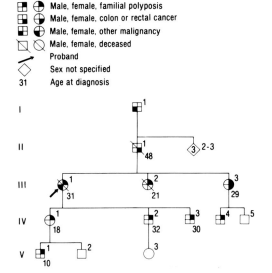

Male, female, familial polyposis
Male, female, colon or rectal cancer
Male, female, other malignancy
Male, female, deceased
Proband
Sex not specified
31 Age at diagnosis

FIG. 1. Typical pattern of inheritance in familial polyposis, together with ages of onset of polyposis in family members (ref. 32).

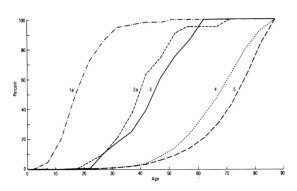

FIG. 2. Computer printout illustrating cumulative percent of incident cases at various ages of familial polyposis, compared with cumulative age incidence of colon cancer in other population groups. Curve 1a shows the onset of nonmalignant polyposis and curve 2a shows the onset of cancer in familial polyposis, in Memorial Hospital registry of high-risk population groups. Curve 3 shows early ages of onset of cancer in 28 affected individuals from Memorial Hospital who have familial colon cancer without polyposis. Curve 4 illustrates the age of onset of colon and rectal cancer in the general population of the U.S., from the Third National Cancer Survey, NCI, and includes white and black males and females combined. Curve 5 illustrates the onset of colon and rectal cancer in males and females in Japan (data supplied by T. Hirayama, *personal communication*). (Modified from Lipkin et al., ref. 30.)

Familial Aggregates Cancer-free for Two or More Generations

Familial aggregates with 41 individuals cancer-free for two or more generations also have been identified and are available for this activity. Additional spouse controls from individuals in the above population groups and medical student volunteers also are available. In addition, measurements have been started on populations at low risk for colorectal cancer in geographic

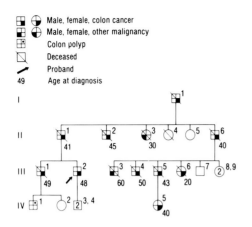

FIG. 3. Typical pattern of inheritance of cancer in a Memorial Hospital familial aggregate highly predisposed to colon cancer without polyposis with ages of onset of cancer in some family members (30).

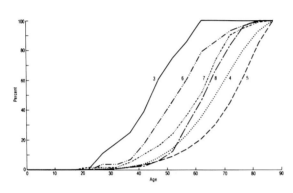

FIG. 4. Computer printout of cumulative percent of incident cases having multiple cancers, including colorectal, from Memorial Hospital series. Curves 3, 4, and 5 show the same population groups seen in Fig. 2. Curve 6 shows the onset of colorectal cancer in individuals with multiple primary cancers and family history of colorectal cancer. Curve 7 shows the onset of colorectal cancer in individuals with multiple primary cancers and family history of cancer other than colorectal. Curve 8 shows onset of colorectal cancer in individuals with multiple primary cancers and no family history of cancer. (Modified from Lipkin et al., ref. 30.)

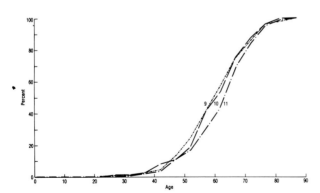

FIG. 5. Computer printout of cumulative percent of incident cases from Memorial Hospital series having primary colorectal cancer without a second malignancy. Curve 9: primary colorectal cancer and family history of colon cancer. Curve 10: primary colorectal cancer and family history of cancer other than colorectal. Curve 11: primary colorectal cancer and no family history of cancer. (Modified from Lipkin et al., ref. 30.)

areas that include Medellin in Colombia, South America, and other regions in Japan for further comparison with the high-risk groups.

The development of these population registries has enabled us to call up individuals and familial aggregates in the above categories for measurements of phenotypic abnormalities associated with high frequency and early age of development of colorectal cancer. Verification of individual and family history of previous colorectal cancer and other pathological findings is made routinely by obtaining pathology records, death certificates, and by consulting physicians of record of family members indicated.

Proliferative Abnormalities in Colonic Epithelial Cells

Modifications in cell proliferation associated with a genetic predisposition to large bowel cancer have been found not only during the growth of benign and malignant neoplasms but also before the appearance of clinically detectable lesions.

During the progressive stages of abnormal development, cell phenotypes are seen in which epithelial cells gain an increased ability to proliferate and to accumulate in the mucosa (4,8,11,12,22,25,28). The identification of these changes has aided our understanding of events that occur during neoplastic transformation of cells in colorectal cancer.

In the normal human colon, these cells proliferate in the lower and mid-regions of the colonic crypts as shown in Fig. 6. About 15% to 20% of the proliferating cells are in DNA synthesis simultaneously, and they migrate to the surface of the mucosa to be extruded. Our earlier studies in humans showed that the colonic mucosa is replaced by new cells in 4 to 8 days (26,27). During migration of these cells, the number that continue to proliferate decreases as they progress to the luminal region of the crypts; they undergo terminal differentiation within hours, and the proliferation ceases as they migrate to the crypt surfaces (27).

However, in subjects with familial polyposis, patches of flat mucosa are found having colonic epithelial cells that fail to repress DNA synthesis during migration to the surface of the mucosa (4,8,11,12,22,25). This is illustrated in Figs. 6 and 7 and occurs in normal-appearing colonic epithelial cells before as well as after the cells develop adenomatous changes and begin to accumulate as polyps.

Observed in over 80% of random biopsy specimens (26,27), a failure of cells to repress DNA synthesis has now been shown to occur with higher frequency in patients with familial polyposis than in population groups at low risk for colorectal cancer (Table 1). More recently, a significant increase in abnormal proliferative activity has also been noted in the colonic mucosa of strongly colon-cancer-prone families without polyposis (Table 1). This finding, in a highly cancer-prone population group that does not develop the early warning signals provided by the appearance of adenomas, has led to newer measurements. Thus, our current work is now focusing on the (ϕ_p, ϕ_h) labeling distribution (28) and related measurements in other high-, average-, and low-risk populations to develop discriminatory indices to identify affected and at-risk subjects in colon-cancer-prone families who carry an abnormal gene predisposing them to neoplasia. To facilitate this work, the data from specific population groups are analyzed using computer-assisted methods to evaluate differences between population groups of interest. Examples of the types of computer-generated outputs that are now possible, related to (ϕ_p, ϕ_h) and other indices, are shown in Figs. 8 and 9.

In the disease familial polyposis, the further modifications of proliferative activity believed to occur prior to the development of malignancy also are shown in Fig. 6. Following the failure of cells that have inherited the germinal mutation to repress DNA synthesis during migration in the colonic crypts, additional events take place, giving rise to new clones from the original cell population. An early event leads to the development of the well-known adenomatous cells that proliferate and accumulate near the surface of the mucosa (Fig. 6). In familial polyposis, according to this concept, additional changes then occur in the cells, giving rise to modifications in cell surface and related properties that lead to invasive malignancy. This concept allows for a contribution of endogenous or exogenous carcinogenic

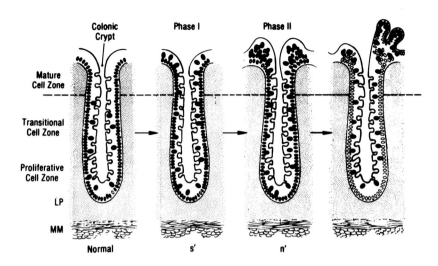

FIG. 6. A sequence of events *(left to right)* to account for the location of abnormally proliferating colonic epithelial cells before and during the formation of polypoid neoplasms in humans. The diagram at the left shows the location of proliferating and differentiating epithelial cells in normal colonic crypt. Dark cells illustrate thymidine labeling in cells that are synthesizing DNA and preparing to undergo cell division. As cells pass from the proliferative zone through the transitional zone, DNA synthesis and mitosis are repressed, and migrating epithelial cells leave the proliferative cell cycle to undergo normal maturation before they reach the surface of the mucosa. The development of a phase I proliferative lesion in the colonic epithelial cells as they fail to repress the incorporation of thymidine ³H into DNA and begin to develop an enhanced ability to proliferate is shown next. The mucosa is flat, and the number of new cells born equals the number extruded without excess cell accumulation in the mucosa. Then the development of a phase II proliferative lesion in colonic epithelial cells is depicted. The cells incorporate thymidine ³H into DNA and also have developed additional properties that enable them to accumulate in the mucosa as neoplasms begin to form. The diagram at the right shows the further differentiation of abnormally retained proliferating epithelial cells into pathologically defined neoplastic lesions, including adenomatous polyps and villous papillomas (25).

or promoter elements interacting with the cells having a hereditary predisposition to neoplasia. It also allows for the introduction of preventive measures to inhibit the steps leading to malignant transformation of the cells.

COMPARISON OF CARCINOGEN-INDUCED PROLIFERATIVE ABNORMALITIES AND PATHOLOGIC CHANGES IN COLONIC MUCOSA

Proliferative and pathologic abnormalities in colonic epithelial cells similar to those observed in humans have now been observed to be induced in rodent colonic epithelial cells. Rodent strains have different susceptibilities to the induction of colon cancer as occurs among humans. In rodents, the cell transformations can be induced by 1,2-dimethylhydrazine (DMH), methylazoxymethanol (MAM), N-methyl-N'-nitro-N-nitrosoguanidine (MNNG), and N-methyl-N-nitrosourea (MNU) (7,13,23,36). Tumor nodules develop in mice following exposure to DMH. The main site of activity is the distal colon, the same distribution noted to occur in humans. In mice, multifocal tumors ranging from adenomatous polyps to metaplasias and carcinomas grow from the mucosa and then protrude into the lumen of the rectosigmoid. Early focal atypias and hyperplasias located mainly on the folds, adenomatous polyps, and carcinomas, appear to be part of the progressive pathologic changes in mice and rats that

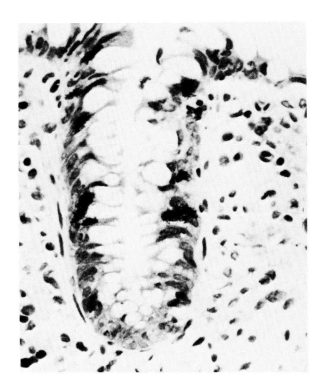

FIG. 7. Thymidine ³H incorporation into epithelial cells near the crypt surface of flat colonic mucosa in a biopsy specimen from a high risk subject. (Data from Hasegawa et al., ref. 21.)

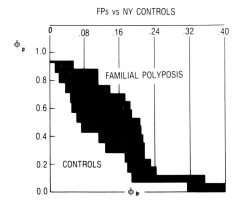

FIG. 8. Diagram of computer-generated curves comparing crypt column occupancy fractions of tritiated thymidine-labeled epithelial cells in a high-risk and a low-risk group. Abscissa ϕ_h records the fraction labeled cells found within the upper 40% of assayed crypt columns adjacent to and including the lumenal surface. The ordinate ϕ_p records the fraction of all individuals in a given group whose measured ϕ_h values equal or exceed the abscissa value. Significant differences are present between high- and low-risk groups ($p < .005$). (Data from Lipkin et al., ref. 28.)

develop following administration of DMH. These changes are accompanied by an increased proliferative activity in the cells. DMH and MNNG both induce an extension of the proliferative zone of the flat mucosa toward the surfaces of the colonic crypts as seen in Fig. 10.

Thus, some of the colonic epithelial cells of rodents exposed to repeated injections of DMH also develop the capacity to continue to synthesize DNA throughout most of their life-span. Thymidine-labeled cells show an increase in both their position up from the crypt base and their total number; these cells also show a shift into expanding adenomas and carcinomas. The tumors that develop manifest a proliferation of neoplastic epithelial cells near the surface of the lesion, with a continued expansion into the colonic lumen.

A failure of colonic epithelial cells to repress DNA synthesis also occurs in epithelial-cell-renewing tissues in other human diseases. Among these are ulcerative colitis (17). In

TABLE 1. *Labeling distribution percent of TdR³H-labeled cells in upper third of colonic crypts (L.D. μ 1/3) in flat normal appearing mucosa of high- and low-risk populations*

Pop. group	No. of individuals	Ratio of mean value of (L.D. μ 1/3) in test group to mean value in control group (C)
Familial polyposis		
Symptomatic (FP$_s$)[a]	18	2.49[b]
Asymptomatic (FP$_a$)[c]	11	2.68[b]
Polyp-free branch	10	1.22[d]
Nonfamilial colon cancer	13	1.41[d]
Normal subjects	15	1.00[d]

[a]Affected individuals.

[b]Percentage of labeled cells significantly greater than normal subjects, nonfamilial colon cancer cases, or polyp-free and cancer-free branches of families ($p < 0.05$).

[c]Possible carriers (about 50% risk of developing disease).

[d]Percentage of labeled cells not significantly greater than normal subjects.

```
UNIFIED   CODE   FOR   PATIENT   I.D.


Digit #      Explanation
--------     -----------

1,2          Location
3,4,5        Clinical category and sub-category
6,7,8        Patient #
9,10         Tissue Section


** LOCATION

Code      Location
----      --------
00        Unspecified
01        Memorial Hospital, New York
02        Nebraska
03        Salt Lake City, Utah
04        Japan
05        Medellin, Colombia
06        Loma Linda, California
07        B.I.
08        Philadelphia
09        China
```

FIG. 9. Computer output illustrating a portion of the patient identification code, used to record information on subjects in high- and low-risk populations. The digits shown, and others that follow, classify subjects according to geographic location, clinical disease or nondisease categories, patient number, and location and types of colonic biopsy and other specimens under study.

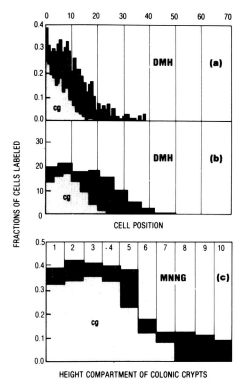

FIG. 10. Extension of proliferative compartment of colonic crypts toward lumenal surface of crypts, after repeated exposure to chemical carcinogens. (*cg*) Control groups; (*black areas*) carcinogenic groups. (**a**) Fraction of cells labeled at various cell positions within colonic crypts, 1 hr after injection of thymidine ³H, and after start of weekly 1,2-dimethylhydrazine (DMH) injection into mice (20 μg/g) (36). (**b**) Fractions of cells labeled at various cell positions within colonic crypts, 125 days after beginning of DMH treatment in mice (7). (**c**) Fraction of cells labeled in segments of colonic crypt after rectal installation of N-methyl-N-¹-nitro-N-nitrosoguanidine (MNNG) in rats (23).

atrophic gastritis, a condition associated with the development of malignancy of the stomach, epithelial cells also fail to repress DNA synthesis and undergo abnormal maturation as they migrate through the gastric mucosa (15,42). Analogous changes are found in the stomachs of rodents after exposure to a chemical carcinogen (14). A similar event occurs in precancerous disease of the human cervical epithelium (39) and in the cervixes of rodents, after introduction of a chemical carcinogen (21). Thus, during the development of neoplasms in organs that contain renewing epithelium other than the colon, persistent DNA synthesis occurs in cells that normally would be terminal or end cells. As occurs in the colon in familial polyposis, similar pathological changes accompany this development and also lead to atypias, dysplasias, and malignancy.

Studies of Cutaneous Cells of Individuals with Familial Polyposis

Phenotypic expressions of the genetic defect leading to familial polyposis have also been found in cutaneous cells. Increased heteroploidy in cutaneous epithelial cells derived from individuals with Gardner's syndrome has been reported (10). Several recent studies have shown differences in the distribution of the cytoskeletal protein actin within cultured skin fibroblasts from individuals with familial polyposis when compared to normal subjects (24).

Immunologic Studies

An immunologic abnormality has recently been reported in individuals from colon-cancer-prone families without polyposis (3). When cancer-free individuals from families predisposed to large bowel cancer, but without familial polyposis, were studied to determine the nature of their cell-mediated immune capacities, 44% showed failure of potentially normal lymphocytes to react to an allogeneic stimulus. This *in vitro* defect in recognitive immunity was similar to that seen in individuals with established malignancies. Several patients with Gardner's syndrome also showed the defect in recognitive immunity. These findings, as well as those noted above, are being applied in evaluations of asymptomatic individuals in familial aggregates having the various disorders leading to large bowel cancer in order to develop the risk factor profiles described below.

Examination of Fecal Contents

In familial polyposis and related disorders, still other studies are in progress to identify constituents of fecal contents that may be abnormal and to examine their potential carcinogenic activity on cells in the colon. A group of compounds currently under examination consists of the bile acids and their bacterial conversion products. Accordingly, several recent reports have compared the fecal neutral sterols and bile acids in patients with familial polyposis to those of controls (16,29,35,38). Individuals with familial polyposis excreted significantly higher amounts of cholesterol and lower levels of the degradation products of cholesterol, which are mainly coprostanol and coprostanone. This is illustrated by our recent data on fecal cholesterol degradation in these high-risk subjects (Table 2). Nondegradation of cholesterol has also been found in a minor fraction of individuals in the general population, whose background and related characteristics have not been defined (40).

Current results also have suggested differences in metabolic activity of fecal microflora in members of familial polyposis aggregates when compared to age- and sex-matched controls who have consumed similar Western style diets. Differences in metabolic activity of fecal microflora have previously been shown in population groups at increased risk for large bowel neoplasia (16,35). Thus, newer studies also are in progress to extend these findings to individuals in the familial colon-cancer-prone groups in order to further assess the utility of these variations in metabolic activity of fecal microflora and in cholesterol and its metabolites.

Recently, an additional and potentially important lead to the identification of factors involved in colon cancer development was provided by detection of mutagenic activity in the feces of humans (37). Studies of this type analyzed mutagenic activity with the well-known Ames assay (1). Wilkins et al. (41) had shown that fecal specimens from the U.S. population were more mutagenic than those from South African Blacks. Bruce and Dion (5) and Wilkins et al. (41) have also described that much of the mutagenic activity in humans, as detected with the Ames test, is due to the presence of a single compound. Recent findings on fecal mutagenic activity in subjects with familial polyposis and familial colon cancer without polyposis are shown in Table 3 (M. Lipkin and T. D. Wilkins, *unpublished data*). The findings have not thus far revealed striking differences between high-risk groups and controls, and larger numbers of subjects are being studied. Thus, in addition to the evaluation of cellular and secretory parameters, a variety of approaches to the analysis of fecal contents of individuals in high- and low-risk groups for cancer of the large intestine are under way.

Development of Risk-Factor Profiles

These current findings have led to the development of a risk factor profile previously described characterizing the first of the high-risk populations with increased susceptibility to colorectal cancer (31). Further risk-factors profiles are being developed for the other population groups with increased susceptibility to cancer of the large intestine.

TABLE 2. *Fecal neutral sterols in subjects at high risk for cancer of the large intestine and in controls*

Pop. groups	No. of individuals	Age	Sex M	Sex F	Cholesterol (mg/g dry feces)	% Degradation
Familial polyposis						
Symptomatic (FP$_s$)	9	12–51	5	4	13.29 ($\pm$1.65)	20.4[a] ($\pm$8.1)
Asymptomatic FP$_a$)						
Low converters	5	17–46	3	2	12.85 ($\pm$2.83)	11.2[a] ($\pm$5.8)
High converters	9	12–23	5	4	1.6 ($\pm$0.23)	90.2 ($\pm$2.8)
Familial colon cancer						
Symptomatic (FCC$_s$)	5	31–59	1	4	16.42 ($\pm$1.97)	32.6[a] ($\pm$7.7)
Asymptomatic (FCC$_a$)						
Low converters	9	7–43	2	7	15.34 ($\pm$1.87)	25.1[a] ($\pm$5.6)
High converters	4	23–59	1	3	3.92 ($\pm$1.88)	82.4 ($\pm$6.7)
Normal subjects	31	10–62	17	14	3.2 ($\pm$0.50)	84.9 ($\pm$2.2)

Average values ($\pm$SE) of cholesterol and degradation products in each population group are shown. In the last column for each population group, the average percent degradation is shown where a given patient's percent degradation is defined as degradation products $\div$ by total neutral sterols $\times$ 100. A tentative lower limit of 60% for degradation of cholesterol in the control group has been derived from the mean value minus 2 SD. Low converters have been defined as having percent degradation below 60% and high converters having values above.

[a]The percent degradation of cholesterol differs significantly from the controls ($>$.001) with Student's *t*-test.

From Lipkin et al. (29), with permission.

TABLE 3. *Fecal mutagens in high risk populations*

Pop. groups	No. of individuals	Age	No. with high activity M	No. with high activity F	Elevated mutagenic ratios TA 98	98 S	100	100 S
Familial polyposis								
Symptomatic (FP$_s$)	11	22	1			2.0		
Asymptomatic (FP$_a$)	8							
Familial colon cancer								
Symptomatic (FCC$_s$)	2	70	1					2.0
Asymptomatic (FCC$_a$)	27	39		1	2.4		1.5	
		60		1				2.0
		28	1				$>$9.0	
		63		1	1.9			
		41	1		2.1			
		36		1	2.3			
		41	1		3.2		2.6	2.2
		28	1		2.3			1.9
Normal subjects	9			1	2.4			

From T. D. Wilkins and M. Lipkin *(unpublished data)*.

In current measurements, we are carrying out multivariate analyses of these various risk factors in subjects who have been affected by cancer and in those who are unaffected and at high risk, in the population groups above. Simultaneous measurements are underway in subjects in families that have been cancer-free for two and more generations as well as others in the general population. Dietary and related variables are being analyzed. We are attempting to determine whether these findings represent general trends within the high-risk population groups or whether any of them may be an absolute marker for identifying individuals destined to develop cancer of the large intestine. In this context, subjects in these populations, in whom neoplastic lesions occur at early ages, are being identified for future prospective analyses. A concurrent program of long-term surveillance of these individuals is also being developed.

REFERENCES

1. Ames, B. N., McCann, J., and Yamasaki, E. (1975): Method of detecting carcinogens and mutagens with the Salmonella Mammalian-microsome mutagenicity test. *Mutat. Res.*, 31:374.
2. Anderson, D. E., and Romsdahl, M. D. (1977): Familial history: A criteria for screening. In: *Genetics of Human Cancer*, edited by J. J. Mulvihill, R. W. Miller, and J. F. Fraumeni, pp. 257–262. Raven Press, New York.
3. Berlinger, N. T., Lopez, C., Vogel, J., Lipkin, M., and Good, R. A. (1977): Defective recognitive immunity in family aggregates of colon carcinoma. *J. Clin. Invest.*, 59:761–769.
4. Bleiberg, H., Mainguet, P., and Galand, P. (1972): Cell renewal in familial polyposis: comparison between polyps and adjacent healthy mucosa. *Gastroenterology*, 63:240–245.
5. Bruce, W. R., and Dion, P. (1980): Studies related to fecal mutagen. *Am. J. Clin. Nutr.*, 33:2511–2512.
6. Bussey, H. J. R. (1975): *Familial Polyposis Coli*. The Johns Hopkins University Press, Baltimore.
7. Chang, W. W. L. (1978): Histogenesis of sym 1-2 DMH-induced neoplasms of the colon in the mouse. *J. Natl. Cancer Inst.*, 60:1405–1418.
8. Cole, J. W., and McKalen, A. (1963): Studies on the morphogenesis of adenomatous polyps in the human colon. *Cancer*, 16:998–1002.
9. Correa, P., and Haenszel, W. (1978): The epidemiology of large-bowel cancer. *Adv. Cancer Res.*, 26:1–141.
10. Danes, B. (1977): Brief communication; the Gardner syndrome, a family study in cell culture. *J. Natl. Cancer Inst.*, 58:771.
11. Deschner, E. E., Lewis, C. M., and Lipkin, M. (1963): *In vitro* study of human rectal epithelial cells. I. Atypical zone of H₃ thymidine incorporation in mucosa of multiple polyposis. *J. Clin. Invest.*, 42:1922–1928.
12. Deschner, E. E., and Lipkin, M. (1970): Study of human rectal epithelial cells *in vitro*. III. RNA, protein and DNA synthesis in polyps and adjacent mucosa. *J. Natl. Cancer Inst.*, 44:175–185.
13. Deschner, E. E., and Long, F. C. (1977): Colonic neoplasms in mice produced with six injections of 1,2-dimethylhydrazine. *Oncology*, 34:255–257.
14. Deschner, E. E., Tamua, K., and Bralow, S. P. (1979): Early proliferative changes in rat pyloric mucosa induced with N-methyl-N'-nitro-N-nitrosoguanidine. *Front. Gastrointest. Res.*, 4:25–31.
15. Deschner, E. E., Winawer, S., and Lipkin, M. (1972): Patterns of nucleic acid and protein synthesis in normal human gastric mucosa and atrophoic gastritis. *J. Natl. Cancer Inst.*, 48:1567–1574.
16. Drasar, B. S., Bone, E. S., Hill, M. F., and Marks, C. G. (1975): Colon cancer and bacterial metabolism in familial polyposis. *Gut*, 16:824–825.
17. Eastwood, G. L., and Trier, J. S. (1973): Epithelial cell renewal in cultured rectal biopsies in ulcerative colitis. *Gastroenterology*, 64:383–390.
18. Fraumeni, Jr., J. F. (1977): Clinical patterns of familial cancer. In: *Genetics of Human Cancer*, edited by J. J. Mulvihill, R. W. Miller, and J. F. Fraumeni, pp. 223–235. Raven Press, New York.
19. Gardner, E. J. (1951): A genetic and clinical study of intestinal polyposis: A predisposing factor for carcinoma of the colon and rectum. *Am. J. Human Genet.*, 3:167–176.
20. Gardner, E. J., and Richards, R. C. (1953): Multiple cutaneous and subcutaneous lesions occurring simultaneously with hereditary polyposis and osteomatosis. *Am. J. Human Genet.*, 5:139.
21. Hasegawa, I., Matsumira, Y., and Tojo, S. (1976): Cellular kinetics and histological changes in experimental cancer of the uterine cervix. *Cancer Res.*, 36:359–364.
22. Iwana, T., Utsunomiya, J., and Sasaki, J. (1977): Epithelial cell kinetics in the crypts of familial polyposis of the colon. *Jpn. J. Surg.*, 7:230–234.

23. Kikkawa, N. (1974): Experimental studies on polypogenesis of the large intestine. *Med. J. Osaka Univ.*, 24:293–314.

24. Kopelovich, L., Lipkin, M., Blattner, W., Fraumeni, Jr., J. F., Lynch, H., and Pollack, R. (1980): Organization of actin-containing cables in cultured skin fibroblasts from individuals at high risk of colon cancer. *Int. J. Cancer*, 26:301–307.

25. Lipkin, M. (1974): Phase I and phase 2 proliferative lesions of colonic epithelial cells in diseases leading to colon cancer. *Cancer*, 34:878–888.

26. Lipkin, M. (1977): Growth kinetics of normal and premalignant gastrointestinal epithelium. In: *Growth Kinetics and Biochemical Regulation of Normal and Malignant Cells*, edited by B. Drewinko and R. M. Humphreys, pp. 562–589. Williams & Wilkins Co., Baltimore.

27. Lipkin, M. (1978): Susceptibility of human population groups to colon cancer. *Adv. Cancer Res.*, 27:281–304.

28. Lipkin, M., Blattner, W., Fraumeni, Jr., J. F., Lynch, H., and Deschner, E. E. (1983): Tritiated thymidine (ϕ_p,ϕ_h) labeling distribution as a marker for hereditary predisposition to colon cancer. *Cancer Res. (in press)*.

29. Lipkin, M., Reddy, B. S., Weisburger, J., and Schechter, L. (1981): Nondegradation of fecal cholesterol in subjects at high risk for cancer of the large intestine. *J. Clin. Invest.*, 67:304–307.

30. Lipkin, M., Scherf, S., Schechter, L., and Braun, D. (1980): Memorial Hospital Registry of populations at high risk for cancer of the large intestine. *Preventive Med.*, 9:335–345.

31. Lipkin, M., Sherlock, P., and DeCosse, J. (1980): Risk factors and preventive measures in the control of cancer of the large intestine. *Curr. Prob. Cancer*, 4(10):1–57.

32. Lipkin, M., Winawer, S. J., and Sherlock, P. (1981): Early identification of individuals at increased risk for cancer of the large intestine, part I: Definition of high risk population. *Clin. Bull.*, 11(1):13–21.

33. Lynch, H. T. (1976): *Cancer Genetics*. PP. 1–639. Charles C. Thomas Co., Springfield.

34. Morson, B. C., and Bussey, H. (1970): Predisposing causes of intestinal cancer. *Curr. Prob. Surg.*, 63:1–50.

35. Reddy, B. S., Mastromarino, A., Gustafson, C., Lipkin, M., and Wynder, E. S. (1976): Fecal bile acids and neutral sterols in patients with familial polyposis. *Cancer*, 38:1694–1698.

36. Thurnherr, N., Deschner, E. E., Stonehill, E., and Lipkin, M. (1973): Induction of adenocarcinomas of the colon in mice by weekly injections of 1,2-dimethylhydrazine. *Cancer Res.*, 33:940–945.

37. Varghese, A. J., Land, P., Furrer, R., and Bruce, W. R. (1977): Evidence for the formation of mutagenic N-nitroso compounds in the human body. Abst. *Proc. A.A.C.R.*, 18:80.

38. Watne, P. L., Lai, H. S., Mance, T., and Core, S. (1976): Fecal steroids and bacterial flora in polyposis coli patients. *Am. J. Surg.*, 131:42–.

39. Wilbanks, G. D., Richart, R. M., and Terner, J. Y. (1967): DNA content of cervical intraepithelial neoplasm studied by two-wave length Feulgen cytophotometry. *Am. J. Obstet. Gynecol.*, 98:792–799.

40. Wilkins, T. D., and Hackman, A. S. (1974): Two patterns of neutral steroid conversion in the feces of normal North Americans. *Cancer Res.*, 34:2250–2254.

41. Wilkins, T. D., Lederman, M., and Van Tassel, R. L. (1981): Isolation of a mutagen producer in the human colon by bacterial action. In: *Banbury Report 7: Gastrointestinal Cancer*, edited by W. R. Bruce, P. Correa, M. Lipkin, S. Tannenbaum, and T. D. Wilkins, pp. 205–212. Cold Spring Harbor Laboratory, Cold Spring Harbor, New York.

42. Winawer, S., and Lipkin, M. (1969): Cell proliferation kinetics in the gastrointestinal tract of man. IV. Cell renewal in intestinalized gastric mucosa. *J. Natl. Cancer Inst.*, 42:9–17.

43. Woolf, C. M., Richards, R. C., and Gardner, E. J. (1955): Occasional discrete polyps of the colon showing inherited tendency in kindred. *Cancer*, 8:403–408.

Precancerous Lesions of the Gastrointestinal Tract, edited by P. Sherlock, B. C. Morson, L. Barbara, and U. Veronesi. Raven Press, New York © 1983.

Markers for Increased Risk of Colorectal Cancer

B. C. Morson

Department of Pathology, St. Mark's Hospital, London EC1V 2PS, England

When considering problems of premalignancy, it is essential to define exactly what is meant by this term. A distinction can be made between a precancerous condition and a precancerous lesion (21). The former is best regarded as a clinical state associated with a significantly increased risk of cancer, whereas a precancerous lesion is a histopathological abnormality in which cancer is more likely to occur than in its apparently normal counterpart. In many clinical conditions with an increased risk of cancer there is also an identifiable precancerous lesion, but this is not invariably so.

In the colorectum there are five groups of patients among whom both clinical as well as histological markers for increased cancer risk can be identified. These are patients with colorectal adenomas, those who have had one cancer removed by partial removal of the large bowel, familial polyposis families, colorectal cancer families, and certain patients with chronic ulcerative colitis. The magnitude of the risk is very variable and attempts to measure this have immense importance for cancer prevention. The aim must be to identify markers for especially high cancer risk because of the administrative, economic, and technical problems involved in screening large numbers of persons, most of whom are not destined to get colorectal cancer.

The histological marker for increased risk that is common to all these patients is epithelial dysplasia or atypia, and the criteria used by pathologists in its recognition are fundamentally no different from those applied to premalignancy in the skin, cervix, liver, urothelium, and other epithelial-lined cavities. The colorectal adenoma is a form of localized, polypoid dysplasia and is the precancerous lesion common to all the groups of patients mentioned above, except those with ulcerative colitis. In this disease dysplasia is nearly always diffuse and arises in a flat as often as a polypoid mucosa, but the histology is fundamentally the same. As in other organs dysplasia in the colon can be graded as mild, moderate, or severe with the latter being equated with carcinoma *in situ*, although this is not an expression favoured for the colon because of its emotive meaning for some (14). There is now ample evidence from clinical, histological, experimental, and epidemiological research that the majority of colorectal cancers have passed through what is now known as the adenoma-carcinoma sequence (14), but which might be more accurately called the dysplasia-carcinoma sequence in order to conform with the life history of malignant disease as we see it in other epithelial organs.

Colorectal polyps, as observed endoscopically and radiologically are very common. It must be emphasized that only those identified by the histopathologist as belonging to the adenoma group of tumours have any malignant potential. This is still a large number of persons and further refinement of the magnitude of the cancer risk is required. In the present state of knowledge it would appear that risk of malignant change is closely related to size of adenoma, being negligible in tumours 1 cm or less in diameter but becoming greater with increasing size over this critical point. Most adenomas are small and experience suggests that only a minority of them grow to sufficient size for the cancer risk to become significant. It follows that polyps over 1 cm in diameter which have been detected by endoscopic or radiological examination should always be removed. It has also been shown that histological type of adenoma is important; villous and tubulo-villous adenomas have greater potential for malignant change than tubular adenomas. When epithelial dysplasia is graded as severe, the malignant potential is greatest. Severe dysplasia is mostly found in the larger adenomas and in those with a villous component in their histological structure (16).

Unfortunately many patients with colorectal adenomas have minor clinical symptoms or no symptoms at all. On the assumption, however, that all adenomas (and cancers) bleed, which is almost certainly correct, an improved method has been introduced for the detection of occult blood in the stools (6,20). The impregnated guaiac slide (hemoccult) test answers many of the criticisms of the older methods of testing for occult blood. Further study will be needed to evaluate the application of this test in the development of mass screening programmes, but it could be argued that a positive hemoccult test places a patient in an "increased risk group" for colorectal adenoma or cancer and this should be followed at least by sigmoidoscopy and barium enema, if not by colonoscopy. The numbers of patients considered to be at risk by this method might be very large with a consequent strain on existing resources of money and expertise. Preliminary data, however, suggest that a screening test based on the potential for polyps and cancers to bleed has considerable promise in the detection of the adenoma-carcinoma sequence at a curable stage.

One important reason why patients who have had a bowel resection for cancer should be advised to submit to indefinite follow-up and periodic investigation is that they are at increased risk from a second primary cancer, which is usually manifest many years after the original operation (5). In these patients the concept of the adenoma-carcinoma sequence is the basis on which risk is evaluated. Thus, the risk is highest in those who had one or more adenomas as well as the cancer in the first operation specimen. The magnitude of the risk increases with time after about 5 years post-operative and on the average the second cancer is discovered about 11 years after the first (7).

There is evidence that the greater the number of colorectal adenomas in a patient the greater the risk of cancer (16). This arithmetical approach becomes of great significance in patients with more than 100 adenomas because, by definition, they are then found to have the hereditary disease known as familial polyposis coli. The cancer risk in such patients is known to be almost inevitable. It happens that whereas it is not unusual to come across individuals with up to 10 adenomas, it is rare to see them with more than this number unless they have familial polyposis, in which case they usually have many thousands of adenomas, including those of microscopic dimensions (microadenomas).

In the past it has become customary to regard polyposis as a wholly separate disease on the assumption that the adenomas present in this condition differ from those found as isolated lesions. Apparent differences have been reported (1,9), but these have failed to stand up to closer scrutiny, and the only differences between the adenomas of polyposis and nonpolyposis patients would appear to be the number of tumours and possibly the mode of inheritance. This being so, it would seem reasonable, therefore, to regard polyposis, with its heavy concentration of adenomas, as a fruitful field for the study of the adenoma-carcinoma sequence.

In the investigation, treatment, and follow-up of polyposis families the important objective is to get affected individuals treated before they develop cancer. Cancer prevention has limited scope in the propositus group, as two-thirds of these patients already have cancer when first seen. The incidence of malignancy among the siblings, however, is considerably less than that found in propositus family members and the reduction is even greater among the children of affected members. The records of the St. Mark's Hospital Polyposis Register show a dramatic decrease in malignant disease among call-up family members as compared with the propositus group. When polyposis is diagnosed before cancer has occurred, the adenoma-carcinoma sequence can be broken by surgical removal of the adenomas. This may be effected by either total proctocolectomy or colectomy and ileorectal anastomosis. The former makes certain that no further adenomas are produced, but leaves the patient with the permanent handicap of an ileostomy; the latter demands half-yearly review for the destruction of any polyps in the rectum. Moertel et al. (13) report that this procedure carries a heavy risk of subsequent malignancy in the rectum, which they estimate to be an accumulative 59% at 23 years after operation. This has not been confirmed by Schapp and Volpe (19), who record only 1 case of subsequent rectal carcinoma although 30 patients had been followed up for 10 years or more. Bussey (4) has also reported a lower figure, 3.6% at 25 years. Cancer prevention can be said to have been highly effective in the cooperative polyposis family up to the present and should be even more so in the future. Indeed with a complete record of all polyposis families and their total cooperation, it should be possible to reduce the incidence of associated cancer of the colon and rectum to a negligible figure. The good results obtained in the St. Mark's Hospital series not only provide evidence that the destruction of adenomas is an effective method of cancer prevention but also point the way to a possible reduction of the incidence of intestinal cancer in the general population.

There are valuable opportunities for cancer prevention among so-called colorectal cancer families (10,11). Every patient with colorectal cancer should be questioned for evidence of a family history of adenomas or cancer of the colon or rectum. A positive history should lead to careful documentation of all relatives, particularly siblings and children of affected members, in the same way that construction of a family pedigree provides the essential information required for the care of a polyposis family. In the St. Mark's Hospital cancer family register there are 70 families with 2 affected members, 18 with 3, and 10 with 4. The age of onset of colorectal cancer in these patients is significantly younger than in the general population and they have an increased incidence of multiple tumours. These patients have not got polyposis, but there is evidence that the incidence of adenomas is increased compared with patients without a family history, giving further support to the concept of the adenoma-carcinoma sequence (H. J. R. Bussey et al., *unpublished data*). Members of cancer families, particularly siblings, should be invited for investigation or at least warned never to neglect symptoms relating to the large bowel. Parents, one of whom has had a cancer or is at increased risk because of the family history, should be encouraged to have their children examined, but current information suggests that this is unnecessary until about the age of 20 years.

Most patients with ulcerative colitis never develop carcinoma of the large bowel. However, it is established that such tumours are more common in colitics than in the general population and tend to occur at an earlier age. Many published studies have confirmed that the cancer risk is largely confined to those with extensive colitis, a history of symptoms for more than 10 years, and histological evidence of severe dysplasia in colorectal biopsies. It is probable that carcinoma as a complication of colitis could be largely eliminated by advising proctocolectomy for all patients with extensive colitis, either early in the course of the disease for acute symptoms or after 10 years in patients with mild disease (2). This policy would greatly increase the number of patients undergoing major surgery, most of whom are not destined to get colorectal cancer. These operations have a mortality and morbidity both in the short- and the long-term (17,18), and excision of the rectum can lead to sexual dysfunction (3,12). The presence of a stoma can cause physical, psychological, and social disability. An alternative policy reserves operation for a patient with ill health due to colitis or when the large intestine shows evidence of neoplastic potential, as judged by the presence of consistent and severe epithelial dysplasia in colorectal biopsies (15).

A prospective study has now shown that the cancer risk in colitis can be minimized by careful follow-up of all patients with a long history of extensive disease and prophylactic proctocolectomy performed when evidence of severe dysplasia is established (8). This is a small and manageable population of patients, like polyposis and colorectal cancer families, among whom a cancer prevention programme is a proven success.

The information made available in recent decades by *cancer* registries has been of enormous value in defining large populations, usually at a national level, who are at increased risk from different varieties of malignant disease. Has the time now arrived for the establishment of official *precancer* registers on a regional or national basis? This would certainly be practicable for polyposis coli families, colorectal cancer families, and colitics at increased risk, and there is now incontrovertible evidence that this would lead to cancer prevention. But there is also the prospect that the registration of patients with isolated large bowel adenomas or even those with a positive stool hemoccult test might be beneficial and cost-effective. If cancer prevention is to be more than a political or professional slogan, then it is time consideration was given to such proposals by our public health authorities.

REFERENCES

1. Birbeck, M. S. C., and Dukes, C. E. (1963): Electron microscopy of rectal neoplasms. *Proc. R. Soc. Med.*, 56:793–798.
2. Bonnevie, O., Binder, V., and Anthonisen, P. (1974): The prognosis of ulcerative colitis. *Scand. J. Gastroenterol.*, 9:81–91.
3. Burnham, R., Lennard-Jones, J. E., and Brooke, B. N. (1977): Sexual problems among married ileostomists. *Gut*, 18:673.
4. Bussey, H. J. R. (1975): *Familial Polyposis Coli*. Johns Hopkins University Press, Baltimore.
5. Bussey, H. J. R., Wallace, M. H., and Morson, B. C. (1967): Metachronous carcinoma of the large intestine and intestinal polyps. *Proc. R. Soc. Med.*, 60:208–210.
6. Greegor, D. H. (1972): Detection of colorectal cancer using quaiac slides. *Cancer*, 22:360–363.
7. Heald, R. J., and Lockhart-Mummery, H. E. (1972): The lesion of the second cancer of the large bowel. *Br. J. Surg.*, 59:16–19.
8. Lennard-Jones, J. E., Morson, B. C., Ritchie, J. K., Shove, D. C., and Williams, C. B. (1977): Assessment of the individual risk by clinical and histological criteria. *Gastroenterology*, 73:1280–1289.
9. Leuchtenberger, C., Leuchtenberger, R., and Liebv, E. (1956): Studies of cytoplasmic inclusions containing desoxribose nucleic acid (DNA) in human rectal polypoid tumours including familial hereditary type. *Acta Genet. Statist. Med.*, 6:291–297.
10. Lovett, E. (1976): Family studies in cancer of the colon and rectum. *Br. J. Surg.*, 63:13–18.
11. Lovett, E. (1976): Familial cancer of the gastro-intestinal tract. *Br. J. Surg.*, 63:19–22.
12. May, R. E. (1966): Sexual dysfunction following rectal excision for ulcerative colitis. *Br. J. Surg.*, 53:29–30.
13. Moertel, C. G., Hill, J. R., and Adson, M. A. (1970): Surgical management of multiple polyposis. *Arch. Surg.*, 100:521–526.
14. Morson, B. C., editor (1978): *The Pathogenesis of Colorectal Cancer*. Monograph, Vol. 10 of *Major Problems in Pathology*. W. B. Saunders Company, Philadelphia.
15. Morson, B. C., and Pang, L. S. C. (1967): Rectal biopsy as an aid to cancer control in ulcerative colitis. *Gut*, 8:423–434.
16. Muto, T., Bussey, H. J. R., and Morson, B. C. (1975): The evolution of cancer of the colon and rectum. *Cancer*, 36:2251–2270.

17. Ritchie, J. K. (1971): Ileostomy and excisional surgery for chronic inflammatory disease of the colon: a survey of one hospital region. Part 1—Results and complications of surgery. Part 11—The health of ileostomists. *Gut.* 12:528–540.
18. Ritchie, J. K. (1972): Ulcerative colitis treated by ileostomy and excisional surgery: fifteen years experience at St. Mark's Hospital. *Br. J. Surg.*, 59:345–351.
19. Schaupp, W. C., and Volpe, P. A. (1972): Management of diffuse colonic polyposis. *Am. J. Surg.*, 124:218–222.
20. Winawer, S. J., Sherlock, P., Schottenfeld, D., and Miller, D. (1976): Screening for colon cancer. *Gastroenterology*, 70:783–789.
21. World Health Organization (1964): *Prevention of Cancer: Report of a WHO Expert Committee, Geneva.* WHO Technical Series No. 276.

Precancerous Lesions of the Gastrointestinal Tract, edited by P. Sherlock, B. C. Morson, L. Barbara, and U. Veronesi. Raven Press, New York © 1983.

Rectal Cell Renewal as Biological Marker of Cancer Risk in Ulcerative Colitis

Guido Biasco, Mario Miglioli, Andrea Minarini, Andrea Dalaiti, Giulio Di Febo, Giuseppe Gizzi, and Luigi Barbara

Department of Gastroenterology, The University of Bologna, S. Orsola Hospital, 40138 Bologna, Italy

In recent years several studies have been devoted to the epithelial cell proliferation of the colon in cancerous and precancerous conditions (7–11,15). These works have shown that cytoproliferative abnormalities can precede alterations of the mucosa detectable by conventional microscopic examination (15). These abnormalities can therefore be considered phenotypic markers of increased colorectal cancer risk (16).

The analysis of the cytoproliferative pattern has been mainly performed on the colorectal mucosa of patients with isolated polyps, patients with familial polyposis, symptom-free relatives of familial polyposis patients, patients with a history of cancer, as well as some symptom-free individuals from geographic areas having high-risk frequencies of colorectal cancer (9–11).

However, few studies have been devoted to patients affected by ulcerative colitis (U.C.). This is surprising because in U.C. patients the risk for colorectal cancer is higher than that of the general population (12); moreover, an altered renewal of the rectal cells has been observed in this disease (4,13). The recognition of proliferative abnormalities and the precise definition of their biological significance would therefore be useful for detecting, among U.C. patients, those at particularly high risk for cancer.

CELL TURNOVER RATE

The gastrointestinal mucosa is characterized by the existence of a cell renewing system in which the cells continuously lost from the surface are replaced by newly formed cells from the crypts (17).

In the colonic mucosa of patients with active U.C., cellular exfoliation is enhanced compared to normals (6). The physiological reaction to this event is an increased cell turnover rate. Autoradiographic studies of rectal biopsies after incubation with tritiated thymidine in patients with active U.C. have clearly shown the existence of this adaptive response (4,13) and its relation to the inflammatory status of the mucosa (3) (Fig. 1 a–c). The turnover time (ToT) of the tissue is in fact increased during the active stages of the disease and returns to quite normal during remission (Fig. 2). Additionally with the double labeling technique it has been shown that the duration of the S phase (dS) is normal and does not change even during the active stage of the disease (3). Therefore in U.C. the alteration of cell production rate, which is calculated by the ratio $dS/labeling\ index\ (L.I.) \times 100$ (14), can be assessed

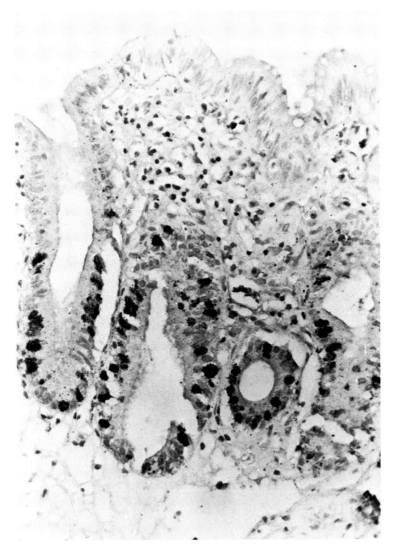

FIG. 1 *(above and following pages)* Proliferative patterns of the rectal epithelial cells in patients with ulcerative colitis (U.C.) and in a normal subject. Autoradiography after incubation with tritiated thymidine. **a:** Active U.C. in patient with short clinical history: high number of labeled cells in the crypts.

by the evaluation of the L.I. only. The L.I. must, however, be determined in the proliferative compartment, whose extension can be obtained from the model proposed by Cleaver for the small bowel (5).

DISTRIBUTION OF THE PROLIFERATING CELLS IN THE CRYPTS

In the normal human colon the proliferative compartment is located in the lower two-thirds of the crypts (15,17). Several works have suggested that the presence of proliferating

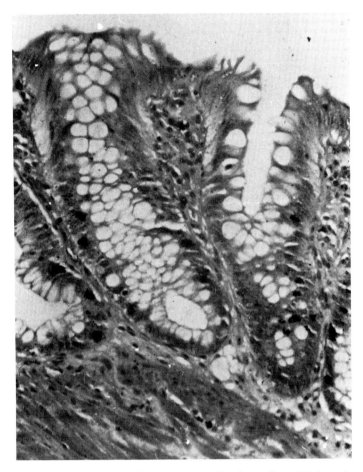

FIG. 1 *(continued)* **b:** Quiescent U.C. in patient with short clinical history: low number of labeled cells in the crypts.

cells in the upper third of the crypts and along the luminal surface can indicate the existence of a failure of the mechanisms repressing DNA synthesis during migration to the surface and can represent the first expression of the proneness of the mucosa toward neoplastic transformation (15). In fact, this deviation is frequently found in histologically normal mucosa of patients with polyps or malignancies of the colon and it has been described in the colon of mice following the injection of 1,2-dimethylhydrazine (DMH) before the development of intestinal neoplasms (9–11,15).

The upward extension of the proliferating cells can follow two different patterns (7):

1. scattered proliferating cells in the upper third of the crypts, but persistence of most of these in the lower third (stage 1 abnormality); and
2. shift of the area of maximal proliferation to the middle and/or upper portions of the crypts (stage 2 abnormality).

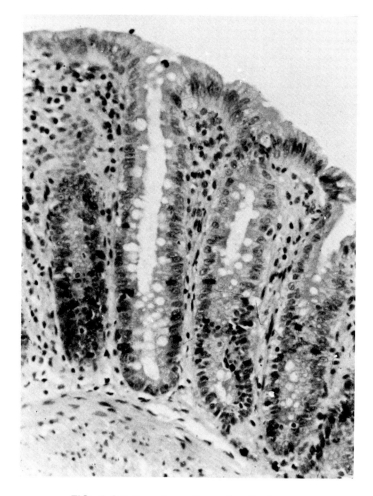

FIG. 1 *(continued)* **c:** Normal subject.

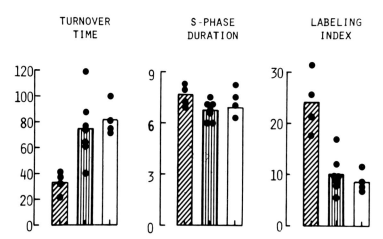

FIG. 2. Turnover time (ToT) (hr), S-phase duration (dS) (hr), and labeling index (L.I.) (%) of the rectal epithelial cells in ulcerative colitis (U.C.). Evaluation by H_3-thymidine double labeling technique. *(Diagonally striped columns)* Active U.C.; *(vertically striped columns)* quiescent U.C.; *(open columns)* normal subject.

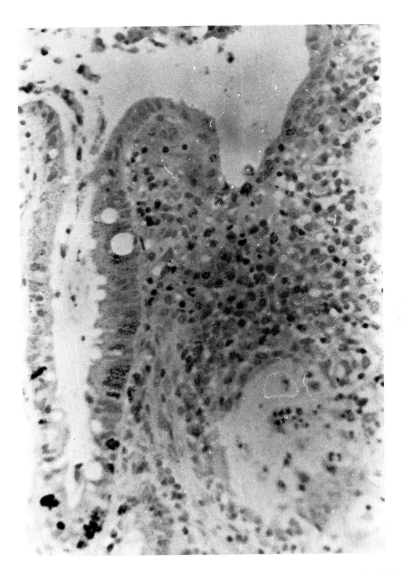

FIG. 3 *(above and following page)* Proliferative patterns of the rectal epithelial cells in patients with ulcerative colitis (U.C.) Autoradiography after incubation with tritiated thymidine. **a:** Active U.C. in patient with short clinical history: stage 1 abnormality.

The biological and clinical significance of stage 1 abnormality is actually under discussion. Particularly a rapid upward migration of the cells has been demonstrated in active U.C. (13), hence in these patients the alteration might be related to an increased migration rate, which does not allow the cell to complete the proliferative cycle (Fig. 3a). This hypothesis is supported by the correlation existing between L.I. and the percentage of replicating cells in the upper portion of the crypts (Fig. 4).

On the other hand, stage 2 abnormality cannot be explained on the same basis. It does not seem to be related to mucosal inflammation (Fig. 3b) and it is observed only in patients with longstanding U.C. (over 10 years) (2), that is, in patients at particularly high risk for

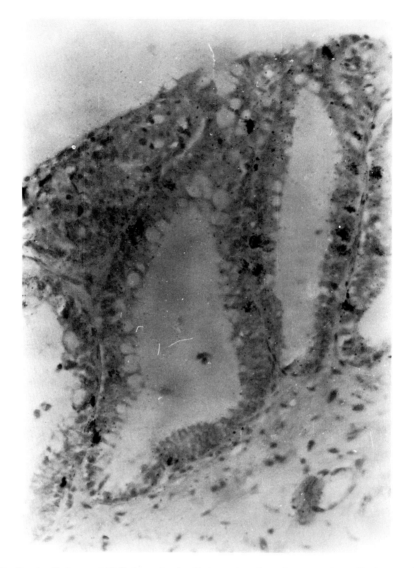

FIG. 3.   b: Quiescent U.C. in patient with longstanding disease: stage 2 abnormality.

colorectal cancer (12) (Fig. 5). Moreover, it has been demonstrated that the colonic cells of patients with longstanding clinical history do not respond to stimuli inhibiting DNA synthesis (1). For these reasons it is likely that stage 2 abnormality represents a true defect in the mechanisms regulating cell proliferation. It must be noted also that stage 2 proliferative abnormality is not related to the extent of U.C. (Table 1). Therefore, it is conceivable that the higher cancer risk of patients with universal colitis compared to partial colitis may be due to the fact that in the former a greater area of mucosa is at risk.

CONCLUSIONS

Alterations of the renewal of colorectal mucous cells can be observed in patients with U.C. Some of these represent physiological reactions to the mucosa inflammatory damage and

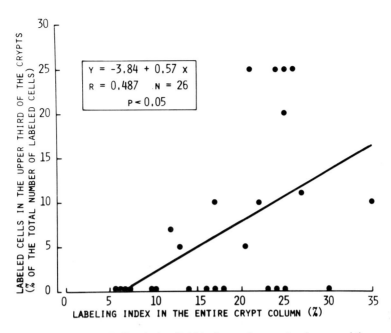

FIG. 4. Comparison of the labeling index (L.I.) in the entire crypt column and the percentage of labeled cells in the upper third. Rectal mucosa of patients with ulcerative colitis (U.C.) and normal distribution of labeled cells in the crypts or stage 1 abnormality.

TABLE 1. *Distribution of proliferating cells in 42 U.C. patients with various extent of the disease*

	Extensive U.C. (%)	Left-sided U.C. (%)	Proctosigmoiditis (%)
Stage 2 abnormality	4 (40)	4 (40)	2 (20)
Stage 1 abnormality	6 (37)	5 (31)	5 (31)
Normal pattern	6 (37)	6 (37)	4 (25)

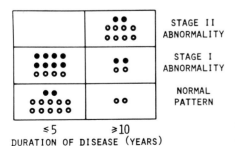

FIG. 5. Relationship between distribution of proliferating cells, duration of the ulcerative colitis (U.C.) and inflammatory status of the mucosa in rectal biopsies of 40 patients.

are reverted to normal when inflammation subsides. On the contrary other abnormalities do not seem related to the presence of inflammation and may represent an increased susceptibility of the mucosa towards malignant transformation.

However, the clinical and biological significance of the latter, particularly of the so-called stage 2 abnormality, must be the subject of further study in order to clarify (a) its value and specificity in the identification of U.C. patients at particularly high risk for colorectal cancer; (b) their extension in the diseased colorectal mucosa. From a clinical standpoint this is very important because if these abnormalities are shown to have a high diffusion in the affected mucosa, their identification on random biopsies would be easy, thus balancing the complexity of the autoradiographic methods; and (c) to what extent they depend on the frequency, duration, and severity of the abnormalities of cell renewal caused by the relapses of the disease. As far as this last point is concerned it would be interesting to evaluate the influence of medical treatment.

REFERENCES

1. Alpers, D. H., Philpott, G., Grimme, N. L., and Margolis, D. M. (1980): Controls of thymidine incorporation in mucosal explants from patients with chronic ulcerative colitis. *Gastroenterology*, 78:470–478.
2. Biasco, G., Miglioli, M., Minarini A., Vallorani, V., Morselli, A. M., Dalaiti, A., and Barbara, L. (1982): Rectal cell proliferation and cancer risk in ulcerative colitis: A preliminary report. *Ital. J. Gastroenterol.*, 14:76–79.
3. Biasco, G., Santini, D., Marchesini, F., Di Febo, G., Baldi, F., Miglioli, M., and Barbara, L. (1979): Kinetics of the mucous cells of the rectum in patients with chronic ulcerative colitis. In: *Frontiers of Gastrointestinal Research: Gastrointestinal Cancer, Advances in Basic Research*, edited by P. Rozen, S. Eidelman, and T. Gilat, pp. 65–72. S. Karger, Basel.
4. Bleiberg, H., Mainguet, P., Galand, P., Chretien, J., and Dupont Mairesse, N. (1970): Cell renewal in human rectum. In vitro autoradiographic study on active ulcerative colitis. *Gastroenterology*, 58:851–855.
5. Cleaver, J. E. (1967): Cell renewal in the small intestine. In: *Thymidine Metabolism and Cell Kinetics*, edited by A. Neuberger and E. L. Tatum, pp. 207–214. North Holland Publishing Company, Amsterdam.
6. Croft, D. N., and Cotton, P. B. (1973): Gastrointestinal cell loss in man: its measurement and significance. *Digestion*, 8:144–160.
7. Deschner, E. E. (1980): Cell proliferation as a biological marker in human colo-rectal neoplasia. In: *Colorectal Cancer: Prevention, Epidemiology and Screening*, edited by S. Winawer, D. Schottenfeld, and P. Sherlock, pp. 133–142, Raven Press, New York.
8. Deschner, E. E. (1980): Cell renewal in precancerous and tumor states of the gastrointestinal mucosa. *Acta Endosc.*, X:139–150.
9. Deschner, E. E., Lewis, C. M., and Lipkin, M. (1963): In vitro study of human rectal epithelial cells. I. Atypical zone of H_3-thymidine incorporation in mucosa of multipla polyposis. *J. Clin. Invest.*, 42:1922–1928.
10. Deschner, E. E., and Lipkin, M. (1975): Proliferative patterns in colonic mucosa in familial polyposis. *Cancer*, 35:413–418.
11. Deschner, E. E., Winawer, S. J., Long, F. C., and Boyle, C. C. (1978): H_3-thymidine labeled colonic epithelial cells and mucosa in mice and man. *Dig. Dis.*, 23(4):305–311.
12. Devroede, G. F., Taylor, W. F., Saver, W. G., Jackman, R. G., and Strickler, G. B. (1971): Cancer risk and life expectancy of children with ulcerative colitis. *N. Engl. J. Med.*, 285:17–21.
13. Eastwood, G. L., and Trier, J. S. (1973): Epithelial cell renewal in cultured rectal biopsies in ulcerative colitis. *Gastroenterology*, 64:383–390.
14. Galand, P. (1967): Comparaison de deux méthodes autoradiographiques basées sur l'emploi de thymidine tritiée, pour la mesure de la durée de la phase S (phase de synthése d'acide désoxyribonucléique) et de l'interphase des cellules de différents tissus de la souris. *Arch. Biol.*, 78:167–191.
15. Lipkin, M. (1974): Phase I and phase II proliferative lesions of colonic epithelial cells in diseases leading to colonic cancer. *Cancer*, 34:878–888.
16. Lipkin, M. (1980): Measurements of cell proliferation and associated risk factors in the identification of population groups with increased susceptibility to colonic cancer. In: *Cell Proliferation in the Gastrointestinal Tract*, edited by D. R. Appleton, J. P. Sunter, and A. J. Watson, pp. 327–342. Pittman Medical Limited, Tunbridge Wells, Kent.
17. Lipkin, M., Bell, B., and Sherlock, P. (1963): Cell proliferation kinetics in the gastrointestinal tract of man. I. Cell renewal in colon and rectum. *J. Clin. Invest.*, 42:767–776.

Precancerous Lesions of the Gastrointestinal Tract, edited by P. Sherlock, B.C. Morson, L. Barbara, and U. Veronesi. Raven Press, New York © 1983.

Proliferative Screening of Ulcerative Colitis Patients

Eleanor E. Deschner

Memorial Sloan-Kettering Cancer Center, New York, New York 10021

Several proliferative patterns have become recognized in the colorectal mucosa of individuals with and without gastrointestinal disease (4). Specific alterations in proliferative behavior are believed related to the development of colonic neoplasia because they have been induced in the mucosa of rodents treated with chemical carcinogens (2,3).

Since the extent of the inflammatory disease within the colon and the duration of the disease are factors believed to be associated with the incidence of malignancy among patients with ulcerative colitis, a technique has been sought that would describe the character of the mucosa of such patients prior to the development of invasive cancer. An *in vitro* procedure allowing the incorporation of tritiated thymidine (^{3}HTdR) to proceed into newly formed DNA has been employed to determine the proliferative pattern characteristic of that biopsy and to provide an assessment of the relative risk for neoplasia of each patient (4).

At present three proliferative patterns have been described in the normal appearing colorectal mucosa. The normal type of cell proliferation is seen in individuals free of gastrointestinal disease and in untreated animals. This is characterized by cell proliferation in the lower two-thirds of the crypts with the lower third functioning as the major zone of DNA synthesis. The second pattern has been seen in patients with familial polyposis, symptom-free relatives of familial polyposis patients, patients with a history of cancer, and patients with an isolated polyp (4). This pattern is characterized by an extension of the proliferative cells to the surface but with the lower third of the gland remaining as the major zone of DNA synthesis (stage 1 defect). A third pattern reported by Maskens and Deschner (5) showed normal appearing crypts with an altered distribution of DNA synthesizing cells such that the basal portion of the gland is no longer the major site of cell renewal (stage 2 defect) (5). This pattern was first described in patients with a history of colorectal cancer. It is believed to be a further, more critical step in the evolution of the mucosa toward the neoplastic state.

Eighteen patients with ulcerative colitis, ages 18 to 72, and 8 patients who were symptom free for gastrointestinal disease were obtained for this study. Patients with inflammatory bowel disease were in a state of remission. The duration of the disease spanned a range from 3 months to 41 years.

PROLIFERATIVE ANALYSES

An analysis of the distribution of these labeled cells within the crypt revealed a normal proliferative pattern in tissue from only 2 of 8 control patients. That is, only 25% had DNA synthesis confined to the lower two-thirds of the gland and the basal third remained the major zone of renewal. The remaining 6 showed extension of the proliferative compartment toward the surface (stage 1 defect). None had the stage 2 defect.

Among the ulcerative colitis patients only 5 of the 18 (27.8%) presented with a completely normal proliferative pattern. The remaining 13 patients (72.2%) expressed the stage 1 defect with extension of the zone of DNA synthesis to the upper third and along the surface of colonic crypts. It was, however, only the ulcerative colitis patients who had an additional proliferative defect in their mucosa. Seven patients of these 13 patients (53.9%) in the colitis group demonstrated a shift in the major zone of DNA synthesis to the middle and upper regions of the crypt (stage 2 abnormality). These 7 patients with the stage 2 defect often displayed extremely elevated levels of labeled cells in the upper third of the gland, that is, over 20%.

CRYPT REGENERATION

New crypt development for repopulation of the mucosa following irradiation or carcinogen treatment has been described as occurring from the basal regions of the glands (1,3). Yet lateral budding of the crypts from the middle third of the gland was seen in some ulcerative colitis patients. This observation is believed to be associated with the shift of the major zone of DNA synthesis to the middle and upper zones of the crypts. The significance of this finding is perhaps best clarified by studies of 1,2-dimethylhydrazine (DMH)-induced colon cancer in mice. After as few as three weekly injections of DMH, lateral outpocketing appeared in the upper region of the cryptal wall. This phenomenon was soon followed by the appearance of microadenomas or foci of cellular atypia, which in time became macroscopically visible adenomas (2).

CORRELATIONS AND ASSESSMENTS

The shift in the major zone of DNA synthesis (stage 2 defect) observed in 7 of the 18 ulcerative colitis patients was correlated with the extent and duration of the disease in each. Four of the 7 patients had ulcerative colitis for more than 10 years, a period beyond which risk for colon cancer increases. Approximately equal percentages of patients with the stage 2 defect had universal colitis and limited colitis (5/12 with universal colitis or 41% vs 2/6 with limited colitis or 33%), suggesting a similar risk for colon cancer in both groups.

Proliferative screening of rectal biopsies may be a useful procedure as a part of a thorough program to detect precancerous changes in the mucosa of patients with a longstanding history of ulcerative colitis. The preneoplastic defects in epithelial cell proliferation and crypt regeneration demonstrated here may in a real sense be the prelude to the dysplastic alterations recognized by Morson and Pang (6).

ACKNOWLEDGMENT

Supported in part by grants No. CA 14991, No. CA 08748, and contract No. CP 43366 awarded by the National Cancer Institute (DHEW) and grant No. CA 15429 from NCI through the National Large Bowel Project.

REFERENCES

1. Cairnie, A. B., Millen, B. H. (1975): Fission of crypts in the small intestine of the irradiated mouse. *Cell Tissue Kinet.*, 8:189–196.
2. Deschner, E. E. (1974): Experimentally induced cancer of the colon. *Cancer*, 34:824–828.

3. Deschner, E. E. (1978): Early proliferative defects induced by six weekly injections of 1,2-dimethylhydrazine in epithelial cells of mouse distal colon. *Z. Krebsforsch.*, 91:205–216.
4. Deschner, E. E. (1980): Cell proliferation as a biological marker in human colorectal neoplasia. In: *Colorectal Cancer: Prevention, Epidemiology and Screening*, edited by S. Winawer, D. Schottenfeld, and P. Sherlock, pp. 133–142. Raven Press, New York.
5. Maskens, A. P., and Deschner, E. E. (1977): Tritiated thymidine incorporation into epithelial cells of normal-appearing colorectal mucosa of cancer patients. *J. Natl. Cancer Inst.*, 58:1221–1224.
6. Morson, B. C., and Pang, L. S. C. (1967): Rectal biopsy as an aid to cancer control in ulcerative colitis. *Gut*, 8:423–434.

Precancerous Lesions of the Gastrointestinal Tract, edited by P. Sherlock, B.C. Morson, L. Barbara, and U. Veronesi. Raven Press, New York © 1983.

Dysplasia in Ulcerative Colitis

Robert H. Riddell

Department of Pathology, Laboratory of Surgical Pathology, University of Chicago, Chicago, Illinois 60637

Dysplasia in ulcerative colitis has become increasingly important in the management of patients at risk of developing carcinoma. The clinical group known to be at high risk consists of patients with extensive or total colonic involvement, and the risk undoubtedly increases with time. These two factors supersede all others to the point that other factors are of little practical consideration in the long-term follow-up of patients at risk. While lip-service may be paid to such factors as early age of onset of disease or persistent active disease, two factors alone, namely, extent of disease (extensive or total large bowel disease) and length of history (arbitrarily more than 7 years of disease) justify entry into a cancer-prevention protocol.

The principle behind the use of dysplasia as an additional marker within this high-risk group assumes that invasive carcinoma arises from a morphologically identifiable precursor. This assumption is both necessary and justifiable, for the development of invasive carcinoma from a coexisting, and presumably preexisting lesion has been described in almost every other organ site. Although the uterine cervix is the organ for which the greatest body of data exists, the noncolitic large bowel follows not far behind. The adenoma-carcinoma sequence presents very strong evidence that adenomas are precursor lesions to large bowel carcinomas, and evidence is also accumulating daily as the result of colonoscopic polypectomy, a small proportion of which contain invasive carcinoma. However, such "early" tumors metastasize uncommonly and most are treated adequately by simple polypectomy.

The analogy can be taken one step further in dealing with ulcerative colitis. The major difference is partly one of semantics, for the adenoma in the adenoma-carcinoma sequence corresponds directly to dysplasia in ulcerative colitis. Indeed, the analogy is so similar that the two lesions (adenoma, dysplasia) may be virtually indistinguishable morphologically. One might therefore ask why there is a need to distinguish between adenomas and dysplasia. The answer is twofold. First, true adenomas that are relatively common in the noncolitic population may occur in colitics; conversely, dysplasia in colitics has far greater significance in the likelihood of its being associated with an invasive carcinoma that it can lead to a false sense of security to call such lesions adenomas. An alternative way of expressing the differences is that by definition all adenomas are dysplastic, but in colitis dysplasia may not take the form of an adenoma. The ambiguity of the word adenoma immediately becomes apparent and partly explains the difficulty. In its broad sense it can mean an adenomatous polyp, that is, a noninvasive epithelial neoplasm projecting into the lumen of the bowel. The term adenoma may also be used in a narrower sense as a noninvasive intraepithelial neoplasm without further qualification. Although dysplasia in colitis may fall into either category, it is the latter definition that would usually describe dysplasia. Simply expressed this means that dysplasia in colitis may occur in flat and otherwise featureless mucosa.

Both dysplasia and adenomas may, because they are both neoplastic by definition, give rise directly to invasive adenocarcinomas, often without a stage of morphological *in situ* carcinoma. As indicated above, the second reason for distinguishing dysplasia from adenomas is because of their mode of behaviour. Adenomas can be removed colonoscopically, and careful follow-up with removal of any further adenomas that develop appears to be effective prophylaxis in preventing the later development of invasive carcinoma (5). Morphologically similar changes in a patient with ulcerative colitis are far more sinister. The evidence suggests that the presence of dysplastic mucosa found on routine biopsy is a much more sensitive indicator of synchronous invasive carcinoma. In several studies this figure is in the region of 30% (2–4,6–8) and rises to over 60% if the biopsy is from an endoscopically visible lesion (1). This raises a further question of why, if a carcinoma is present, it is not detected clinically pre-operatively? The problem is that small (? "early") carcinomas in colitis tend to be flat, plaque-like, or slightly nodular at a time when they may already have infiltrated into, or even through, the muscularis propria and may therefore readily escape detection by all of the usual clinical methods used for their detection. The overlying mucosa is usually not ulcerated, and biopsy of such lesions (as well as more obvious carcinomas) may show only the overlying dysplasia, but not the underlying invasive carcinoma (1). Even *in situ* carcinoma is not usually present in the overlying mucosa. As a result of the difficulty in detecting such carcinomas clinically, and because of the relatively high sensitivity of dysplasia as a marker of invasive carcinoma, the mere presence of dysplasia has to be treated with caution. The wisdom in keeping dysplasia separate from adenoma can therefore be better appreciated.

The final major problem arising is that if the argument regarding the separation of dysplasia and adenoma is accepted, why not just report the presence or absence of dysplasia? Although logical, this presents practical difficulties that occur in the diagnosis of dysplasia in colitis but not in the diagnosis of adenomas in noncolitis. In the latter situation, diagnosis is virtually never a problem because the adenomatous mucosa exhibits all of the hallmarks of neoplasia, such as enlarged crypts with large cells containing enlarged hyperchromatic nuclei that are invariably stratified and accompanied by some degree of mucin loss. These changes are usually most marked at the surface. The obvious contrast between neoplastic and normal crypts can often be made in the same histologic section, when the difference between neoplastic and nonneoplastic crypts becomes emphasized.

In contrast, the distinction between dysplastic and nondysplastic mucosa in colitis is much more difficult for several reasons. First, the change from dysplastic to nondysplastic is often not abrupt, as in adenomas, but is a spectrum in which any lines that are drawn are necessarily arbitrary and therefore subjective. This becomes readily apparent on review of the literature. The lack of uniformity in classification and terminology is a major factor in the general inability to compare results from different institutions (10).

The problems with terminology are reflected by the variety of definitions applied to a term such as "dysplasia", and the variety of terms used (e.g., atypia, papillary hyperplasia, precancer, premalignant change, carcinoma *in situ*).

To instill a little order into the terminology and classification of the changes that may be seen in inflammatory bowel disease, an international group of pathologists with an interest in the subject have met regularly and exchanged slides. The group consists of Drs. C. Ahren (Sweden), H. Appelman (Ann Arbor), C. Fenoglio (New York), H. Goldman (Boston), R. Haggitt (Memphis), S. R. Hamilton (Baltimore), B. C. Morson (London), P. Correa (New Orleans), R. H. Riddell (Chicago), S. C. Sommers (New York), J. H. Yardley (Baltimore), and a clinician-statistician, D. Ransohoff (Cleveland). This has resulted in the development of a system that potentially all could agree on and utilize. It seems to be practical and to have significance in patient management.

The crux of the system is in the definition of *dysplasia*, which is defined as an unequivocal noninvasive neoplastic epithelial proliferation of the large bowel mucosa in a patient with inflammatory bowel disease. Biopsies (or resected material) are classified as positive, negative, or indefinite for dysplasia. Because the adjectives "unequivocal" and "neoplastic" imply that the mucosa may give rise directly to an invasive carcinoma (carcinoma infiltrating into the submucosa or beyond), a positive diagnosis of dysplasia cannot be taken lightly. If there is any doubt at all by the observer as to whether or not the changes present are neoplastic, the diagnosis is changed to that of "indefinite for dysplasia." This latter category covers a broad range of changes that at one extreme falls just short of changes that can be described as unequivocally neoplastic while at the other end includes changes that are probably the result of inflammation but perhaps a little more exuberant than those usually seen. The "indefinite" category also includes those biopsies that the observer cannot classify as belonging to either of the other two subgroups in the indefinite category (probably reactive, probably neoplastic) irrespective of the reason. They may include the extremes of regeneration, chronic active disease with nuclear features beyond those usually associated with repair but not really neoplastic, or quiescent disease with nuclei far larger than those usually associated with quiescent disease and often accompanied by some degree of mucus depletion, which might represent transition to dysplasia. It also includes other patterns that are unusual and cause concern because even though they have not been observed to give rise directly to invasive carcinoma, their behaviour is not known. The importance of this category is that it is not just a hedge for genuine ignorance but demands further biopsies within a relatively short period of time [usually months (see below)] so that the behaviour of these lesions can be followed closely and progress to dysplasia or regression documented. Dysplasia involving only one part of the crypt (usually sparing the crypt bases, but sometimes only involving the crypt base with apparent maturation of the epithelium as the lumenal surface is approached) is included with dysplasia providing it satisfies the definition for dysplasia.

The category of dysplasia has itself also been divided into "low grade" (Fig. 1) and "high grade" (Fig. 2), largely to facilitate patient management. However, the influence of biopsies on patient management must be discussed in the light of the alternatives available. Most "routine" follow-up of patients relies heavily on colonoscopy with multiple biopsies, and this is usually carried out roughly at annual intervals. Assuming the latter to be about the least amount of follow-up that is desirable given our current lack of objective data, biopsy

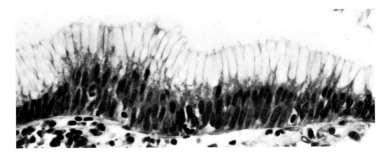

FIG. 1. Low-grade dysplasia in ulcerative colitis in which the nuclei are markedly increased in number, hyperchromatic, and show mild loss of nuclear polarity. However, they are largely confined to the basal half of the cells and there is still moderate mucin production. H.-E. ×400.

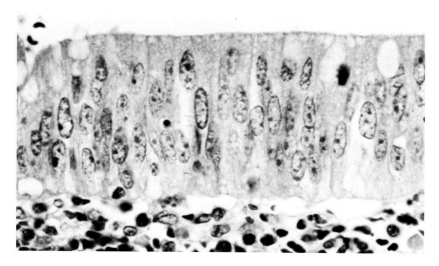

FIG. 2. High-grade dysplasia in which there is much greater loss of polarity and mucin. The open vesicular nuclei with small nucleoli may also be seen in low-grade dysplasia. H.-E. ×400.

can only result in a recommendation for follow-up colonoscopy at the same interval, follow-up at a shorter interval, or a recommendation for colectomy (usually proctocolectomy).

A series of biopsies reflecting changes that may be seen in quiescent, active, or resolving colitis, or biopsies that seem most likely to be the result of these processes, do not justify any increase in surveillance.

Management of patients with equivocal biopsies (indefinite for dysplasia) cannot simply be dismissed, neither are such biopsies sufficient to justify colectomy. Follow-up at shorter intervals is therefore appropriate to elicit the exact nature of the suspicious biopsy. In those instances where the changes are most likely an exuberant reaction to acute inflammation, the time interval between colonoscopies probably does not need to be reduced. Where there is greater uncertainty, short-interval follow-up (often after a few months) is indicated. Medical treatment of active disease may lead to resolution of the lesion. If the lesion persists it can be carefully followed to ensure that it does not ultimately become neoplastic.

At the other end of the spectrum, a biopsy or biopsies yielding high-grade dysplasia (i.e., unequivocally neoplastic and including those biopsies previously included under moderate or severe dysplasia or *in situ* carcinoma) justify recommendation for colectomy in view of the high risk of the patient having a carcinoma as described previously. Clearly, if nothing is to be advocated in the face of a biopsy yielding high-grade dysplasia, then there is no point in having the patient in a cancer-prevention protocol.

The most controversial and difficult issues regard the management of biopsies that show low-grade dysplasia, and also the problem of true adenomas in a patient with colitis. Patients that have biopsies showing low-grade dysplasia (i.e., unequivocal neoplastic change but with relatively little dysplasia) pose a problem because arguments can be made for a variety of different courses of management. The most serious is the recommendation that the patient undergo proctocolectomy because the ability to form mucosa that can give rise directly to an invasive carcinoma (dysplasia) has been demonstrated. This is particularly true if the biopsy was taken from an endoscopic lesion, as this could prove to be an invasive carcinoma on resection (1). At the other extreme an argument can be made that there is no information regarding the behaviour of these biopsies, therefore the patient should be followed to gain information as to the true significance of such biopsies. The obvious counterargument is that the development of an unequivocally neoplastic lesion could itself be regarded as an endpoint, particularly as the patient is under surveillance because of a recognized tendency to develop such neoplasms. There is also the possibility that small carcinomas are present that went unrecognized endoscopically. A further difficulty is that if such patients are merely followed, what is to be the endpoint for these patients particularly when it is known that even invasive carcinomas may not be detected even if biopsied (1)? The situation is perhaps analogous to following an adenoma in the noncolitic just to see if it will ultimately become invasive. A final argument against prophylactic proctocolectomy under these circumstances is that the diagnosis of dysplasia, particularly low grade, is still sufficiently subjective that it should be confirmed before the irrevocable step of recommending proctocolectomy is taken. This may be achieved either by repeating the biopsies to confirm that a persistently dysplastic abnormality is present or, to obtain confirmation of the dysplasia, by referring the biopsy for a further opinion. The problem with rebiopsy is that dysplasia is usually patchy, so that the area of dysplasia that was previously biopsied may be missed (9). Does the lack of confirmation negate the first biopsy? This inevitably leads one to question the reliability and reproducibility of a diagnosis of dysplasia, but this is only part of the problem. Although uncommon, an embarrassing situation sometimes arises when colectomy is carried out for dysplasia, for numerous blocks may fail to reveal any dysplasia at all. Furthermore, this situation also arises, albeit rarely, when biopsy has revealed an invasive adenocarcinoma. The only possible explanations are that the lesion was completely removed by the biopsy, that the remainder of the lesion was present in the resected specimen but not observed or sampled, that the biopsy was somehow confused with that from another patient, or that the lesion regressed. Nevertheless, it only requires one encounter with a situation such as this to cause a fall in the confidence that clinicians have in their pathologists, to say nothing of the fall in the pathologists' self-confidence.

The reproducibility of a diagnosis of dysplasia, even when high grade, is not perfect. The problem is much less when dealing with high-grade dysplasia than low-grade dysplasia. Nevertheless, even among the group of "self-confessed experts" described above, there was some variability, and certainly enough to suggest that pathologists less familiar with the problem might be open to even greater error. As a result, it is recommended that whenever colectomy is considered based almost entirely on the diagnosis on dysplasia or biopsy (or biopsies), that confirmation of the dysplasia should be obtained from a second interested pathologist (not necessarily one of the pathologists in the group above, although any would be willing to add their own opinion if required).

When one makes the transition from high-grade to low-grade dysplasia the "spread" in pathological diagnoses becomes greater, but the advice regarding confirmation of the dysplasia when colectomy is contemplated remains the same.

The final problem with dysplasia regards the management of what appears to be a true adenoma in a patient. The major concern of such adenomas is that it may represent part of a larger area of dysplasia. If the latter is the case then it will be impossible to excise the lesion completely colonoscopically, as the dysplastic mucosa will run into the stalk and the adjacent mucosa. When the possibility of this situation is encountered endoscopically, the polyps should be snared if possible and multiple biopsies taken of the adjacent mucosa, particularly in patients who are in the adenoma-bearing age range. If the adjacent mucosa proves to be dysplastic as well as the polyp, then polypectomy will not remove the entire lesion, and colectomy is recommended. However, there is theoretically no reason why colitic patients in the adenoma-bearing age group (for the sake of convenience, over 45 years old) should not be as susceptible to (or more susceptible to) adenoma formation as the noncolitic population. The management of such lesions is currently controversial. At one extreme, if such a lesion occurs in a 30-year-old patient with a 16-year history of colitis, it can be argued that he has demonstrated the potential of his large bowel to form neoplastic lesions and is therefore in a very high risk category for the subsequent development of carcinoma. In addition it would seem likely that these lesions are in some way a result of the colitic process and it is unlikely that he will continue for the next 50 years without producing more of these lesions. Logically one could argue that the wisest course of action would be excision of the large bowel to ensure as far as one can the patient's longevity irrespective of the presence or absence or dysplasia in the mucosa adjacent to the polyp.

At the other end of the spectrum might be a 68-year-old patient with a 10-year history of colitis who has two typical adenomas excised from his sigmoid colon but no other evidence of dysplasia. Why should these not be just simple adenomas and treated as such? The possibility that these may have been potentiated by the colitic process cannot be denied, but it currently seems most reasonable to treat such patients conservatively and just follow them very carefully clinically. The lack of dysplasia in the mucosa adjacent to the polyp would support this interpretation.

The most difficult patients to manage are those intermediate between these two examples, for example, a 42-year-old patient with an adenoma but no other evidence of dysplasia and a 12-year history of colitis. Arguably he could be treated conservatively. However, if he has two or three such lesions, the possibility that these are not simple adenomas but part of the colitic process is increased, and the chance that other undiscovered lesions are present also has to be borne in mind. Under these circumstances it is difficult to escape suggesting colectomy. In such patients a variety of other factors tend to affect this decision, such as the activity of disease, the amount of time lost at work in the previous year or two, the clinician's impression of the patient's attitude towards colectomy, and, of course, the patient's willingness to undergo the operation. It is apparent from these examples that clinical judgment still has a large role to play in determining when a patient should undergo colectomy.

In summary, the development of a classification system for dysplasia in inflammatory bowel disease that is reasonably reproducible and has direct implication for patient management provides the means by which many of the questions raised in this chapter might be answered.

REFERENCES

1. Blackstone, M. D., Riddell, R. H., Rogers, B. H. G., and Levin, B. (1981): Dysplasia-associated lesion or mass (DALM) detected by colonoscopy in long-standing ulcerative colitis: An indication for colectomy. *Gastroenterology*, 80:366–376.
2. Cooke, M. G., and Goligher, J. C. (1975): Carcinoma and epithelial dysplasia complicating ulcerative colitis. *Gastroenterology*, 68:1127–1136.
3. Dickson, R. J., Dixon, M. F., and Axon, A. T. R. (1980): Colonoscopy and the detection of dysplasia in patients with longstanding ulcerative colitis. *Lancet*, ii:620–622.
4. Fuson, J. A., Farmer, R. G., Hawk, W. A., and Sullivan, B. H. (1980): Endoscopic surveillance for cancer in chronic ulcerative colitis. *Am. J. Gastroenterol.*, 73:120–126.
5. Gilbertson, V. A., and Nelms, J. M. (1978): The prevention of invasive cancer of the rectum. *Cancer*, 41:1137–1139.
6. Lennard-Jones, J. E., Morson, B. C., Ritchie, J. K., Shore, D. C., and Williams, C. D. (1977): Cancer in colitis: Assessment of the individual risk by clinical and histological criteria. *Gastroenterology*, 73:1280–1289.
7. Myrvold, H. E., Kock, N. G., and Ahren, C. (1974): Rectal biopsy and precancer in ulcerative colitis. *Gut*, 15:301–306.

8. Nugent, F. W., Haggitt, R. C., Colcher, H., and Kutteruf, G. C. (1979): Malignant potential of chronic ulcerative colitis. Preliminary report. *Gastroenterology*, 76:1–5.

9. Riddell, R. H., and Morson, B. C. (1979): Value of sigmoidoscopy and biopsy in the detection of carcinoma and premalignant change in ulcerative colitis. *Gut*, 20:575–580,

10. Yardley, J. H., Bayless, T. M., and Diamond, M. P. (1979): Cancer in ulcerative colitis. (Editorial) *Gastroenterology*, 76:221–225.

Precancerous Lesions of the Gastrointestinal Tract, edited by P. Sherlock, B.C. Morson, L. Barbara, and U. Veronesi. Raven Press, New York © 1983.

Colorectal Cancer and Malignancy in Fistulae Complicating Crohn's Disease

H. Thompson, S. Gyde, and R. N. Allan

General Hospital and University of Birmingham, Birmingham B4 6NH, United Kingdom

An increased incidence of malignancy complicating Crohn's disease has been reported in the literature by various authors since 1968 (2–6,9,11,12). Weedon et al. (12), in a highly selected group of patients starting their Crohn's disease before the age of 21, found that the incidence of colorectal cancer was 20 times greater than the calculated number in the general population. There was no excess shown for carcinoma of the small intestine. In 1978 Greenstein et al. (4) drew attention to the risk of carcinoma developing in the bypassed segment either in the small intestine or colon and to the risk of malignancy developing in fistulous tracts.

Gyde et al. (6) have recently reported an increased incidence of colorectal cancer in the extended Birmingham series, which comprised 513 patients (243 males and 270 females) under long-term review between 1944 and 1976. The mean interval since diagnosis was 14.5 years. The age and sex distribution among the patients studied is summarised in Table 1.

STATISTICAL METHODS

Since the majority of patients in the series were resident in the West Midlands Region for the duration of their illness, the cancer incidence rates for the region have been used to assess the level of risk. Age-specific incidence rates for 52 anatomical sites in males and 53 in females were computed from notifications recorded by the Birmingham Cancer Registry for the midpoint of the study between the years 1960 and 1962 inclusive, together with the Registrar Generals Census Population figures for the region, which were centered on 1961.

TABLE 1. *Crohn's disease: distribution of series by sex at age of onset and diagnosis*

Group	Age	% of group	
		Onset	Diagnosis
Male	<30 years	62.6	58.4
	30+ years	37.4	41.6
Female	<30 years	64.1	55.6
	30+ years	35.9	44.4
Total	<30 years	63.3	57.0
	30+ years	36.7	43.0

The survival experienced by the series was expressed as patient years at risk grouped by sex, age at diagnosis, and interval from diagnosis. By applying the appropriate age- and sex-specific incidence rates to the patient years at risk, the number of tumours that might be expected to occur in the series was computed. The corresponding observed number of tumours was ascertained from the clinical records of the patients with Crohn's disease corroborated by scanning the Registry files. The Poisson distribution was used to test the significance of the differences between observed and expected numbers.

The analysis was carried out initially for the series as a whole and for the group of patients with extensive colitis (disease extending proximally for at least as far as the hepatic flexure). The patient years at risk were corrected for those patients who had undergone panprocto-colectomy in whom the risk of developing cancer of the large intestine and rectum had been eliminated. A similar correction was made for those patients treated by colectomy and ileorectal anastomosis where the risk of developing carcinoma of the large intestine had been eliminated and the risk of developing carcinoma of the rectum remained.

RESULTS

The mean age at onset of symptoms was 29.3 years with a mean duration of symptoms of 2.5 years before diagnosis. Nearly half of the patients (45%) had involvement of the ileum with or without extension into the right colon; a third (34%) had extensive involvement of the colon with or without distal ileal involvement. During the period of review, the cancer risk in the large intestine and rectum was eliminated by panproctocolectomy in 17.3% of patients and eliminated in the large intestine following colectomy and ileorectal anastomosis in 9.4%

CANCER MORBIDITY IN ALL SITES

Up to the termination date of the survey (Dec. 31, 1976) 31 tumours were diagnosed in the series. Eighteen of these tumours occurred in the digestive system: 1 in the pharynx; 1 in the parotid gland; 1 in the oesophagus; 4 in the stomach; 1 in the pancreas; 1 in the small intestine; and 9 in the colon (Table 2).

Taken all together these 18 tumours were significantly in excess ($p < 0.001$) of the 5.39 tumours that might have been expected to occur during the review period. There was no statistical evidence of increased cancer risk outside the gastrointestinal tract.

In the 9 cancers observed in the large intestine representing a highly significant excess $p < 0.001$, cancer usually occurred at the site of macroscopic disease (7 of 9 cases) and usually in patients with extensive colitis of longstanding (6 of 9 cases). There was a fourfold increased incidence of carcinoma of the colon and rectum (observed = 9, expected = 2.26, O/E = 4).

The risk rose to 24-fold when the analysis was restricted to patients with extensive colitis (Table 3). This suggests extensive colitis may be an important risk factor in Crohn's disease as well as ulcerative colitis.

Correction of the patient years at risk for surgical resection increased the cancer risk but not greatly (Table 3).

Only 2 of the 9 patients who developed cancer of the large intestine are still alive (2 and 8 years later). Four of them died from metastatic disease at intervals of 1 and 4 years after resection, 1 died post-operatively, and 2 others died of incidental causes 9 and 18 years later. All but 2 of the patients were diagnosed as having cancer only after they had developed symptoms related to the cancer.

TABLE 2. *Crohn's disease: cancer morbidity—digestive system (513 patients)*

Site	Total[b]		
	E	O	P
All sites	18.67	31	†
Digestive system[a]	5.39	18	‡
Upper tract	2.53	8	†
Lower tract	2.26	9	‡
Remainder digestive system	0.60	1	—
Remainder other sites	13.28	13	—

[a]Upper: buccal cavity, throat, oesophagus to distal ileum. Lower: colon, rectum, and all reticulum cell sarcomas. Remainder digestive system: liver, gall bladder, pancreas, appendix.
[b]O = observed number; E = expected number; P = probability.

TABLE 3. *Crohn's disease: cancer morbidity with particular reference to large intestine[a]*

Patients	Patient-years at risk	E	O	O/E	P
Whole series (*n* = 513)	All	2.26	9	4.0	‡
	Adjusted for colectomy/PPC[b]	2.07	9	4.3	‡
Extensive colonic involvement (*n* = 174)	All	0.39	5	12.8	‡
	Adjusted for colectomy/PPC[b]	0.21	5	23.8	‡
Other	All	1.87	4	2.1	

[a]The cancer risk in patients with Crohn's disease is shown for the whole series and for those patients with extensive colitis and others separately. The patient-years at risk are shown for all patients in each group and adjusted for patients who have been treated by colectomy/PPC. The expected number of cancers in the matched population (E) are compared with the number of cancers observed in each group (O) and the significance of ratio (O/E) is shown in the final column.
[b]PPC, panproctocolectomy.

Most of the tumours were clearly visible, ulcerating, stenosing or polypoid lesions. Keighley et al. (8) described a case of multiple colorectal cancers in 1 of the patients included in this series with Crohn's disease.

Some of the tumours were occult, diffusely infiltrating lesions and were only discovered after extensive examination of the specimen, but all showed the characteristic appearance of infiltrating adenocarcinoma.

Precancerous changes synonymous with moderate and severe dysplasia were occasionally encountered in the series. Malignancy in the form of several minicancers was identified following the diagnosis of severe dysplasia in rectal biopsies from 1 patient.

The absolute numbers of patients developing cancer remains small, but since this study closed we have observed a further 5 cancer cases in the series of 513 patients, namely, 2 in the upper digestive tract and 3 in the lower digestive tract. These additional cases strengthen the observations on the cancer risk.

There was no statistical evidence of an increased incidence of lymphoma in Crohn's disease, although there was 1 lymphoma of the caecum that was identified concurrently with regional ileitis. One other lymphoma of the colon complicating Crohn's disease has occurred outside the series.

The incidence of carcinoma of the small intestine as a complication of Crohn's disease is much more difficult to assess, since the frequency of carcinoma of the small intestine is low in the general population. Gyde et al. (6) reported 1 case of carcinoma of the small intestine in the recent study, but the incidence did not reach statistical significance. Hawker et al. (7) reported 3 cases of carcinoma of the small intestine complicating Crohn's disease encountered over an 18-year period (1963–1981) in the General Hospital, Birmingham. Two were located in the ileum and 1 in the jejunum. A total of 61 cases have been recorded in the literature and the association has become highly significant. Dysplasia may be present in the adjacent mucosa and an endometriosis-like pattern is sometimes encountered in the wall of the infiltrated intestine.

The Birmingham series also includes 3 cases of carcinoma developing in fistulae associated with Crohn's disease. These are briefly documented below.

Case 1: Carcinoma Developing in a Rectovaginal Fistula

A woman age 23 (1) presented with Crohn's disease in 1956; it was treated by right hemicolectomy. She developed an ischiorectal abscess and low perianal fistula in 1959. Two years later she developed an abscess in the vagina. Five years later she complained of passing air per vagina. At the age of 45 she presented in 1978 with tenderness and swelling of the wall between the vagina and rectum. Biopsy revealed microscopic foci of carcinoma cells permeating lymphatic channels with intestinal epithelium lining a fistulous tract. Proctectomy was carried out. Detailed examination of the specimen revealed a carcinoma situated between the rectum and vagina, which was arising from a rectovaginal fistula. The cancer was of intestinal type and there was no evidence of primary carcinoma of the rectum, vagina, cervix uteri, or any other related structure. There was one lymph node metastasis and she died 2 years later from metastatic carcinoma confirmed by necropsy.

Case 2: Carcinoma Developing in Cystic Caecostomy Remnants

A 32-year-old male (J. G. Gray, *personal communication*, 1980) was discharged from the Army in 1945 with a diagnosis of ulcerative colitis. There was an earlier history of dysentery while serving in the Army in North Africa in 1942.

In 1947, he was admitted as an emergency into the hospital with acute exacerbation of his symptoms, and caecostomy was performed. Although his health improved, he was never really free from symptoms and he also developed perianal disease. Panproctocolectomy was carried out in 1953. The existing caecostomy was excised and the hole in the abdominal wall was closed. An ileostomy was fashioned just above the previous stoma. A diagnosis of ulcerative colitis was established on pathological examination of the colectomy specimen.

Over the ensuing years the patient remained in good health apart from an intermittent and minimal discharge at the site of his previous caecostomy.

In September 1977 he was admitted as an emergency with haemorrhage from the abdominal wall. Clinical examination revealed induration of the abdominal wall in the right iliac fossa with an area of superficial ulceration at the site of his previous caecostomy. Biopsy established a diagnosis of mucin-secreting adenocarcinoma. Wide excision of the abdominal tumour was carried out and the observation was made that the tumour was restricted to skin and subcutaneous fat. The peritoneum, liver, and abdominal contents were free from carcinoma. He developed a recurrence in the right iliac fossa in 1978. Excision showed that this also consisted of moderately differentiated adenocarcinoma of large bowel type. Radiotherapy was instituted, but he developed a further recurrence.

The original colectomy specimen was reviewed by two independent gastrointestinal pathologists who made a diagnosis of Crohn's disease of the colon.

More detailed examination of the abdominal tumour mass confirmed that this was a mucin-secreting adenocarcinoma of large intestine type with argentaffin cells and a mucin-secretion pattern consistent with an origin in colonic mucosa. Cystic remnants of colonic mucosa were identified in the vicinity of the caecostomy site. It would appear, therefore, that remnants of colonic mucosa persisted at the caecostomy site with slight intermittent discharge and cyst formation eventually giving rise to invasive adenocarcinoma of the intestinal type. The residual remnants of colonic mucosa showed dysplasia.

Case 3: Carcinoma Developing in Remnants of Ileorectal Fistula

A female age 19 presented with Crohn's disease in 1964; this was followed by laparotomy and appendicectomy. She was referred to the Gastrointestinal Unit as intractable Crohn's disease in 1976, when she was 31 years old, with a fistula from mid-ileum to rectum, rectovaginal fisula, and anal stenosis. Intestinal resections, namely, right hemicolectomy and subsequent panproctocolectomy revealed Crohn's disease and superimposed tuberculosis (confirmed bacteriologically). She recovered following antituberculous treatment.

She died 3 years later at the age of 34 with pelvic adenocarcinoma (featuring signet ring cells), which had developed from cystic remnants of the previous Crohn's fistulous tract leading from mid-ileum to rectum. Full necropsy failed to demonstrate a primary tumour in any other structure or organ.

Other Cases

There has also been a case in a male age 27 who had a panproctocolectomy for Crohn's disease of 12 years duration. Detailed examination revealed a small infiltrating carcinoma of sigmoid colon closely related to a fistulous tract.

Simpson (10) also described malignancy developing in fistulae associated with Crohn's disease and he has drawn attention to dysplasia of the rectum, colon, and fistulae in patients with longstanding Crohn's disease.

CONCLUSIONS

1. The incidence of colorectal carcinoma is four times greater than expected in patients with Crohn's disease.
2. Patients with extensive colitis of longstanding are at greatest risk.
3. Carcinoma of the small intestine is a recognised complication of Crohn's disease.
4. Carcinoma is a well-documented complication of longstanding fistulae associated with Crohn's disease.

REFERENCES

1. Buchmann, P., Allan, R. N., Thompson, H., and Alexander-Williams, J. (1980): *Am. J. Surg.*, 140:462–463.
2. Darke, S. G., Parks, A. G., Grogono, J. L., and Pollock, D. J. (1973): Adenocarcinoma and Crohn's Disease. A report of 2 cases and analysis of the literature. *Br. J. Surg.*, 60:169–175.
3. Fielding, J. F., Prior, P., Waterhouse, J. A., and Cooke, W. T. (1972): Malignancy in Crohn's Disease. *Scand. J. Gastroenterol.*, 7:3–7.
4. Greenstein, A. J., Sachar, D., Pucillo, A., et al. (1978): Cancer in Crohn's disease after diversionary surgery. *Am. J. Surg.* 135:86–90.
5. Greenstein, A. J., Sachar, D. B., Smith, H., et al. (1980): Cancer complicating Crohn's Disease. *46:403–407.*
6. Gyde, S. N., Prior, P., Macartney, J. C., Thompson, H., Waterhouse, J. A. H., and Allan, R. N. (1980): Malignancy in Crohn's disease. *Gut*, 21:1024–1029.
7. Hawker, P., Gyde, S. N., Thompson, H., and Allan, R. N. (1982). Adenocarcinoma of the small intestine complicating Crohn's disease. *Gut*, 23:188–193.
8. Keighley, M. R. B., Thompson, H., and Alexander-Williams, J. (1975): Multifocal colonic carcinoma and Crohn's disease. *Surgery*, 78:534–537.
9. Perrett, A. D., Truelove, S. C., and Massarella, G. R. (1968): Crohn's disease and carcinoma of the colon. *Br. Med. J.*, 2:466–468.
10. Simpson, S., Traube, J., and Riddell, R. H. (1981): The histologic appearance of dysplasia (precarcinomatous change) in Crohn's disease of the small and large intestine. *Gastroenterology*, 81:492–501.
11. Thompson, H. (1976): Malignancy in Crohn's disease in the management of Crohn's disease. In: *Proceedings of Workshop in Crohn's Disease*, edited by I. I. Weterman, A. S. Penna, and C. C. Booth. Excerpta Medica, Amsterdam, pp. 146–149.
12. Weedon, D. D., Shorter, R. G., Ilstrup, D. M., Huizenga, K. A., and Taylor, W. F. (1973): Crohn's disease and cancer. *N. Engl. J. Med.*, 289:1099–1103.

Precancerous Lesions of the Gastrointestinal Tract, edited by P. Sherlock, B.C. Morson, L. Barbara, and U. Veronesi. Raven Press, New York © 1983.

Surveillance of Patients Operated for Colorectal Cancer

*A. Montori and **L. Risa

*Via di Villa Ada, 10, 00199 Rome, Italy and **Via C. Lorenzini, 11, 00137 Rome, Italy

Considering the proper surveillance of patients operated for colorectal neoplasia, it is necessary to note the following: First, the choice of study is not easy even though we deal with selected patients having been operated surgically or endoscopically, because we need to consider sensitivity and the specific and predictive value of the research and determine its cost-benefit ratio.

Second, the methodology for studying these patients must be directed toward simplifying clinical research and trying to reduce the number of examinations performed. We must determine when to perform clinical studies considering the development of precancerous lesions and colorectal cancer. Obviously, the surveillance of patients operated for colorectal cancer will be different than that applied to patients treated endoscopically for adenomatous polyps.

Finally, we cannot forget the problem of the "drop-out." In our experience the number of patients who return for regular check-up is low (about 25%); it is important to focus on the real motivations that explain this phenomenon and it is necessary to inform and update family physicians. In this way we hope to improve the number of controlled patients.

The examinations we suggest for a good check-up are coloscopy, double-contrast enema, echography, computerized tomography (CT), laboratory tests, colonic cytology, and guaiac test (Table 1).

Concerning endoscopy we prefer total coloscopy to discover metachronous lesions such as cancer and polyps, which in our experience have a 50% chance for local recurrence. In this regard we think it more useful to increase the number of physicians able to perform total coloscopy rather than shorten the length of the instruments.

In our opinion the use of short- or middle-range fiberscopes would add to the number of useless examinations and may increase a false negative examination, thereby reducing its diagnostic effectiveness.

Postoperative coloscopy in patients treated for colorectal cancer enables us to examine the anastomosis site and identify local recurrences or the presence of polyps or metachronous cancer (Table 2).

In our study of 204 patients followed for 6 months to 18 years, we noted a local recurrence in 4% and growth of a metachronous cancer in 7%; we also identified 71 adenomatous polyps, one of which was an invasive cancer (Table 3). Furthermore, we discovered that (a) the percentage of local recurrences is lower, if in the carcinoma of the sigmoid, we perform a left hemicolectomy instead of a simple resection of the sigmoid; and (b) there is a difference

TABLE 1. *Surveillance of patients operated for colorectal cancer*

Coloscopy
Double-contrast enema
Echography or computerized tomography
Laboratory tests
Colonic cytology
Fecal occult blood

TABLE 2. *Aims of postoperative coloscopy*

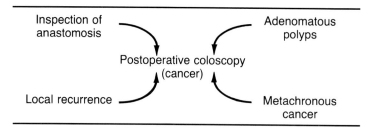

TABLE 3. *Postoperative endoscopy in colonic carcinoma (retrospective study on 5 years)*

No. of patients	Local recurrences	Adenomatous polyps	Metachronous cancer
204	8 (4%)	71 1 Ca in adenoma	14 (7%)

Surveillance time: 6 months–18 years.

in the percentage of local recurrences following low resection of the rectum, if the anastomosis is done by a Stapler device (0% in our series) instead of handplaced sutures (3%).

In 19% of these patients the double-contrast enema gave a negative response, whereas in 58% the same examination showed a neoplastic lesion, making essential the coloscopy with histological examination. In 23% diagnosis was made only by coloscopy (Table 4). For these reasons we prefer to perform endoscopic examinations, choosing radiology only when doubt remains after endoscopy.

Considering these results of the periodic examinations of patients who underwent surgery for cancer and of high risk patients treated for cancer in an adenoma by endoscopic polypectomy, we advise a definite program of control; this consists of a total coloscopy 3 to 6 months after the operation, repeated every 6 months for 5 years and yearly thereafter (Table 5).

This scheme of surveillance entails very frequent and closed controls, especially for the first 5 years after surgery; in fact in our experience all local recurrences were discovered during this period, and some of these as early as 3 to 6 months after surgery.

The most important serum examination is carcinoembryonic antigen (CEA), which has been widely used to check patients who have had surgery for colorectal carcinoma. Other daily serum tests are γ-glutamil transpeptidase (γ-GT), phosphoisomerase, and alkaline phosphatase, which are elevated following hepatic involvement.

TABLE 4. *Postoperative endoscopy in colonic carcinoma*

No. of patients (204)	No. of Ca (22)	
	(n)	(%)
Identified	4	19
Clarified	13	58
By coloscopy only	5	23

TABLE 5. *Endoscopic surveillance (coloscopy)*

Patient operated for
Invasive carcinoma (endoscopic polypectomy) or cancer
Within 3–6 months
Every 6 months for 5 years
Every year for life

There are other serum tests still being studied, the most important of them are CEA-S, pregnancy associated α2-glycoprotein (α2-PAG), IgA/IgM ratio, and A and H plasma antigens (Table 6).

Since we cannot use the CEA level for the early diagnosis of colorectal cancer, obviously it is not even a sensitive index of local recurrence, although it seems quite meaningful in hepatic and extraabdominal spread. Wanebo reports a CEA level more than 5 ng/ml in 50% and more than 20 ng/ml in 22% of patients with local recurrences, as opposed to 90% of subjects with hepatic or extraabdominal metastases with higher than 5 ng/ml CEA and 58% to 76% of patients with higher than 20 ng/ml CEA.

Similar results come from the study by Schillace et al., which involved 69 patients operated for polyps or colorectal cancer. These subjects had a CEA level of more than 2,5 ng/ml correlated with local recurrences in 40%; other subjects, about 10%, had values in the normal range correlated with local recurrences. On the other hand CEA levels higher than 20 ng/ml were found in 18% of patients with local recurrences and in 55% of subjects with distant metastases; these results confirm that CEA control is a sensitive test to display hepatic and extraabdominal spread.

Concerning the guaiac test, its usefulness for screening is well known; this test is positive in 1% to 4% of cases, half of which are patients with neoplastic lesions. Keeping in mind these items, the guaiac test should be utilized in postoperative control of these patients because if it is negative, the instrumental examination should be done less frequently.

During the period 1975 to 1981 we performed 1,866 endoscopic polypectomies; 1,560 (83.3%) of these were neoplastic polyps, and the histological results showed a carcinoma ex-adenoma in 27 subjects (1.7%). This last percentage is lower than all other reported figures, which are about 6%. In patients who had undergone endoscopic removal of all polyps, the demonstration of new polyps occurred more frequently during the first 20 months of follow-up. The periodic examinations we perform on patients who have undergone endoscopic polypectomy for adenomatous polyp, with or without severe dysplasia, or for multiple polyposis consists of one control 6 months after the operation, repeated after a year

TABLE 6. *Surveillance for patients operated for colorectal cancer: laboratory tests*

Guaiac test	α_2-PAG
CEA, CEA-S	IgA/IgM ratio
γ-GT	IgA
Phosphoisomerase	A and H plasma antigens
Alkaline phosphatase	Glycosiltransferase
	^{14}C-fucose
	α_2, α_3-fucosyltransferase
	Leucocyte-migration-inhibition test

TABLE 7. *Endoscopic surveillance (coloscopy)*

Patient operated for
Adenomatous polyp
6 months
After 18 months
Every 5 years
Multiple polyposis or adenomatous
polyp with severe dysplasia
After 6 months
After 18 months
Every 3 years

and subsequently every 3 years. This last period has to be extended to 5 years in subjects with adenomatous polyp without severe dysplasia (Table 7).

On the basis of these results we can say that postoperative surveillance of patients operated for colorectal cancer has to be performed following the established scheme, the methods and time of which we have suggested above.

We can conclude that this kind of approach increases early diagnosis of local recurrences and metachronous lesions.

REFERENCES

1. Bauer, C. H., Reutter, W. G., Erhart, K. P., Kottgen, E., and Gerok, W. (1978): Decrease of Human Serum Fucosyltransferase as an Indicator of successful Tumor Therapy. *Science*, 201:1232–1233.
2. Bertario, L., Severini, A., Mantero, M., Pizzetti, P., and Spinelli, P. (1979): Diagnosis of asymptomatic colorectal cancer using a stabilized guaiac test (Hemoccult) for detecting occult blood in stools. Preliminary results. *Ital. J. Gastroenterol.*, 11:53–55.
3. Burnett, D., Booth, S. N., Cove, D. H., Howell, A., Sturde, D., and Bradwell, A. R. (1977): Pregnancy-associated α_2-glycoprotein. *Lancet*, 1:257–258.
4. Burtin, P., Pinset, C., Chany, E., Fondaneche, M. C., and Chavanel, G. (1978): Leucocyte-migration-inhibition test in patients with colorectal cancer: clinicopathological correlations. *Br. J. Cancer*, 37:685–691.
5. Devidsohn, I., Ni, L. Y., and Stejkal, R. (1971): Tissue, isoantigens A, B and H in carcinoma of the stomach. *Arch. Pathol.*, 92:456–464.
6. Evans, J. T., Mittleman, A., Chu, M., and Holyoke, E. D. (1978): Pre- and postoperative uses of CEA. *Cancer*, 42:1419–1422.
7. Fazio, V. W. (1979): Early Diagnosis of Anorectal and Colon Carcinoma. *Hospital Medicine*, 1:25–35.
8. Kuhn, H. A., Ottenjann, R., Thaler, H., and Gheorghiu, T. H. (1977): Screening for Colorectal Cancer with Haemoccult. *Leber Magen Darm*, 7:32–35.
9. Lev, R. (1978): On controlling colorectal cancer. *Curr. Top.*, 621.
10. Ma, J., De Boer, W. G. R. M., Ward, H. A., and Nairn, R. C. (1980): Another oncofoetal antigen in colonic carcinoma. *Br. J. Cancer*, 41:325–328.

11. Martin, Jr., E. W., Cooperman, M., King, G., Rinker, L., Carey, L. C., and Minton, J. P. (1979): A retrospective and prospective study of serial CEA determinations in the early delection of recurrent colon cancer. *Am. J. Surg.*, 137:167–169.

12. Martin, Jr., E. W., Kibbey, W. E., Di Vecchia, Anderson, G., Catalano, P., and Minton, J. P. (1976): Carcinoembryonic antigen, clinical and historical aspects. *Cancer*, 37:62.

13. Montori, A., Messinetti, S., Viceconte, G., and Di Curzio, B. (1976): Endoscopic and surgical treatment of the colonic polyps. *Acta Hepatogastroenterol.*, 23(6):459–466.

14. Montori, A., Viceconte, G., Miscusi, G., Viceconte, G. W., and Pastorino, C. (1976): The operative colonoscopy. Reprinted from Proceedings of the 2nd Asian Pacific Congress of Endoscopy, 279–282. Singapore, 27–29 May 1976.

15. Milano, G., Cooper, E. H., Goligher, J. C., Giles, G. R., and Neville, A. M. (1978): Serum prealbumin, retinol-binding protein, transferrin and albumin levels in patients with large bowel cancer. *J. Natl. Cancer Inst.*, 61:687–691.

16. Miller, S. F. (1978): The detection of asymptomatic colorectal cancer. *A.F.P.*, 18:89–92.

17. Montgomery, B. J. (1979): New screening test for colorectal cancer developed in Canada. *Med. News*, 242:1005–1006.

18. Norgaard-Pedersen, B., and Axelsen, N. H. (1978): Carcinoembryonic proteins: Recent progress. *Scand. J. Immunol. (Suppl.)*, 8(8):172–178.

19. Rittgers, R. A., Steele, G., Zamcheck, N., Loowenstein, M. S., Sugarbaker, P. H., Mayer, R. J., Lokich, J. J., Mattz, J., and Wilson, R. E. (1978): Transient carcinoembryonic antigen (CEA) elevations following resection of colorectal cancer: A limitation in the use of serial CEA Levels as an indicator for second-look surgery. *J. Natl. Cancer Inst.*, 61:315–318.

20. Rouger, Ph., Riveau, D., Samon, Ch., and Loygue, J. (1979): Plasma blood group changes in gastrointestinal tract carcinoma. *J. Clin. Pathol.*, 32:907–911.

21. Schillaci, A., Cosinelli, M., Nicolini, V., Gallo, P., and Stipa, S. (1981): Preliminary results in treatment of large bowel neoplasia: Immunological and clinical follow-up. *Folia Oncol., (Suppl.)*, 4:404–410.

22. Slater, G., Papatestas, A. E., Shafir, M., and Aufses, Jr., A. H. (1980): Serum immunoglobulins in colorectal cancer. *J. Surg. Oncol.*, 14:167–171.

23. Sopranzi, N., Ponzini, D., Di Paola, M., Inserra, A., and Colizza, S. (1980): Serial CEA levels in colorectal carcinoma on adjuvant immuno (chemo) therapy. Further follow-up—Modulation of adjuvant treatment. *J. Surg. Oncol.*, 13:169–176.

24. Sugarbaker, P. H., Zamcheck, N., and Moore, F. D. (1976): Assessment of serial carcinoembryonic antigen (CEA) assay in postoperative detection of recurrent colorectal cancer. *Cancer*, 38:2310–2315.

25. Wanebo, H. J. (1981): Are carcinoembryonic antigen levels of value in the curative management of colorectal cancer? *Surgery*, 89:290–295.

26. Welch, J. P., and Donaldson, G. A. (1974): Recent experiences in the management of cancer of the colon and rectum. *Am. J. Surg.*, 127:258–266.

27. Winawer, S. J., Andrews, M., Flehinger, B., Sherlock, P. D., Schottenfeld, D., and Miller, D. G. (1980): Progress report on controlled trial of fecal occult blood testing for detection of colorectal neoplasia. *Cancer*, 45:2959–2964.

28. Winawer, S. J., Leidner, S. D., Hajdu, S. I., and Sherlock, P. (1978): Colonscopic biopsy and cytology in the diagnosis of colon cancer. *Cancer*, 42:2848–2853.

29. Winawer, S. J., and Sherlock, P. (1976): Approach to screening and diagnosis in colorectal cancer. *Semin. Oncol.*, 3:387–397.

30. Winawer, S. J., and Sherlock, P. (1977): Detecting early colon cancer. *Hosp. Pract.*, 12:49–56.

31. Winawer, S. J., Sherlock, P., and Miller, D. G. (1979): Current Diagnosis of Large Bowel Cancer. *Continuing Education*, 3:56–60.

32. Winawer, S. J., Sherlock, P., Schottefeld, D., and Miller, D. G. (1976): Screening for colon cancer. *Gastroenterology*, 70:783–789.

33. Winawer, S. J., Weston, E., Hajdu, S., Edelnan, M., Sherlock, P., Stearns, Jr., M., and Miller, D. (1978): Sensitivity of diagnostic techniques in patients with positive fecal occult blood screening tests. *Gastrointest. Endosc.*, 24:2013 (Abstr. A/S/G/E).

34. Wood, C. B. (1980): Prognostic factors in colorectal cancer. *Rec. Adv. Surg.*, 12:259–280.

35. Wood, C. B., Horne, C. H. W., Towler, C. M., Bohn, H., and Blumgard, L. H. (1978): The value of pregnancy-associated α_2-glycoprotein in patients with colorectal cancer. *Br. J. Surg.*, 65:653–656.

36. Wood, C. B., Ratcliffe, J. G., Burt, R. W., Malcolm, A. J. H., and Blumgart, L. H. (1980): The clinical significance of the pattern of elevated serum carcinoembryonic antigen (CEA) levels in recurrent colorectal cancer. *Br. J. Surg.*, 67:46–48.

37. Zamcheck, N. (1976): A summary of the present status of CEA in diagnosis, prognosis and evaluation of therapy of colonic cancer. *Bull. Cancer*, 63:463–472.

Precancerous Lesions of the Gastrointestinal Tract, edited by P. Sherlock, B.C. Morson, L. Barbara, and U. Veronesi. Raven Press, New York © 1983.

Principles of Screening Adapted to Precancerous Conditions of the Gastrointestinal Tract

R. Lambert

Centre D'Epidemiologie, C.N.R.S.L.P. 5440, Faculté De Médecine de Lyon, 69003 France

The objective of a screening program concerning cancer is to reduce the morbidity and mortality from that cancer. The disease proposed must fulfill the following criteria: have serious consequences when fully advanced, be easily detected at an early preclinical stage when an effective treatment can be proposed, and have a significant prevalence in the population at this early stage. It is necessary to evaluate the utility of the screening system (cost and benefits, adverse effects, etc.). Indeed its value as a progress in cancer control is controversial and the evaluation through early or late outcomes is subject to bias (the lead time and length bias). The experimental evaluation of a screening system requires a randomized study with a nonscreened control group. Such studies are time-consuming and costly; this is why they are rare (2,22,40).

Precancerous lesions can be detected through screening in two different conditions: they can be a by-product of a screening system adapted specifically to the detection of cancer and they can also be detected through a screening system specifically designed for the precancerous lesions. In any event, the screening of precancerous lesions concerns risk factors rather than a disease. The benefit may be very small and difficult to assess. The main difficulties lie in the high prevalence of such lesions in the population, and in assessing the precancerous character of a dysplastic lesion, and therefore establishing the sequence "precancer to cancer." Furthermore, the detection of these lesions is more difficult than that of cancer at an early stage, and their management is controversial.

RELATIONSHIP BETWEEN PRECANCEROUS AND CANCEROUS LESIONS

Precancerous conditions in the gastrointestinal tract must be considered as risk factors rather than as diseases. When considering their significance, the following points will be examined: persons exposed to the risk according to genetic and environmental factors, prevalence of the lesions in the population, and morphological characters of the lesions and their potential evolution.

Esophagus

Persons at Risk

There are examples of high-risk populations for esophageal cancer, in northeast Iran or in Linxian, Honan province in China (3–5,9,44). In these areas the whole of the population is exposed to the risk. The precursor lesions could be caused by a carcinogen or by environmental factors, including thermal injury, coarse food, and vitamin deficiency. In other countries alcohol and tobacco introduce a risk factor for a small part of the population. These observations concern the *epidermoid carcinoma* of the esophagus. A high risk for *adenocarcinoma* of the lower esophagus is also observed in persons with chronic peptic esophagitis and Barrett's epithelium (71). In these instances, the precancerous condition is associated with a disease.

Prevalence of the Lesions

Studies in Iran and China (5,9,44) demonstrate that the precancerous condition (a very peculiar type of esophagitis) is present in a high percentage of the adult population (around 85% from the age group 20–30 years to the old-age group). However, most lesions are characterized as mild esophagitis and the percentage of severe lesions (atrophy or dysplasia) is around 10%. These observations are of little significance when the usual risk factors observed in occidental countries are considered. Indeed the prevalence of precancerous lesions (dysplasia) in persons exposed to the risk (high consumption of alcohol, high smoking) is not known. In regard to esophageal reflux, the risk factor is limited to the small percentage of patients with chronic peptic esophagitis and development of a columnar lined epithelium (Barrett). It is estimated that 10% of patients with chronic esophagitis are involved (71).

Morphology of the Lesions

Esophagitis, in the high-risk populations of Iran and China is characterized by inflammation (lymphocyte and plasma cell infiltration) of the submucosa. Erosions are not present; the lesion is not similar to peptic esophagitis (9,44). Esophagitis by itself is not a precancerous condition; the groups with mucosal atrophy or dysplasia (around 10%) are exposed to the high risk. This is still a significant percentage of the adult population (around 8%) in these countries. The lesion involves the middle and lower third of the esophagus. In persons at high risk for esophageal cancer in occidental countries, the precancerous lesions are multifocal in the upper digestive and lower respiratory tract (37,53). Hyperplasia, parakeratosis, and acanthosis may be observed. The dysplasia with cell atypia is a dyschromic area very similar to the four fundamental types of preinvasive carcinoma (42,43): (a) type 1 limited protruded area with a whitish colour; (b) type 2 multifocal depressed areas with a reddish colour; (c) type 3 associating protruded and depressed lesions; and (d) type 4 corresponding to a flat mucosa normal in appearance. The characterization of the dysplasia as mild, moderate, and severe is based on multiple biopsies and there is no sharp macroscopic difference between severe dysplasia and a preinvasive carcinoma. In the Barrett's esophagus, the columnar epithelium is easily distinguished from an epidermoid mucosa; however, the precancerous condition (dysplasia) is detected only by systematic sampling of the mucosa. Dysplasia is present in about 15% (71) of patients with a junction type of gastric epithelium in the esophagus (this type of epithelium is present in approximately 75% of patients with a Barrett's esophagus).

The Dysplasia-Cancer Sequence

The data collected in China by the coordinating group for the research (3–5) on esophageal cancer show that marked dysplasia introduces a high risk of progression to cancer (about 25% in a 4-year period). However, in one-third of the patients marked dysplasia is stabilized; in one-fourth there is regression to mild dysplasia. The endoscopic survey of esophagitis

(9,44) stresses two groups of persons at risk: those with atrophy (about 10%) and those with dysplasia (about 8%). The respective role of the sequences "esophagitis-atrophy-cancer" and "esophagitis-atrophy-dysplasia-cancer" is not known. As concerning precursors lesions of esophageal cancer in occidental countries, the term *precancerous condition* should be limited to severe dysplasia. Epithelial alterations such as acanthosis and simple hyperplasia should not be classified in this group.

Stomach

Persons at Risk

Atrophic gastritis is the main precursor of gastric cancer. The significance of chronic atrophic gastritis is examined in two groups (30,66). The common type is gastritis B, characterized by multifocal lesions and associated with antral and fundal atrophy. The second condition, the A type of gastritis, is more rare and is the usual precursor of gastric cancer. This bears a relationship with genetic factors associated with pernicious anemia and gastric cancer (14,24,69). The risk for cancer is higher than in the type B gastritis, but it accounts only for a small percentage of cases in the incidence of gastric cancer. The type A gastritis involves mainly the fundus. Atrophic gastritis is a risk factor not a disease. On the other hand, an increased risk for cancer is observed in some gastric diseases (gastric ulcer). In the follow-up of chronic benign ulcers, a malignant transformation is observed in 2% to 4% in a 2-year period. This applies to chronic ulcers in the lesser curvature below the cardia, or chronic linear ulcers in the lesser curvature below the angulus. However, the increased risk for gastric cancer in such patients is not limited to the area adjacent to the lesion and every surface having atrophic gastritis is concerned. Individuals with adenomatous polyps of the stomach are exposed to a higher risk of malignant transformation, but these lesions are uncommon and most gastric polyps (90%) are of the hyperplastic (nonneoplastic) type (15,38,41). The latter are not precancerous lesions, but they develop in a mucosa with gastric atrophy; therefore, an increased risk for cancer at a distance from the hyperplastic polyp is reported. Gastric cancer observed in persons after partial gastrectomy is in relation to atrophic gastritis and duodeno-gastric reflux in the stomach. Genetic factors have been demonstrated in the type A gastritis. The development of type B gastritis and gastric carcinogenesis is related to environmental factors such as the nitrate, nitrite, nitrosamine sequence and the salt consumption (6,7,25,65).

Prevalence of the Lesions

The prevalence of atrophic gastritis is very high in the population and is age related. It is admitted that in an adult population the prevalence of type B gastritis reaches 20% whereas the prevalence of type A gastritis is limited to 5% (66). The chronic gastric ulcer or the gastrectomized stomach introduce a higher risk for gastric cancer, more especially related to the presence of chronic atrophic gastritis in such patients. On the other hand, the prevalence of atypical epithelium foci or borderline lesions (45–47,51,68) with dysplasia in association with atrophic gastritis is very low. In a recent study (48) concerning the pathology of 16,606 stomachs, only 40 specimens with isolated dysplastic lesions were observed, whereas 115 specimens demonstrated such lesions at a distance from a gastric cancer or ulcer. Therefore, the screening for such lesions will be of little significance in the control of gastric cancer.

Morphology of the Lesions

Atrophic gastritis is a diffuse lesion of the gastric mucosa, its macroscopic appearance at endoscopy is characteristic only in a small percentage of cases. Sampling of the mucosa with histological typing is required to characterize the stage of the lesions. Marker enzymes and mucin may be of some help in determining the stage of cellular atypia (39). Examining the mucosa with higher optical systems, will indicate minute abnormalities in the mucosal architecture. Islets of intestinal metaplasia have a rather characteristic appearance (villous structure). As for atypical epithelial foci, they cover a very limited surface of the mucosa and two main types are described (45–48,68): the protruded or elevated type associated with mild moderate or severe dysplasia and the depressed dyschromic type, which is more often associated with severe dysplasia. Individualization of dysplastic lesions in a flat mucosa is much more difficult and is obtained from the study of an operative specimen on serial sections.

The Dysplasia-Cancer Sequence

It is evident that gastric cancer may result in some cases from the progression of cellular atypia in elevated or depressed types of dysplasia. However, it was suggested recently (48) that this concerns only a very small percentage of cancers. Generally the cancers arise directly from cellular atypia in an atrophic gastric mucosa. The sequence "normal mucosa-atrophy-cancer" is responsible for most cases of gastric cancer; the sequences "normal mucosa-dysplasia-cancer" and "normal mucosa-adenoma-cancer" are uncommon. Therefore, the main precursor of gastric cancer is gastric atrophy in a flat mucosa in the absence of any specific morphological marker (to focus mucosal sampling at endoscopy). Islets of intestinal metaplasia are markers of a higher risk for gastric cancer but do not represent precancerous lesions. The term *precancerous lesion* should be reserved for severe cellular atypia. Mild lesions have the tendency to regress.

Colon and Rectum

Persons at Risk

That the disease may be genetically predetermined is manifest in a small percentage (5%) of cases when familial aggregation is observed (1). The following categories are described: (a) inherited familial adenomatosis of the colon and rectum associated with an autosomal dominant genetic defect; and (b) inherited nonpolyposis cancer occurring when multiple cases are observed in a family. The latter condition has the following characteristics: absence of concentration of the tumors in the distal colon, higher percentage of tumors in the right colon, occurrence at an earlier age, and increased risk for other primary tumors in organs such as stomach, breast, ovary, uterus (endometre). In both conditions, the genetic transmission concerns adenomatous polyps and their malignant potential. In the common situation (95%) neoplastic lesions of the colon (adenoma and cancer) occur sporadically. There is room for a genetic factor demonstrated by an increased risk (three- or fourfold) in close relatives of patients with colorectal cancer (35) for the same disease. However, the role of environmental factors is predominant (36,54). The epidemiological correlation with cancer of the breast and genital organs is present in females (59). Patients with chronic inflammatory bowel disease are also at high risk for colorectal cancer (10). Other morbid associations such as cholecystectomy (70) are of no practical importance.

Prevalence of the Lesions

Cancer of the colon and rectum is a major cause of illness and death in highly developed countries (58). The cumulative incidence rate reaches 4% to 5% in these countries for the life-span 0 to 74 years (67). Familial aggregation of cases does not account for a significant percentage in the prevalence of the disease. On the other hand, the prevalence of the lesion reputed as the precursor of most cases of colon cancer, viz., the adenomatous polyp, is very high, representing about 10% of the adult population. If diminutive adenomatous polyps are considered, the prevalence of such lesions in the population will be very high—50% to 60% (8,56).

Persons at high risk of cancer among ulcerative colitis patients include those with a disease in evolution for more than 10 years and who have lesions throughout the entire colon. Such cases do not account for a significant percentage in the prevalence of precancerous lesions.

Morphology of the Lesion

The adenomatous polyp is the most representative precancerous lesion in the colon and rectum (12,13,19,29,31,34,55). The macroscopic appearance of the polyp is characteristic when its size is over 5 mm, the shape being sessile or pediculated (63). However, nonneoplastic polyps (hyperplastic or inflammatory) may have the same macroscopic appearance and the diagnostic requires histological analysis. Diminutive polyps are detected in the colon and rectum; their size is less than 5 mm and they are often sessile. The percentage of adenomatous lesions is far from being low, when diminutive polyps have been examined with biopsies (18,49). Serial histological sections of the mucosa on operative specimens show that microadenoma undetectable at endoscopic examination of a flat mucosa are common in patients with patent polyps or cancers (33,52). The adenomatous polyp may be considered as a dysplastic lesion and its malignant potential is correlated with the degree of cellular atypia. The stage of dysplasia may, as usual, be characterized as mild, moderate, or severe or may be described according to a 5-stage scale (29). Only the polyps with severe dysplasia can be considered as precancerous lesions. The percentage of severe dysplasia among polyps varies from 20% to 60% according to series studies (16,63,76). Severe dysplasia increases in frequency when the polyp is large and when there are multiple polyps; however, the precancerous condition can be observed in diminutive lesions. Furthermore, cancer may develop from a flat colonic mucosa without any known precursor polyps. The ulcerative colitis model is often cited as an example of the "*de novo* carcinoma."

The Dysplasia-Cancer Sequence

The malignant potential of adenomatous polyps in the colon is well established (19). However, not all polyps will develop cellular atypia and the prevalence of adenoma is by far much higher than that of cancer. Furthermore, certain cancers will develop in the absence of precursor adenomas. Therefore, if the sequence "normal mucosa-adenoma-dysplasia-cancer" is the common route in colorectal carcinogenesis, there is also room for a sequence "normal mucosa-cellular-atypia-cancer." However, the distinction between a microadenoma in a flat mucosa and foci of cellular atypia is without practical significance.

SELECTION OF PERSONS AT RISK AND DETECTION OF PRECANCEROUS LESIONS

Selection of persons at risk for having precancerous lesions in the gastrointestinal tract raises no difficulties (ethical or cost efficiency) when it is based on a questionnaire on environmental and genetic risk factors. Case findings of precancerous lesions through this method deserves more emphasis in the education of the physician. Usually the screening of a population (or a group in the population) for cancer is based on a selection test fulfilling the sensitivity and specificity criteria. Acceptability, low cost, and absence of adverse effects are also important factors. A diagnostic test, proposed only to "positive" persons, characterizes the lesion with an histological grading of cellular atypia. It is suggested that the first step of the system (the selection test) be completed by a questionnaire. The state of the art for esophageal, gastric, and colorectal precancerous conditions is summarized below.

Esophagus

A method allowing the screening of large groups in the population has been developed in China using cytology on smears collected with a rubber balloon. The validity of this procedure as a selection test for cancerous lesions has been demonstrated, resulting in selection of cases with a good prognosis in nonrandomized trials (77). As for precancerous lesions the efficiency is confirmed in areas where esophagitis has a very high incidence and when cellular atypia and dysplasia have a high prevalence (5–10%). The method could not be proposed in countries where the prevalence of these abnormalities is very low. Therefore, under most conditions there is no selection test adaptable to the screening system other than the questionnaire.

The diagnostic test is based on a very careful endoscopic study, either with the flexible or (rarely) with the rigid endoscope. The latter instrument is well adapted to the analysis of multifocal lesions in the aerodigestive tract, but it requires anesthesia. In both cases the help of the dye staining method is acknowledged. In this method the hypochromic character of the dysplastic lesion when the Lugol solution is applied, and blue staining of dysplasia or preinvasive carcinoma when the Toluidine blue is applied following an acetic lavage are characteristic.

Stomach

The selection tests for gastric atrophy based on hyperchlorhydria do not fulfill the criteria of simplicity if the gastric secretory test is applied. A similar objection will be made to the tests using enzymes analysis in the gastric juice. On the other hand, the use of AZUR A resin with a urine sample has been abandoned owing to the lack of specificity. The increase in fasting gastrinemia points is found in too small a percentage of cases. Therefore, there is no satisfactory test for the selection of gastric atrophy. The detection of borderline lesions and atypical epithelial foci through tests proposed for early gastric cancer with good results on nonrandomized trials (20,21,23,26,28) (gastrocamera, indirect minature X-ray examination) is of no practical importance, because these lesions are very rare. On the other hand, the diagnostic step of the screening system is adequately achieved by the measurement of acid secretion under pentagastrin (estimation of the parietal acid output) and by a careful endoscopic study of the gastric mucosa with multiple sampling.

Colon

The guaiac test for fecal occult blood has been designed (sensibility and specificity) as a selection test in the screening for colorectal cancer (17,60,61,74,75). The prevalence of polyps is about 10% in the adult population, whereas the prevalence of a positive guaiac test in the same population varies between 1% and 3%. Therefore, most patients with polyps will not be detected. However the false negatives involve more often small and diminutive polyps (severe dysplasia is less frequent in such lesions). The guaiac test is not a good selection test for polyps.

The diagnostic tool well adapted to the diagnosis of these precancerous lesions is coloscopy. Coloscopy yields a higher incidence of these polyps than that of the double contrast enema. However these can hardly be classified as "screening techniques" in the average-risk population. Flexible sigmoidoscopy is a rather simple and efficient procedure among diagnostic tests (32,50,72,73), but one needs to consider the changing distribution of sites of colorectal cancers in countries with a high risk (57), which tend to be shifting more primarily.

TREATMENT AND SURVEILLANCE OF PRECANCEROUS LESIONS

In the critical study of a screening program the management of precancerous lesions of the gastrointestinal tract raises still more problems than their detection. Dysplasia does not mean precancer and the high risk of transformation is limited to severe dysplasia. Some lesions progress towards more atypia, but others are stabilized, and still others return to a less atypical structure. In addition, the treatment of multifocal lesions is an obstacle to a nonaggressive therapy without adverse effects in patients in good health. This is why the discovery of diffuse precancerous lesions will result in a surveillance program with repeated endoscopies rather than in a radical treatment. The management of polyps raises less difficulties.

Esophagus

The detection of precancerous lesions without confirmation of preinvasive carcinoma in a very high risk area, such as China or Iran, justifies a surveillance with yearly explorations of the esophagus. It has been suggested that a primary prevention of cancer by introducing vitamin supplements in the diet could be attempted through a randomized trial in the Linxian country (44). The detection of similar lesions in a patient exposed to the alcohol-tobacco risk results in repeated endoscopic examination of the esophagus, with histological sampling of the dysplastic areas. The rhythm of surveillance is based on the severity of dysplasia: 6-month intervals are used for severe dysplasia, 2- to 3-year intervals for mild to moderate dysplasia. The surveillance should include the larynx and pharynx. Suppression of the risk factors may reduce the progression of the lesions towards an increasing cellular atypia. In occidental countries a similar surveillance program is proposed to patients with chronic peptic esophagitis. The operation preventing chronic reflux is recommended in these patients, but it will not suppress the surveillance program.

Stomach

There is no treatment proposed to prevent the development of cellular atypia and dysplasia in the operated or nonoperated stomach with atrophic gastritis. The reduction in the incidence of gastric cancer in most countries is linked to environmental factors, resulting in a spontaneous primary prevention. On the other hand, a gastric polyp should be removed with a diathermic snare (62), the risk of cancer being limited to the adenomatous one. Finally, all cases of chronic gastric ulcers not healing under medical therapy should be promptly surgically treated. The surveillance program of a dysplastic lesion in the stomach is adapted to the severity of cellular atypia. Severe lesions should be controlled at 3- to 6-month intervals. The acceptance of the endoscopic control for mild dysplasia is very low.

Colon

The management of colonic polyps is well codified. The lesions must be removed with a diathermic snare or destroyed by electrocoagulation. The endoscopic polypectomy does not add a significant risk to the usual risk of colonoscopy (11,76,116). There is still some controversy about the surveillance program after polypectomy. If the patient has only one or two adenomatous polyps and if there is no risk added by the familial history, surveillance at 3-year intervals is satisfactory. If there are multiple polyps or if there is a family history, the rhythm of surveillance is yearly. The treatment of an intramucosal carcinoma by endoscopic polypectomy is considered as satisfactory. On the other hand, when the stalk is invaded, even if the section is in a normal mucosa, there is a risk of recurrence, and surgery is advised in adults in good health condition. Finally, the management of villous flat polyps in the rectum is now improved by the use of LASER photocoagulation.

PRECANCEROUS LESIONS OF THE GASTROINTESTINAL TRACT AND SCREENING PROGRAMS

Precancerous lesions of the gastrointestinal tract are not diseases. They are considered as risk factors for cancer. There is reasonable evidence that a questionnaire oriented to family history (familial aggregation of cancers) and to environmental factors (alcohol, tobacco) should be more systematically applied by the physician interviewing a patient (consulting for any class of symptoms). The questionnaire method would offer a strong basis to a campaign of prevention for an improved control of gastrointestinal cancer. Persons selected on the basis of the questionnaire will be investigated. It should be recalled that more gastric and esophageal precancerous lesions are multifocal and diffuse. Therefore, surveillance and staging of dysplasia will be the consequence of screening rather than an operative procedure. On the other hand, the colonic precancerous adenomatous lesion is easily controlled by endoscopic polypectomy.

There are very few screening programs adapted specifically to the detection of precancerous lesions, usually the expected benefit would be less than the adverse effect. An exception is the screening program for the detection of esophagitis and dysplasia in high-risk areas, as in Linxian in China (3–5). The blind cytology is the selection test proposed to patients. The progressive decrease in the incidence of stomach cancer in most countries does not justify extensive studies on the screening for atrophic gastritis. On the other hand, at the level of colon and rectum, proctoscopy and pansigmoidoscopy have been proposed, and abandoned, as the initial selection test for screening colon cancer. The cost effectiveness of the procedure was poor. When the detection of the adenomatous polyp and its treatment is taken into account, a new estimation of the procedure is possible. Indeed the Minnesota study demonstrated that polypectomy reduced the incidence of cancer by 85% in the examined area. Limited screening programs for the detection of adenomatous polyps could be offered to restricted groups, if included in a polyphasic screening. Furthermore, the use of a 30-cm sigmoidoscope, less expensive, less dangerous (biopsy possible but not polypectomy), and adapted to the general practitioner, could modify the cost effectiveness ratio of the procedure.

Finally screening programs designed for cancer at an early stage will detect some precancerous conditions. As an example, a trial of the guaiac test for fecal occult blood will detect not only carcinoma cases but also some polyps in the colon and rectum. The latter represent a very small fraction of the lesions expected in the screened population. However, the detected lesions will be treated and will interfere in the final evaluation of the benefit and adverse effects of the screening program.

CONCLUSIONS

Progress in health care can be expected from case findings of precancerous conditions in the gastrointestinal tract of patients who answered a questionnaire. The detection of the lesion results in surveillance rather than in therapy in the stomach and esophagus. Advice on diet and familial survey will complete the case findings. In the colon and rectum, endoscopic polypectomy is proposed when polyps are detected; their adenomatous structure is demonstrated only after polypectomy. The indication for a screening design aimed at precancerous conditions is limited to very restricted areas in the world. Finally a by-product of screening programs adapted to cancer is the detection of persons with precancerous lesions. Their management must be included in the evaluation of screening programs.

REFERENCES

1. Anderson, D. E. (1980): Risk in families of patients with colon cancer: In: *Colorectal cancer; Prevention, Epidemiology and Screening*, edited by S. J. Winawer, D. Schottenfeld, and P. Sherlock, pp. 109–116. Raven Press, New York.
2. Cole, P., and Morrison, A. S. (1978): Basic issues in cancer screening. In: *Screening in Cancer*, edited by A. B. Miller, pp. 7–39. UICC, Geneva.
3. Coordinating Group for Research on Esophageal Cancer (1973): The early detection of carcinoma of the oesophagus. *Scientic Sinica*, 16:457–463.
4. Coordinating Group for Research on Esophageal Cancer (1975): Studies on the relationship between epithelial dysplasia and carcinoma of the esophagus. *Chin. Med. J.*, 1:110–116.
5. Coordinating Group for Research on Esophageal Cancer (1976): Early diagnosis and surgical treatment of esophageal cancer under rural conditions. *Chin. Med. J.*, 2:113–116.
6. Correa, P., Cuello, C., and Montes, G. (1979): Pathogenesis of gastric carcinoma. The role of the microenvironment. In: *Gastric Cancer*, edited by C. J. Pfeiffer, pp. 9–12. Springer Verlag, Berlin.
7. Correa, P., Haenzel, W., Cuello, C., Tannenbaum, S., and Archer, M. (1975): A model for gastric cancer epidemiology. *Lancet*, ii:58–59.
8. Correa, P., Strong, J. P., Reif, A., and Johnson, W. D. (1977): The epidemiology of colorectal polyps, prevalence in New Orleans and international comparisons. *Cancer*, 39:2258–2264.
9. Crespi, M., Grassi, A., Amiri, G., Munoz, N., Aramesh, B., Mojtabai, A., and Casale, I. (1979): Oesophageal lesions in northern Iran: a premalignant condition? *Lancet*, ii:217–220.
10. Devroede, G. (1980): Risk of cancer in inflammatory bowel disease. In: *Colorectal Cancer; Prevention, Epidemiology and Screening*, edited by S. J. Winawer, D. Schottenfeld, and P. Sherlock, pp. 325–334. Raven Press, New York.
11. Deyle, P. (1980): Results of endoscopic polypectomy in the gastrointestinal tract. *Endoscopy (Suppl.)*, 12:35–46.
12. Doll, R. (1980): General epidemiologic considerations in etiology of colorectal cancer. In: *Colorectal Cancer; Prevention, Epidemiology and Screening*, edited by S. J. Winawer, D. Schottenfeld, and P. Sherlock, pp. 3–12. Raven Press, New York.
13. Ekelund, G. R. (1980): Cancer risk with single and multiple adenomas: synchronous and metachronous tumors. In: *Colorectal Cancer; Prevention, Epidemiology and Screening*, edited by S. J. Winawer, D. Schottenfeld, and P. Sherlock, pp. 151–156. Raven Press, New York.
14. Elsborg, L., and Mosbech, J. (1979): Pernicious anemia as a risk factor in gastric cancer. *Acta Med. Scand.*, 206:315–318.
15. Elster, K. (1976): Histologic classification of gastric polyps. In: *Current Topics in Pathology of the Gastrointestinal Tract*, edited by B. C. Morson, pp. 78–93. Springer Verlag, Berlin.
16. Fruhmorgen, P., Laudage, G., and Matek, W. (1981): Ten years of colonoscopy. *Endoscopy*, 13:162–168.
17. Gilbertsen, V., McHugh, R. B., Schuman, L. M., and Williams, S. E. (1980): The colon cancer control study: an interim report. In: *Colorectal Cancer; Prevention, Epidemiology and Screening*, edited by S. J. Winawer, D. Schottenfeld, and P. Sherlock, pp. 261–266. Raven Press, New York.
18. Grangvist, S., Gabrielsson, N., and Sudelin, P. (1979): Diminutive colonic polyps. Clinical significance and management. *Endoscopy*, 11:36–42.

19. Hill, M. J., Morson, B. C., and Bussey, H. J. R. (1978): Aetiology of adenoma-carcinoma sequence in large bowel. *Lancet*, i:245–247.
20. Hirayama, T. (1975): Epidemiology of cancer of the stomach with special reference to its recent decrease in Japan. *Cancer Res.*, 35:3460–3463.
21. Hirayama, T. (1978): Outline of stomach cancer screening in Japan. In: *Screening in Cancer*, edited by A. B. Miller, pp. 264–278. UICC, Geneva.
22. Hoey, J., and Lambert, R. (1981): *Elements d'épidémiologie pour le clinicien.* C.N.R.S., Paris.
23. Ichikawa, H. (1978): Mass screening for stomach in Japan. In: *Screening in Cancer*, edited by A. B. Miller, pp. 279–299. UICC, Geneva.
24. Ihamaki, T., Varis, K., and Siurala, M. (1979): Morphological, functional and immunological state of the gastric mucosa in gastric carcinoma families. *Scand. J. Gastroenterol.*, 14:801–812.
25. Joossens, J., and Geboers, J. (1981): Nutrition and gastric cancer. *Nutr. Cancer*, 2:256–261.
26. Kajitani, T. (1979): *Treatment Results of Stomach Carcinoma in Japan, 1963–1966.* WHO CC Monograph No. 2, Japan.
27. Kawai, K. (1978): Screening for gastric cancer in Japan. *Clin. Gastroenterol.*, 7:605–622.
28. Kidokoro, T., Haysashida, Y., Urabe, M., Wanatabe, K., Maekawa, K., and Kumagai, K. (1981): Progress of gastric carcinoma diagnosis and long term surgical results of early carcinoma. *Acta Endosc.*, II:133–154.
29. Kosuka, S. (1975): Premalignancy of the mucosal polyps in the large intestine. I. Histologic gradation of the polyps. *Dis. Colon Rectum*, 18:483.
30. Lambert, R. (1972): Chronic gastritis. A critical study of the progressive atrophy of the gastric mucosa. *Digestion*, 7:82–126.
31. Lambert, R. (1981): Epidemiology of colorectal carcinogenesis. In: *Falk Symposium No. 31*, edited by R. Malt, pp. 1–12. MTP Press Limited.
32. Lambert, R., Olive C., Melange, M., and Chabanon, R. (1978): Flexible rectosigmoidoscopy in the detection of tumoral colonic lesions. *Endoscopy*, 10:284–288.
33. Lev, R., and Grover, R. (1981): Precursors of human colon carcinoma: a serial section study of colectomy specimens. *Cancer*, 47:2007–2015.
34. Lipkin, M., Sherlock, P., and De Cosse, J. (1980): Risk factors and preventive measures in the control of cancer of the large intestine. *Curr. Prob. Cancer*, 4:1–57.
35. Lovett, E. (1976): Family studies in cancer of the colon and rectum. *Br. J. Surg.*, 63:13–18.
36. Lyon, J. L., Gardner, J. W., and West, D. W. (1980): Cancer incidence in Mormons and non Mormons in Utah during 1967–1975. *J. Natl. Cancer Inst.*, 65:1055–1061.
37. Mandard, A. M. (1981): Les lésions précancéreuses de l'oesophage humain. *Acta Endosc.*, 10:81–88.
38. Martin, E., Roset, F., and Lopez, C. (1981): Les lésions précancéreuses de l'estomac. *Acta Endosc.*, 10:89–106.
39. Matsukura, N., Susuki, K., Kawachi, T., Kinebachi, M., Sugimura, T., Itabashi, M., Hirota, T., and Kitaoka, H. (1980): Distribution of marker enzymes and mucin intestinal metaplasia in human stomach. *J. Natl. Cancer Inst.*, 65:231–240.
40. Miller, D. G. (1981): Principles of early detection of cancer. *Cancer*, 47:1142–1145.
41. Ming, S. C., and Goldman, H. (1965): Gastric polyps: a histogenic classification and its relation to carcinoma. *Cancer*, 18:721–726.
42. Monnier, Ph., Savary, M., Pasche, R., and Anani, P. (1981): Intramucosal carcinoma of the oesophagus: endoscopic morphology. *Endoscopy*, 13:185–191.
43. Monnier, Ph., Savary, M., and Pasche, R. (1981): Apport du bleu de toluidine en cancérologie bucco-pharyngo-oesophagienne. *Acta Endosc.*, 11:299–310.
44. Munoz, N., Grassi, A., Shenquiong, Crespi, M., Wang Guo Quing, and Li Zhang Gai (1982): Precursor lesions of oesophageal cancer in high-risk populations in Iran and China. *Lancet*, April, 876–879.
45. Nagayo, T. (1971): Histological diagnosis of biopsied gastric mucosae with special reference to that of borderline lesions. *Gan.*, 11:245–250.
46. Nagayo, T. (1975): Microscopical cancer of the stomach. A study on histogenesis of gastric carcinoma. *Int. J. Cancer*, 16:52–60.
47. Nagayo, T. (1980): Dysplastic changes of the digestive tract related to cancer. *Acta Endoscop.*, 10:69–80.
48. Nagayo, T. (1981): Dysplasia of the gastric mucosa and its relation to the precancerous stage. *Gan.*, 72:813–823.
49. Nishisawa, M., Okada, T., Sato, F., Kariya, A., Mayma, S., and Nakamura, K. (1980): A clinicopathological study of minute polypoid lesions of the colon based on magnifying fiber colonoscopy and dissecting microscopy. *Endoscopy*, 12:124–129.
50. Nivatvongs, S., and Fryd, D. (1980): How far does the proctosigmoidoscope reach. A prospective study of 1000 patients. *N. Engl. J. Med.*, 302:380–382.
51. Oehlert, W. (1979): Biological significance of dysplasias of the epithelium and of atrophic gastritis. In: *Gastric Cancer*, edited by C. J. Pfeiffer, pp. 91–103. Springer Verlag, Berlin.
52. Oohara, T., Ogino, A., and Tohma, H. (1981): Histogenesis of microscopic adenoma and hyperplastic (metaplastic) gland in non polyposis coli. *Dis. Colon Rectum*, 24:375–384.

53. Pasche, R., Savary, M., and Monnier, P. (1981): Multifocalité du carcinome épidermoîde sur les voies digestive et respiratoire distale: technicité du diagnostic endoscopique. *Acta Endosc.*, 11:277–285.
54. Phillips, R. L. (1975): Role of life style and dietary habits in risk of cancer among seventh day adventists. *Cancer Res.*, 35:3513–3522.
55. Potet, F. (1981): Pathologie précancéreuse du colon. *Acta Endosc.*, 10:123–138.
56. Restrepo, C., Correa, P., Duque, E., and Cuello, C. (1981): Polyps in a low risk colonic cancer population in Columbia, South America. *Dis. Colon Rectum*, 24:29–36.
57. Rosato, F. E., and Marks, G. (1981): Changing site distribution patterns of colorectal cancer at Thomas Jefferson University Hospital. *Dis. Colon Rectum*, 24:93–95.
58. Schottenfeld, D. (1980): Fundamental issues in cancer screening. In: *Colorectal Cancer; Prevention, Epidemiology and Screening*, edited by S. J. Winawer, D. Schottenfeld, and P. Sherlock, pp. 167–174. Raven Press, New York.
59. Schottenfeld, D., and Berg, J. W. (1971): Incidence of multiple primary cancers. IV. Cancers of the female breast and genital organs. *J. Natl. Cancer Inst.*, 46:161–169.
60. Schottenfeld, D., Winawer, S. J., and Miller, D. J. (1978): Screening and early diagnosis of large bowel cancer. In: *Screening in Cancer*, edited by A. B. Miller, pp. 307–327. UICC, Geneva.
61. Schwartz, F. W., Holstein, H., Brecht, J. G. (1980): Preliminary report of fecal occult blood testing in Germany. In: *Colorectal Cancer; Prevention, Epidemiology and Screening*, edited by S. J. Winawer, D. Schottenfeld, and P. Sherlock, pp. 267–270. Raven Press, New York.
62. Seifert, E., and Elster, K. (1975): Gastric polypectomy. *Am. J. Gastroenterol.*, 63:451–456.
63. Shinya, H., and Wolff, W. I. (1979): Morphology, anatomic distribution and cancer potential of colonic polyps. *Ann. Surg.*, 190:679–683.
64. Snyder, D. N., Heston, J. F., Meigs, J. W., and Flannery, J. T. (1977): Changes in site distribution of colorectal carcinoma in Connecticut 1940–1973. *Dig. Dis. Sci.*, 22:791–797.
65. Stemmermann, G. N. (1981): The impact of epidemiology upon the diagnosis and management of gastric disease: the experience of the Hawaï Japanase. *Acta Endosc.*, 11:103–122.
66. Strickland, R. G., and Mackay, R. (1973): A reappraisal of the nature and significance of chronic atrophic gastritis. *Am. J. Dig. Dis.*, 18:426–440.
67. Stukonis, M. K. (1979): *Cancer Cumulative Risk.* I.A.R.C., technic report, no. 79/004, Lyon.
68. Sugano, H., Nakamura, K., and Takagi, K. (1971): An atypical epithelium of the stomach. A clinicopathological entity. *GAN*.11:257–269.
69. Varis, K., Ihamaki, T., Harkunen, M., Samloff, I. H., and Siurala, H. (1979): Gastric morphology, function and immunology in first degree of probands with pernicious anemia and controls. *Scand. J. Gastroenterol.*, 14:129–139.
70. Vernick, L. J., Kuller, L. H., Lohsoonthorn, P., Rycheck, R. R., and Redmond, C. (1980): Relationship between cholecystectomy and ascending colon cancer. *Cancer*, 45:392–395.
71. Wesdorp, I. C. E., Bartelsman, J., Schipper, M. E. J., Offerhaus, J., and Tytgat, G. N. (1981): Malignancy and premalignancy in Barrett's oesophagus: a clinical endoscopical and histological study. *Acta Endosc.*, 11:317–322.
72. Wherry, D. C. (1981): Screening for colorectal neoplasia in asymptomatic patients using flexible fiberoptic sigmoidoscopy. *Dis. Colon Rectum*, 24:521–522.
73. Winawer, S. J., Andrews, M., Flehinger, B., Sherlock, P., Schottenfeld, D., and Miller, D. G. (1980): Progress report on controlled trial of fecal occult blood testing for the detection of colorectal neoplasia. *Cancer*, 45:2959–2964.
74. Winawer, S. J., Andrews, M., Miller, C. H., and Fleisher, M. (1980): Review of screening for colorectal cancer using fecal occult blood testing. In: *Screening in Cancer*, edited by A. B. Miller, pp. 249–260. UICC, Geneva.
75. Winnan, G., Berci, G., Panish, J., Talbot, T. M., Overholt, B. F., and McCallum, R. W. (1980): Superiority of the flexible to the rigid sigmoidoscope in routine proctosigmoidoscopy. *N. Engl. J. Med.*, 302:1011–1012.
76. Wolff, W. I., and Shinya, H. (1975): Endoscopic polypectomy; therapeutic and clinicopathologic aspects. *Cancer*, 36:683–690.
77. Wu Ying Kai and Huang Kuo Chun (1979): Chinese experience in the surgical treatment of carcinoma of the esophagus. *Ann. Surg.*, 190:361–365.

Precancerous Lesions of the Gastrointestinal Tract, edited by P. Sherlock, B.C. Morson, L. Barbara, and U. Veronesi. Raven Press, New York © 1983.

Value of Endoscopy in the Surveillance of High-Risk Groups for Gastrointestinal Cancer

G. N. J. Tytgat, E. M. H. Mathus-Vliegen, and J. Offerhaus

Division of Gastroenterology, University of Amsterdam, Academic Medical Center, Meibergoheef 020-5663634, Amsterdam, the Netherlands

It seems appropriate to realize that at present only few systematic large-scale screening programs exist in gastroenterology, except for Japan, although many gastrointestinal units are initiating endoscopic facilities, based on theoretical considerations. Often, however, such programs are not adequately organized, unless they are conducted within the framework of a research trial. In addition, repetitive endoscopy requires a high degree of motivation of the individual at risk because of its unpleasant or even traumatic nature.

This review is more or less a theoretical analysis of conditions where endoscopic screening might be useful and should be considered. Unequivocal proof of efficacy, feasibility, and cost effectiveness is, however, largely still lacking. Attention will be focused on the one hand on premalignant conditions, being clinical situations associated with an increased risk of carcinomatous degeneration, and on the other hand on premalignant lesions, being histopathological abnormalities leading to or associated with cancer, such as severe dysplasia.

CANCER SCREENING IN THE ESOPHAGUS

In general few esophageal cancers are detected at an early stage. Early detection, however, is possible as shown by ongoing population screening studies in high-incidence areas in China and South Africa, using cytology of exfoliated cell material collected via abrasive balloons or sponges. Cancer screening of the general population is probably not meaningful, except perhaps for such high-incidence areas. There is an increasing awareness of premalignant esophageal conditions, such as endobrachy-esophagus, lye burns, achalasia, and perhaps the Plummer-Vinson syndrome, where endoscopic screening might be meaningful.

Endobrachy-Esophagus

Columnar-lined or endobrachy-esophagus or Barrett's esophagus is increasingly recognized as a premalignant condition. The incidence of malignancy in 913 patients, selected from 15 publications since 1953, was 12.7%. In 100 recently analysed patients in Amsterdam, adenocarcinoma was discovered in 16%. Because of this figure, it seems reasonable to determine if patients with persistent reflux symptoms and/or stricturing have an endobrachy-esophagus and to enter such patients in an annual endoscopic surveillance program. Special endoscopic attention should be given to discrete lesions such as areas of discoloration, flat or polypoid excrescences, shallow ulcerations, areas of friability, and irregular narrowing. Occasionally nonsuspicious-looking Barrett-like mucosa may prove to be composed entirely of superficial spreading adenocarcinoma.

When no focal abnormalities are discernable, biopsies should be taken at increments of 1 to 2 cm and screened for dysplastic changes or malignancy. Preliminary findings suggest that severe dysplasia may be considered a reliable marker. It is uncertain at present if malignant degeneration is linked to a certain type of columnar tissue. Despite a conflicting report (7), it is fair to state that neither antireflux surgery nor prolonged intensive medical therapy (90) seems to be capable of reverting the mucosal condition back to squamous epithelium. Neither is there any evidence in the literature that antireflux surgery protects against possible subsequent malignant degeneration. To what extent the use of vital staining, with lugol or methylene blue, will facilitate the endoscopic screening in the future awaits further study.

Achalasia

The incidence of malignancy in lye burns varies from 0.8% to 4% (2). Usually the delay is over 20 years, although exceptions occur. The later in life the lye was ingested, the earlier underlying condition usually interfering with normal food passage for a long time and because of the enlargement of the esophageal diameter, cancer in a wide esophagus is usually detected rather late. Cancers occur in both medically and surgically treated patients. Wychulis et al. (94) followed 1,318 patients for a mean of 13 years and found 7 carcinomas. The location of the squamous carcinoma was usually in the middle segment of the esophagus. Achalasia symptoms were present for over 20 years. Cancers occurred in 0.59% of patients treated with dilatation and in 0.33% of surgically treated patients. It is unknown at present if malignancy only occurs in patients with ongoing stasis. Because achalasia patients are usually followed up in specialized centres, annual endoscopy with special attention to dysplastic changes or early lesions seems readily feasible. Although no information is available, vital staining with Lugol's solution or methylene blue (45,82,85) may facilitate endoscopic screening and biopsy.

Lye Burns

The incidence of malignancy in lye burns varies from 0.8% to 4% (2). Usually the delay is over 20 years, although exceptions occur. The later in life the lye was ingested, the earlier the carcinoma appeared. Recurrent dysphagia is the usual way of presentation. We are not aware of systematic screening programs at present. Because lye burns often occur at an early age, it seems justified to screen such patients annually with endoscopy and biopsy or cytology, in order to discover malignancies at an early stage, especially in areas of scarring.

Plummer-Vinson Syndrome

The incidence of cancer in the Plummer-Vinson or Paterson-Kelly syndrome varies from 4% to 16% (63) and occurs mainly in females with longstanding anemia and dysphagia. Well known are the dystrophic changes in the oropharynx and upper esophagus with web-formation, causing dysphagia. Chronic iron deficiency is considered of pathogenetic importance. Nowadays this syndrome is hardly ever seen, as longstanding nutritional deficiencies have been eliminated in developed countries.

Tylosis

Tylosis (familial keratosis palmaris et plantaris), a rare autosomal disease, leads to esophageal cancer in at least 30% of patients, usually at a rather early age (63).

Practical Considerations

The mentioned precancerous lesions and conditions only make up a small percentage of the total incidence of esophageal cancer. For practical purposes, screening for dysplasia or early malignancy should be done preferably by annual endoscopy. Systematic endoscopy of the upper digestive tract is also mandatory in patients with dysplastic changes or malignancy in the upper respiratory tract, including the oropharync, trachea, and bronchial tree and vice versa.

The role of endoscopy mainly centers on adequate tissue sampling via multiple target biopsies of suspicious areas or of random sites. Area selection will be facilitated by more widespread use of vital staining.

CANCER SCREENING IN THE STOMACH

Mass screening for stomach cancer in asymptomatic people should be distinguished from cancer screening in high-risk groups.

Cancer Screening in High-Incidence Areas

Cancer screening in high-incidence areas has mainly been performed in Japan. This has led to the recognition of the generally accepted concept of "early gastric cancer." In Japan, with the world's highest mortality from stomach cancer, cancer screening is done either with radiology or with endoscopy, mainly with gastrocamera examination. Endoscopic mass survey in Europe is not considered to be cost effective.

The endoscopic appearance of early gastric cancer has led to the well-known Japanese classification (54). In practice, many endoscopists use a simpler classification (22,36), subdividing the lesions into protruded or elevated, flat or superficial, and excavated or depressed lesions, corresponding to respectively 1 + 11ᵃ, 11ᵇ and 11ᶜ + 111 of the Japanese classification. Because no large-scale endoscopic mass screening studies are available outside Japan, it is difficult to compare the Japanese findings with the available endoscopic data from Europe, obtained by questionnaire and based on endoscopic studies of a large group of symptomatic and asymptomatic patients (47–49). The overall endoscopic detection rate of gastric cancer greatly depends on the expertise of the endoscopist and on the composition of the examined patient material, with positive results varying from 68% to 97% (4,24,57–59,67). Using gastroscopy for population screening in the Western world leads to a detection rate varying from 0.12% to 0.6% (44,47,48,79), without reaching the high figures from Japan. In that country 1 early gastric cancer is found in 67 gastroscopies in specialized clinics such as the Tokyo Women's Medical College, compared with 1 early cancer in 308 to 334 gastroscopies in Europe (47–49). Both in the Japanese and Western European studies, the depressed, excavated type (11ᶜ + 111) is the most common variant of endoscopic presentation (Table 1).

The vast majority of gastric cancers are situated along the lesser curve, antrum, and posterior wall. The distribution of the lesions varies considerably among the different coun-

TABLE 1. *Characteristics of early gastric cancer*

Refs.	No. of examinations	Gastric Ca	Early gastric Ca	Type (%)		
				(I + II[a])	(II[b])	(II[c] + III)
79[a]	2,800	225	16	25		75
31[b,c]	90,557	137	55	19.8		75.6
47-49	872,376	39,168	2,832	32.4	11.5	56.1
3[a,c]	9,276	819	68	26.4	10	63.1
44[a,d]	2,958	166	15	6.6	6.6	85.8
32[a,d]		1,233	437	26.2	5.5	68
36[a,c,d]		937	432	17	26.2	56.8

[a]Endoscopy.
[b]Gastrocamera.
[c]Röentgen.
[d]Gastric resections.

tries (47). Gastric cancer, also in the early stage, can be detected accurately provided multiple biopsies are taken, with positive results varying from 84% to 99% (4,17,24,32,33,36,48,59,67).

Cancer Screening in High-Risk Patients

In view of the dismal outlook of advanced gastric cancer with an overall 5-year survival of less than 10%, one should try to detect such lesions at an earlier stage, especially in those conditions known to be associated with an increased risk of gastric cancer, such as atrophic gastritis with or without intestinal metaplasia, with or without pernicious anemia, gastric polyps, longstanding partial gastric resection, familial gastric cancer, Ménétrier's disease, and perhaps a group of older, particularly male patients with persistent epigastric discomfort.

Atrophic Gastritis, Intestinal Metaplasia, Pernicious Anemia

Atrophic gastritis, with or without intestinal metaplasia, is linked to gastric cancer. In high-incidence areas, gastric mucosal atrophy and intestinal metaplasia are found to be frequent precursors or frequent concomitant abnormalities (53). Gastric cancer is also more prevalent in patients with atrophic gastritis (4,63,66) and in patients with pernicious anemia with frequencies up to 12% (65,84). A prospective follow-up study by Siurala et al. (74,77) revealed that most subjects with normal stomach mucosa still manifested a normal mucosa 15 to 20 years later; of the patients with superficial gastritis which could be followed for a long time, about half ultimately developed atrophic gastritis. Out of 160 patients with atrophic gastritis, ultimately 10 developed gastric carcinoma, all of the intestinal type. Of 45 patients with atrophic gastritis followed up during at least 15 years, 30 remained unchanged, 8 progressed, and 7 regressed. According to Siurala and co-workers, the risk of gastric malignancy in patients with severe atrophic gastritis is 10 times higher than that in a control population (73,75,76,78).

Ordinary chronic atrophic gastritis (type B gastritis) is different from that seen in pernicious anemia (type A gastritis). In the former, glandular atrophy and intestinal metaplasia is more severe in the antrum and less pronounced in the body and fundus area, whereas in the latter the antral mucosa remains essentially normal with atrophic changes limited to corpus and fundus. This corresponds to the more proximal localization of the malignancies in type A gastritis (52,55). Despite the apparent relationship between atrophic gastritis and intestinal metaplasia and the presence of all transitional stages between metaplasia to fullblown carcinoma, including morphological and histochemical signs of intestinalization within the cancer itself, the interpretation of the mere finding of atrophic gastritis and/or intestinal metaplasia in gastric biopsies remains difficult. Indeed, the incidence of atrophic gastritis unquestionably increases with age and may occur in 50% of patients above age 50, of whom only a minority will ultimately die of gastric cancer (72). Therefore some authors (65) are somewhat hesitant to consider atrophic gastritis by itself as a reliable precancerous lesion. The same holds true, to some extent, for intestinal metaplasia occurring in 20% of the general population. Even if over half the biopsies show evidence of intestinal metaplasia, this still does not indicate that cancerous degeneration is present somewhere in the stomach (30).

It is to be expected that in future research our attention will be focused not so much on atrophic gastritis or intestinal metaplasia as on the detection of dysplastic changes as recently stressed by Morson et al. (52) and Ming (50). The latter author distinguishes four grades of dysplasia based on structural and cytological criteria, with the occurrence of grades 1 and 2 in gastritis, Ménétrier's disease, and hyperplastic polyps and the occurrence of grades 3 and 4 in atrophic gastritis, adenoma, and carcinoma. Grade 4 especially deserves vigorous vigilance, because of its occurrence in 25% of gastric carcinoma specimens and absence in benign conditions.

Gastric Polyps

The occurrence rate of gastric polyps in asymptomatic individuals is rather low and usually less than 1% (83). The frequency of polypoid lesions in the stomach is much higher during screening of patients with atrophic gastritis and/or pernicious anemia, the polyposis syndromes or postgastrectomy. Although there is no evidence for direct degeneration of hyperplastic or hyperplasiogenic polyps, their mere presence often serves an indicator function (71), pointing towards increased risk of malignancy in the surrounding polyp bearing gastric mucosa, in which often atrophic gastritis and/or intestinal metaplasia is present. This indicator function of hyperplasiogenic polyps may be as high as 18% (63). A minority of gastric polyps are true adenomas or borderline lesions. Also, adenomas often occur in the stomachs of patients with atrophic gastritis, achlorhydria, or pernicious anemia. Malignant transformation is possible, not only within the adenomatous polyp itself but also in the surrounding gastric mucosa. The bigger the polyps and the higher the number of polyps, the greater the chance for gastric cancer (86). After removal of a single hyperplastic or hyperplasiogenic polyp or, when multiple polyps are present, after removal of four polyps for proper histologic identification, gastroscopic follow-up seems indicated about every 2 years. After removal of adenomatous polyps, endoscopic follow-up should be carried out annually. Removal of lesions with severe dysplasia requires closer follow-up with shorter intervals, at least initially (Table 2).

Screening of Postgastrectomy Patients

Gastric stump cancer is defined as a cancer occurring more than 5 years after surgery for a preferably histologically proven benign condition. The incidence of stump cancer varies markedly, depending on the method of investigation (postmortem, retrospective, prospective). In many studies, the incidence is lower than 5%, but in about one-third of the available literature higher figures, up to 15% (14), are obtained. The incidence of malignancy in a prospective study from Scandinavia (20) and from our group in the Netherlands (29) using gastroscopy reveals an incidence of about 2% in older asymptomatic postgastrectomy pa-

TABLE 2. *Follow-up after gastric polypectomy*

Time interval (years)	1/4	1/2	1	2	3	5
Hyperplastic				X		X
Hyperplasiogenic			X		X	X
Adenomatous						
Complete removal			X		X	X
Incomplete removal	X		X		X	X
Borderline lesions	X	X	X	X	X	X
Early gastric cancer (types I, IIa)	X	X	X	X	X	X

tients. In the latter study, half the malignancies were early intramucosal cancers, undetectable by the naked eye and only discovered by multiple at-random biopsies of the stomal area and the lesser and greater curves. The incidence of malignancy is clearly related to the lagtime between surgery and the development of stump cancer, being on the average 20 to 22 years. In general the risk of cancer in the first 15 years after surgery is less (80) than that in the general population, but it increases two to three times thereafter. With a few exceptions there are no differences between the various partial gastrectomy types. Why the gastric stump is at risk is a matter of speculation. Because two-thirds of the distal stomach, the main site for ordinary gastric cancer, is resected, one would expect only one-fourth of the cancers in the remaining upper part. In fact, the cancer risk is not decreased to one-fourth but is increased on the average two to three times over the incidence in the general population. As in many other premalignant conditions, the development of chronic atrophic gastritis with intestinal metaplasia, together with presumably increasingly severe dysplasia (29), may favour cancerous degeneration. There is some debate as to whether or not dysplasia progresses with time, as suggested by a few of our patients (29). On the other hand, a recent Scandinavian study (81) showed regression of dysplasia in a substantial number of post-gastrectomy patients during a 3-year endoscopic follow-up, starting 20 to 25 years after gastrectomy. In some patients dysplasia regressed despite progression of the atrophic gastritis.

In view of the dismal outlook of stump cancers in the symptomatic stage and because of the poor results with radiology as a detection modality, it seems justified to screen post-gastrectomy patients, especially of the younger age group, starting 15 years after previous gastrectomy, with annual or biannual gastroscopy with multiple biopsies of the stomal area and the lesser and greater curves.

Endoscopists should concentrate on minute abnormalities such as tiny erosive defects, slight thickening, and irregularity of folds and/or areas of nodular irregularity or discoloration. When severe dysplasia is discovered, closer follow-up may be necessary. Other authors (81) suggest a follow-up at 3- to 5-year intervals with multiple biopsies.

Ménétrier's Disease

Although the available evidence on the incidence of cancer in Ménétrier's disease is rather limited and occasionally controversial, with incidences varying from 8% to 42% (13,64), usually in selected material, it is probably wise to follow such patients with annual endoscopy and biopsy of any suspicious area for possible malignant degeneration. Obviously selection of the biopsy sites in such stomachs bearing giant folds or polypoid clusters may cause great difficulty. Perhaps sampling larger quantities of tissue with a snare biopsy technique or with larger biopsy forceps will prove to be helpful in this regard.

Familial Gastric Cancer

Many authors find a four to five times higher gastric cancer incidence in relatives compared to the expected frequency in the general population as summarized by Kopf et al. (34). The first generation is especially at risk. To what extent atrophic gastritis is present in such relatives at risk is rather poorly documented in all these studies. Although prospective studies are lacking, screening relatives of gastric cancer families should be considered, especially in those with immune disorders or with evidence of autoimmune diseases, such as thyroiditis, Addison's disease, or autoimmune gastritis (16).

Practical Considerations

Gastroscopy with multiple target biopsies or target cytology remains at present the most suitable technique for screening patients at risk for gastric malignancy. Biopsies should be obtained from any visible abnormality, such as slight mucosal elevation, areas of discoloration, depressed areas with mucosal roughness, and areas of conspicuously increased friability. When no abnormalities can be detected, at-random biopsies should be obtained from the antrum and from the fundic area in order to look for dysplastic changes (50,52).

CANCER SCREENING IN THE RECTOCOLON

Screening for colorectal cancer is of major importance in view of its high frequency and because the 5-year survival in asymptomatic patients with early lesions is excellent, with figures varying between 90% and 100%. This is in contrast with the poor results obtained in symptomatic patients where the 5-year survival often drops below 50%, owing to the fact that metastases are present in over half the patients at the time of surgery.

Patients with Adenomatous Polyps

Patients with adenomatous polyps are at risk for colonic cancer. Morson pioneered the well-known adenoma-carcinoma sequence, recently rephrased as "adenoma-dysplasia-carcinoma sequence" (27,51). The bigger the size, the higher the number, the more villous in character, and the higher the degree of dysplasia, the higher the risk of ultimate development of colorectal cancer. The risk for synchronous and for metachronous cancer is also higher in patients bearing adenomatous polyps together with a carcinoma (21,35,69). Although no extensive proof is as yet available regarding the reduction in advanced colorectal cancer by large-scale application of colonoscopic polypectomy except perhaps for Gilbertsen and Nelm's study (23), it is logical to expect that screening for and removal of adenomatous polyps will ultimately lower the death rate of colorectal cancer.

There are various schemes for endoscopic follow-up after colonoscopic polypectomy, which is nowadays a routine procedure (Table 3). Patients with a pedunculated or sessile adenomatous polyp should be followed up after the colon is polyp-free about every 2 to 3 years, with one earlier control when completeness of the initial removal is in doubt. When severe dysplasia is present, the patients should be reexamined after 6 months, 2 years, and when polyp-free, after 5 years. An earlier first control is again advised when the initial removal is incomplete or of dubious completeness.

Some physicians and patients prefer to alternate the colonoscopy with barium enema examination. Polyps with superficial cancer, with a noninvolved resection line, should be followed more closely. When cancer approaches the line of resection, one should at first always try to remove a remaining segment of the stalk, whenever possible, to rule out the

TABLE 3. *Follow-up after colonoscopic polypectomy*

Time interval (years)	1/4	1/2	1	2	3	5
Pedunculated adenoma					X	
Sessile or pedunculated but questionable complete removal	X				X	
Adenoma with severe dysplasia						
Complete removal		X		X		X
Incomplete removal or questionable completeness	X			X		X
Adenoma with invasive cancer completely removed[a]	X	X	X	X	X	X

[a]When completeness of removal is questionable, very close follow-up, when surgery is not considered.

presence of residual tumor. When no pedicle remnants can be snared, biopsies obtained from the coagulation crater and surrounding edges may be helpful. For adenomatous polyps with limited superficial malignant infiltration, an expectant attitude may be sufficient (70).

When cancer has deeply penetrated the stalk, has invaded lymphatic structures, or is poorly differentiated, then a subsequent surgical resection of that segment is in order. In that case, there will be about a 5% chance that lymph nodes are involved. It is of paramount importance that the polyp is properly oriented for histological examination. The long axis of the polyp and the coagulation line should, in principle, be clearly recognizable in order to allow accurate analysis. Local recurrence after removal of usually large villous tumors is common and demands for close follow-up at a 3- to 6-month interval. After adequate tissue sampling for histology, such local recurrences are easily removed with fulguration or laser-photocoagulation, which we prefer.

Patients with Genetic Predisposition

Familial Adenomatous Polyposis Syndromes

Several of the genetically determined polyposis syndromes are characterized by a highly malignant potential (8). Family members of such patients should always be carefully studied. In familial polyposis, the presence of polyps is clearly demonstrable in half the patients by age 22. With modern techniques of vital staining or with multiple at-random biopsies, tiny adenomatous foci can occasionally be discovered, which are still practically invisible to the naked eye during routine endoscopic examination. In view of the tremendous cancer risk, nearly all these patients are treated with prophylactic (procto) colectomy upon discovery. In a substantial number of patients the rectal stump is left behind, which necessitates regular, careful, endoscopic follow-up with biopsies, at least every 6 months, if necessary, and with destruction of new polyps with either diathermy fulguration or laser-photocoagulation. Transient spontaneous regression of polyps after ileorectal anastomosis should not disguise the need for lifelong sigmoidoscopic control.

Hereditary, Nonpolyposis Syndromes

The hereditary nonpolyposis syndromes are divided into four groups (1,42): (a) the cancer family syndrome (43); (b) the hereditary gastrocolonic carcinoma; (c) the hereditary site-specific colonic carcinoma (41,43); and (d) the Muir's or Torre's syndrome.

The most frequent variety, the cancer family syndrome, is characterised by increased incidence of adenocarcinoma, mainly in the proximal colon and endometrium, and to a lesser extent in the breast and ovary. The annual risk for a second primary carcinoma after the first and for a third after the second is estimated as, respectively, 3% and 6.9% (42). Screening for colorectal cancer with biannual fecal smears on a high-roughage, meat-free diet and with colonoscopy and/or barium enema has to be started at age 20, in addition to screening for endometrial cancer. Lovett (40) found a threefold increased risk for colonic carcinoma when examining first-degree relatives of a young index case with colon cancer, with death due to colon-carcinoma of 9.3% of the fathers, 7.7% of the mothers, 15.8% of the brothers, and 19.3% of the sisters. Since the initial studies on cancer families, one has the impression that such families are increasingly discovered in many areas of the world.

The relationship between extracolonic and colonic cancers recently led the Lyon group to screen breast cancer patients and controls for the presence of adenomatous lesions in the distal rectocolon using flexible sigmoidoscopy (37). It is intriguing to note that polyps were found to be four times more frequent in the breast cancer group. Obviously, these studies need confirmation before more definite conclusions can be drawn from this observation.

Inflammatory Bowel Disease

In the United States, United Kingdom, and Scandinavian countries in particular, there is a consensus that patients with chronic ulcerative colitis have a 7 to 11 times greater risk of developing colorectal cancer and that such cancers usually become manifest at a rather early age. In addition, the risk seems to be related directly to the duration of the colitis, increasing rapidly after 10 years of evolution. This increased cancer risk is also related to the extent of colonic involvement and usually occurs in patients with total colonic involvement (18,26,38). Colonoscopy has been proposed as a way of identifying patients particularly at risk by obtaining histologic evidence of severe dysplasia. The presence of severe dysplasia appears to carry a 30% to 40% likelihood of cancer being found at subsequent colectomy (19,62). Although it has been found that a high proportion of patients with dysplasia in colonoscopic biopsies also have dysplasia in sigmoidoscopic biopsies (56,61), most experts would agree that it is desirable to obtain multiple biopsy samples from various parts of the colon in order to enhance the chances of finding premalignant abnormalities. Biopsies should be taken preferably from thickened areas, slightly elevated areas, and areas with a velvety or rough appearance of the mucosa or suspicious-looking polypoid lesions or nodular excrescences. In the absence of suspicious visible lesions, biopsies should be obtained preferably with increments of 10 cm throughout the rectocolon, because dysplasia may occur in rather inactive or somewhat atrophic-looking mucosa (5,9,10,28,88,91,95). In general, only patients with a history of chronic ulcerative colitis of 10 or more years duration with involvement of the whole colon are eligible for annual colonoscopic examination with biopsy. Because the tendency to carcinoma in patients with colitis confined to the left half of the colon is only slightly increased, at present this risk does not appear great enough to warrant a special follow-up program for these patients (9), although other authors have a different opinion (87). When suspicious findings are found at colonoscopy, the procedure should perhaps be performed more often in a few selected patients. In others with very normal findings, perhaps an annual rectal biopsy and colonoscopy every 2 years may be sufficient. In addition to the patients with extensive longstanding colitis, patients treated by colectomy with ileorectal anastomosis should also be screened annually for dysplastic changes in the rectal remnant (9,38).

When severe dysplasia is found, authorities differ on whether or not to recommend colectomy. For some, dysplasia, even moderate, constitutes an indication for colectomy

(56). Others advise surgery only for severe dysplasia, preferably found at different sites within the rectocolon and preferably documented on sequential examinations (9,19,38). According to Blackstone et al. (5), the presence of dysplasia associated lesions or masses, especially polypoid structures, should be regarded as a strong indication for surgery.

Not only ulcerative colitis but also longstanding schistosomiasis may favour the development of dysplastic changes with subsequent malignancy (11,12). Recently dysplasia (15) and increased cancer risk (25,89) has also been reported in Crohn's disease, although certainly much less than seen in chronic ulcerative colitis. Indeed the chance of remaining cancer-free was 99.7% after 10 and 97.2% after 20 years of evolution in Weedon et al.'s analysis (89).

Because the increase in malignancy in Crohn's disease is still rather doubtful, and because of the still insufficiently known incidence of dysplasia, clinical screening of patients with Crohn's disease at present cannot be recommended until more pertinent information becomes available (9,10).

Postcolonic Cancer Resection

Patients previously operated for colonic cancer have a threefold increased risk of developing a metachronous malignancy. The risk was even higher when the initial carcinoma was located in the cecum or when adenomatous polyps were present at the time of the initial resection (68).

Males and Females Above the Age of 40

Beyond age 40, the overall risk for colorectal cancer doubles with each decade, reaching a peak incidence between 75 and 80 years. Screening asymptomatic individuals may reveal adenomatous polyps in 4.7% to 9.7% and colonic cancer in 0.12% to 0.3% (35,39,68,69). Obviously, we are still a long way from worldwide routine screening of the older population.

Practical Considerations

Experience with systematic screening for precancerous or cancerous lesions during endoscopy is still rather limited. Gilbertsen and Nelms (23) were the first to show that systematic proctosigmoidoscopy combined with polypectomy when necessary, in over 20,000 individuals, led to a decrease in the expected cancer incidence; after finding 27 carcinomas at the first exam, only 13 instead of the 90 expected cancers were found on follow-up sigmoidoscopy. The cancers that were found during systematic screening were all, but 1, limited to the superficial layers. According to the literature the chance of finding cancers and polyps using sigmoidoscopy beyond age 40 is, respectively, 1.5‰ and 2% to 17% (6,69,93).

During the last years, several investigators (45,60,92) have used flexible instead of rigid sigmoidoscopy. Obviously the yield of abnormalities is higher, about two to three times, because a longer segment of the rectocolon can be investigated. With experience, the flexible sigmoidoscope can usually be introduced beyond the sigmoid, heading for the splenic flexure. The yield for flexible sigmoidoscopy in a group of 1,012 patients was 3.2 times higher than proctosigmoidoscopy (46). There is still some doubt as to whether or not flexible sigmoidoscopy should become the screening method of choice. For patients at high risk of colonic cancer, such as cancer family syndromes and inflammatory bowel disease, total colonoscopy should be preferred instead of limiting the examination to the left colon. One should keep in mind that lesions may be missed during colonoscopy, especially in areas of acute angulation in up to 6% to 8% (69). There may well be a place for flexible sigmoidoscopy in the work-up of patients with positive occult blood testing. Indeed, flexible sigmoidoscopy combined with double-contrast radiology approaches the accuracy of total colonoscopy (92). Such a policy may be applicable in smaller hospitals.

CONCLUDING REMARKS

When reviewing the state of knowledge and actual realization regarding endoscopic cancer screening, it becomes obvious that we still are far from the ideal situation. Some progress, however, has been made because several gastrointestinal units are initiating screening facilities. The problems with patient compliance, especially for endoscopic screening, are formidable. A major issue for the future will be whether or not the society is willing to sponsor large-scale education of the population and to subsidize expensive endoscopic cancer-screening programs. In the meantime, physicians should try to establish if the endoscopic approach is adequate and cost effective.

REFERENCES

1. Anderson, D. E. (1980): Risk in families of patients with colon cancer. In: *Colorectal Cancer: Prevention, Epidemiology and Screening*, edited by S. Winawer, D. Schottenfeld, and P. Sherlock, pp. 109–115. Raven Press, New York.
2. Appelqvist, P., and Salmo, M. (1980): Lye corrosion carcinoma of the esophagus, a review of 53 cases. *Cancer*, 45:2655–2658.
3. Aste, H., Amadori, D., Maltoni, C., Crespi, M., Pugliese, V., Ravaioli, A., Pacini, F., and Cosale, V. (1981): Early gastric cancer detection in areas at different gastric cancer death rate. *Acta Endosc.*, 11:123–130.
4. Berndt, H., Gütz, H. J., and Woft, G. (1977): Wissenschaftliche Grundlagen der Bekämpfung des Magenkrebses. *Arch. Geschwulstforsch.*, 44:67–85.
5. Blackstone, M. O., Riddell, R. H., Rogers, B. H. G., and Levin, B. (1981): Dysplasia associated lesion or mass (DALM) detected by colonoscopy in longstanding ulcerative colitis; an indication for colectomy. *Gastroenterology*, 80:366–374.
6. Bolt, R. J. (1971): Sigmoidoscopy in detection and diagnosis in the asymptomatic individual. *Cancer*, 28:121–122.
7. Brand, D. L., Ylvisaker, J. Th., Gelfand, M., and Pope, C. E. (1980): Regression of columnar esophageal (Barrett's) epithelium after antireflux surgery. *N. Engl. J. Med.*, 302:844–848.
8. Bussey, H. J. R., Veale, A. M. O., and Morson, B. C. (1978): Genetics of gastrointestinal polyposis. *Gastroenterology*, 84:1325–1330.
9. Butt, J. H., Lennard-Jones, J. E., and Ritchie, J. K. (1980): A practical approach to the risk of cancer in inflammatory bowel disease. Reassure, watch or act? *Med. Clin. North Am.*, 64:1203–1220.
10. Butt, J. H., and Morson, B. C. (1981): Dysplasia and cancer in inflammatory bowel disease. *Gastroenterology*, 80:865–868.
11. Chen Ming-Chai, Chuang Chi-Yuan, Chang Pei-Yu, and Hu Jen-Chun (1980): Evolution of colorectal cancer in schistosomiasis—transitional mucosal changes adjacent to large intestine carcinoma in colectomy specimens. *Cancer*, 46:1661–1675.
12. Chen Ming-Chai, Chuang Chi-Yuan, C., Wang Fu-Pan, W., Pei-Yu, C., Yi-Jen, C., Yang-Chuan, T., and Shun-Chuan, C. (1981): Colorectal cancer and schistosomiasis. *Lancet*, 1:971–973.
13. Chusid, E. L., Hirsch, R. L., and Colcher, H. (1964): Spectrum of hypertrophic Gastropathy. *Arch. Int. Med.*, 114:621–628.
14. Clémençon, G., Baumgartner, R., Leuthold, E., Miller, G., and Neiger, A. (1976): Das Karzinom des operierten Magens. *Dtsch. Med. Wschr.*, 101:1015–1020.
15. Craft, C. F., Mendelsohn, G., Cooper, H. S., and Yardley, J. H. (1981): Colonic "Precancer" in Crohn's Disease. *Gastroenterology*, 80:578–584.
16. Creagan, E., and Fraumeni, J. (1973): Familial gastric cancer and immunologic abnormalities. *Cancer*, 32:1325–1331.
17. Dekker, W., and Tytgat, G. N. (1977): Diagnostic accuracy of fiberendoscopy in the detection of upper intestinal malignancy. A follow-up analysis. *Gastroenterology*, 73:710–714.
18. DeVroede, G. J., Taylor, W. F., Sauer, W. G., Jackman, R. J., and Stickler, G. B. (1971): Cancer risk and life expectancy of children with ulcerative colitis. *N. Engl. J. Med.*, 285:17–21.
19. Dobbins, W. O. (1977): Current status of the precancerous lesion in ulcerative colitis. *Gastroenterology*, 73:1431–1433.
20. Dömellöf, L., Eriksson, S., and Janunger, K. G. (1975): Late occurrence of precancerous changes and carcinoma of the gastric stump after Billroth 11 resection. *Acta Chir. Scand.*, 141:292–297.
21. Editorial (1980): Evolution of colonic polyps. *Br. Med. J.*, 1:257–258.

22. Elster, K., Wild, A., and Thomasko, A. (1980): Prognose des Magenfrühkarzinoms. *Dtsch. Med. Wschr.*, 105:949–953.
23. Gilbertsen, V. A., and Nelms, J. M. (1978): The prevention of invasive cancer of the rectum. *Cancer*, 41:1137–1139.
24. Gloor, F. (1976): Das Oberflächenkarzinom (Frükarzinom) des Magens. *Schweiz. Med. Wschr.*, 106:21–27.
25. Greenstein, A. J., Sachar, D. B., Smith, H., Janowitz, H. D., and Aufses, A. H. (1980): Patterns of neoplasia in Crohn's disease and ulcerative colitis. *Cancer*, 46:403–407.
26. Greenstein, A. J., Sachar, D. B., Smith, H., Pucillo, A., Papatestas, A. E., Kreel, I., Geller, S. A., Janowitz, H. D., and Aufses, A. H. (1979): Cancer in universal and leftsided ulcerative colitis: factors determining risk. *Gastroenterology*, 77:290–294.
27. Hill, M. J., Morson, B. C., and Bussey, H. J. R. (1978): Aetiology of adenoma-carcinoma sequence in large bowel. *Lancet*, 1:245–247.
28. Hogan, W. J., Hensley, G. T., and Geenen, J. E. (1980): Endoscopic evaluation of inflammatory bowel disease. *Med. Clin. North Am.*, 64:1083–1102.
29. Huibregtse, K., Offerhaus, J., Verhoeven, T., de Boer, J., van der Stadt, J., and Tytgat, G. N. (1981): Endoscopic screening for malignancy in the gastric remnant. *Acta Endosc.*, 11:171–175.
30. Johansen, A., and Sikjär, B. (1977): The diagnostic significance of intestinal metaplasia in endoscopic gastric biopsies. *Acta Pathol. Microbiol. Scand. (A)*, 85:240–244.
31. Kaneko, E., Nakamura, T., Umeda, N., Fujino, M., and Niwa, H. (1977): Outcome of gastric carcinoma detected by gastric mass survey in Japan. *Gut*, 18:626–630.
32. Kidikoro, T., Haysashida, Y., Urabe, M., Watanabe, S., Maekawa, K., And Kumagai, K. (1981): Progress of gastric carcinoma diagnosis and long-term surgical results of early carcinoma. *Acta Endosc.*, 11:133–144.
33. Kobayashi, S., Yoshii, Y., and Kasugai, T. (1976): Biopsy and cytology in the diagnosis of early gastric cancer. *Endoscopy*, 8:53–58.
34. Kopf, A., Zeitoun, P., and Bonfils, S. (1967): Les formes familiales du cancer de l'estomac. *Arch. Fr. Mal. App. Dig.*, 56:827–840.
35. Kronborg, O. (1980): Polyps of the colon and rectum: approach to prophylaxis in colorectal cancer. *Scand. J. Gastroent.*, 15:1–5.
36. Kurihara, M., Shirakabe, H., Izumi, T., Miyasaka, K., Maruyama, T., Sasaki, Y., Kobayashi, S., and Hamada, T. (1980): X-ray and endoscopy in the diagnosis of small early gastric cancer. In: *International Congress on Diagnosis and Treatment of Upper Gastrointestinal Tumors*, edited by M. Friedman, M. Ogawa, and D. Kisner, pp. 15–24. International Congress Series 542. Excerpta Medica.
37. Lambert, R. (1982): Epidemiology of colorectal carcinogenesis. In: *Falk Symposium No. 31: Colonic Carcinogenesis*, edited by R. O. Molk and R. Williamson, pp. 1–10. Paris, Mai, Société nationale française d'Endoscopie digestive, Palais de Congrès, Porte Maillot.
38. Lennard-Jones, J. E., Morson, B. C., Ritchie, J. K., Shove, D. C., and Williams, C. B. (1977): Cancer in colitis: assessment of the individual risk by clinical and histological criteria. *Gastroenterology*, 73:1280–1289.
39. Lipkin, M., Scherf, S., Schechter, L., and Braun, D. (1980): Memorial Hospital Registry of Population Groups at high risk for cancer of the large intestine: age of onset of neoplasms. *Prev. Med.*, 9:335–345.
40. Lovett, E. (1976): Family studies in cancer of the colon and rectum. *Br. J. Surg.*, 63:13–18.
41. Lynch, H. T., Harris, R. E., Bardawil, W. A., Lynch, P. M., Guirgis, H. A., Swartz, M. J., and Lynch, J. F. (1977): Management of hereditary site-specific colon cancer. *Arch. Surg.*, 112:170–174.
42. Lynch, H. T., Lynch, P. M., and Lynch, J. F. (1980): Analysis of genetics of inherited colon cancer. In: *Colorectal Cancer: Prevention, Epidemiology and Screening*, edited by S. Winawer, D. Schottenfeld, and P. Sherlock, pp. 117–131. Raven Press, New York.
43. Lynch, P. M., Lynch, H. T., and Harris, R. E. (1977): Heriditary proximal colonic cancer. *Dis. Colon Rectum*, 20:661–668.
44. Machado, G., Davies, J. D., Tudway, A. J. C., Salmon, P. R., and Read, A. E. (1976): Superficial carcinoma of the stomach. *Br. Med. J.*, 2:77–79.
45. Mandard, A. M., Tourneux, J., Gignoux, M., Blanc, L., Segol, P., and Mandard, J. C. (1980): In situ carcinoma of the esophagus: macroscopic study with particular reference to the Lugol Test. *Endoscopy*, 12:51–57.
46. Marks, G., Boggs, H. W., Castro, A. F., Gathright, J. B., Ray, J. E., and Sawati, E. (1979): Sigmoidoscopic examinations with rigid and flexible fiberoptic sigmoidoscopes in the surgeon's office: a comparative prospective study of effectiveness in 1,012 cases. *Dis. Colon Rectum*, 22:162–168.
47. Miller, G., and Froelicher, P. (1978): Das Magenfrühkarzinom in Europa. Resultate einer Umfrage von 1978. *Z. Gastroenterol.*, 11:678–683.
48. Miller, G., Froelicher, P., Kaufmann, M., and Maurer, W. (1979): 10 years endoscopic diagnosis of early gastric cancer in Europe. *J. Cancer Res. Clin. Oncol.*, 93:99–107.
49. Miller, G., and Kaufmann, M. (1975): Das Magenfrühkarzinom in Europa. *Dtsch. Med. Wschr.*, 100:1946–1949.
50. Ming, S.-Ch. (1979): Dysplasia of gastric epithelium. *Front. Gastroint. Res.*, 4:164–172.
51. Morson, B. C., and Konishi, F. (1980): Dysplasia in the colorectum. In: *Recent advances in gastrointestinal pathology. Clin. Gastroenterol. Suppl. 1.* W. B. Saunders Co. Ltd., London.

52. Morson, B. C., Sobine, L. H., Grundmann, E., Johansen, A., Nagayo, T., and Serck-Hanssen, A. (1980): Precancerous conditions and epithelial dysplasia in the stomach. *J. Clin. Pathol.*, 33:711–721.

53. Munioz, N., and Matko, I. (1972): Histological types of gastric cancer and its relationship with intestinal metaplasia. *Cancer Res.*, 39:99.

54. Murakami, T. (1971): *Early Gastric Cancer*, pp. 53–55. University of Tokyo Press, Tokyo.

55. Myren, J., and Serck-Hanssen, A. (1974): Gastroscopic biopsies in gastric disease. *Acta Pathol. Microbiol. Scand. (Suppl.)*, 248:137–144.

56. Nugent, F. W., Haggitt, R. C., Colcher, H., and Kutteruf, G. C. (1979): Malignant potential of chronic ulcerative colitis. Preliminary report. *Gastroenterology*, 76:1–5.

57. Ochsner, A., Weed, T. E., and Nuessle, W. R. (1981): Cancer of the stomach. *Am. J. Surg.*, 141:10–14.

58. Olearchyck, A. S. (1978): Gastric carcinoma: a critical review of 243 cases. *Am. J. Gastroenterol.*, 70:25–45.

59. Prolla, J. C., Kobayashi, S., and Kirsner, J. B. (1969): Gastric cancer, some recent improvements in diagnosis, based upon the Japanese Experience. *Arch. Int. Med.*, 124:238–246.

60. Ribet, A., Escourrou, J., Frexinos, J., and Delpu, J. (1980): Evaluation des differentes methodes pour le dépistage des tumeurs colorectales. *Acta Endosc. XVIIth International Congress of the S.M.I.E.R. Brussels, May.*

61. Riddell, R. H. (1976): The precarcinomatous phase of ulcerative colitis. In: *Topics in Pathology*, edited by B. C. Morson, pp. 179–219. Springer Verlag, Berlin.

62. Riddell, R. H., and Morson, B. C. (1979): Value of sigmoidoscopy and biopsy in detection of carcinoma and premalignant change in ulcerative colitis. *Gut*, 20:575–580.

63. Rösch, W., and Elster, K. (1977): Gastrointestinale Präkanzerosen. *Verlag Gerhard Witzstrock, Baden-Baden.*

64. Rösch, W., Fuchs, H. F., Kemmerer, G., and Hermanek, P. (1975): Morbus Ménétrier—eine Präkanzerose? Ergebnisse einer prospektiven Studie. *Leber Magen Darm.*, 5:85–89.

65. Rösch, W., Hermanek, P., and Elster, K. (1973): Gastritis und Magenfrühkarzinom. *Fortschr. Endosk.*, 5:23–25.

66. Schindler, R. (1965): Gastric carcinoma and gastritis. *Am. J. Dig. Dis.*, 10:607–624.

67. Schlag, P., Merkle, P., Wetzel, S., Rödl, W., Meister, H., and Herfarth, Ch. (1978): Diagnostische und Therapeutische Aspekte des Magenfrühkarzinoms. *Dtsch. Med. Wschr.*, 103:773–777.

68. Schottenfeld, D., Winawer, S. J., and Miller, D. G. (1978): Screening and early diagnosis of large bowel cancer. *U.I.C.C. Techn. Rep. Ser.*, 40:309–333.

69. Sherlock, P., Lipkin, M., and Winawer, S. J. (1980): The prevention of colon cancer. *Am. J. Med.*, 68:917–931.

70. Shinya, H., and Wolff, W. I. (1979): Morphology, anatomic distribution and cancer potential of colonic polyps. An analysis of 7000 polyps endoscopically removed. *Ann. Surg.*, 190:679–683.

71. Singer, M., Busse, R., Seib, H. J., Elster, K., and Ottenjann, R. (1975): Endoskopische Polypektomie in oberen Verdauungstrakt. *Dtsch. Med. Wschr.*, 100:2313–2316.

72. Siurala, M., Isokoski, M., Varis, K., and Kekki, M. (1968): Prevalance of gastritis in a rural population. *Scand. J. Gastroenterol.*, 3:211–223.

73. Siurala, M., Lehtola, J., and Ihamäki, T. (1974): Atrophic gastritis and its sequelae results of 19–23 years' follow-up examinations. *Scand. J. Gastroenterol.*, 9:441–446.

74. Siurala, M., and Salmi, H. J. (1971): Long-term follow up of subjects with superficial gastritis or a normal gastric mucosa. *Scand. J. Gastroenterol.*, 6:459–463.

75. Siurala, M., and Seppälä, K. (1960): Atrophic gastritis as a possible precursor of gastric carcinoma and pernicious anemia. *Acta Med. Scand.*, 166:455–474.

76. Siurala, M., Varis, K., and Wiljasalo, M. (1966): Studies of patients with atrophic gastritis—a 10–15 year follow-up. *Scand. J. Gastroent.*, 1:40–48.

77. Siurala, M., and Vuorinen, Y. (1963): Follow-up studies of patients with superficial gastritis and patients with a normal gastric mucosa. *Acta Med. Scand.*, 173:45–52.

78. Siurala, M., Vuorninen, Y., and Seppälä, K. (1961): Follow-up studies of patients with atrophic gastritis. *Acta Med. Scand.*, 170:151–155.

79. Stadelmann, O., Müller, R., Miederer, S. E., Löffler, A., Kozuschek, W., and Elster, K. (1972): Frühdiagnose des Magenkarzinoms—ein Kritischer Rückblick. *Fortschritte der gastroenterologischen Endoskopie*, Vol. 4, p. 53–59. 4e Kongresz für gastroenterologischen Endoskopie, Frankfurt.

80. Stalsberg, H., and Taksdal, S. (1971): Stomach cancer following gastric surgery for benign conditions. *Lancet*, 2:1175–1177.

81. Stokkeland, M., Schrumpf, E., Serck-Hanssen, A., Myren, J., Osnes, M., and Stadaas, J. (1981): Incidence of malignancies of the Billroth 11 operated stomach. A prospective follow-up. *Scand. J. Gastroenterol. (Suppl.)*, 16(67):169–171.

82. Treille, C., Aubert, H., and Rachail M. (1981): L'usage des colorants de muqueuze en endoscopie digestive haute: intérêt, applications pratiques, perspectives. *Acta Endosc.*, 11:369–381.

83. Ueno, K., Oshiba, S., Yamagata, S., Mochizuki, F., Kitagawa, M., and Hisamichi, S. (1976): Histo-clinical classification and follow up study of gastric polyp. *Tohoku J. Exp. Med. (Suppl.)*, 118:23–38.

84. Ungar, B., Strickland, R. G., and Francis, C. M. (1971): The prevalence and significance of circulating

antibodies to gastric intrinsic factor and parietal cells in gastric carcinoma. *Gut*, 12:903–905.

85. Vicari, F. (1980): Progress in the methods of endoscopic diagnosis in gastroenterology. *Endoscopy (Suppl.)*, 19–34.

86. Wangensteen, O. H., and Sosin, H. (1968): How can the outlook in alimentary tract cancer be improved? *Am. J. Surg.*, 115:7–16.

87. Way, J. D. (1980): Role of colonoscopy in surveillance for cancer in patients with ulcerative colitis. In: *Colorectal Cancer: Prevention, Epidemiology and Screening*, edited by S. Winawer, D. Schottenfeld, and P. Sherlock, pp. 387–392. Raven Press, New York.

88. Way, J. D. (1980): Endoscopy in inflammatory bowel disease. *Clin. Gastroenterol.*, 9:2.

89. Weedon, D. D., Shorter, R. G., Ilstrup, D. M., Huizenga, K. A., and Taylor, W. F. (1973): Crohn's disease and cancer. *N. Engl. J. Med.*, 289:1099–1103.

90. Wesdorp, I. C. E., Bartelsman, J., Schipper, M. E. I., and Tytgat, G. N. (1981): Effect of long-term treatment with cimetidine and antacids in Barrett esophagus. *Gut*, 22:724–727.

91. Williams, C. B., and Way, J. D. (1978): Colonoscopy in inflammatory bowel disease. *Clin. Gastroenterol.*, 7:701–717.

92. Winawer, S. J., Leidner, S. D., Boyle, C., and Kurtz, R. C. (1979): Comparison of flexible sigmoidoscopy with other diagnostic techniques in the diagnosis of rectocolon neoplasia. *Am. J. Dig. Dis.*, 24:277–281.

93. Winawer, S. J., Sherlock, P., and Schottenfeld, D. (1976): Screening for colon cancer. *Gastroenterology*, 70:783–789.

94. Wychulis, A. R., Woolam, G. L., Andersen, H. A., and Ellis, F. H. (1971): Achalasia and carcinoma of the esophagus. *JAMA*, 215:1638–1641.

95. Yardley, J. H., Bayless, T. M., and Diamond, M. P. (1979): Cancer in ulcerative colitis. *Gastroenterology*, 76:221–225.

Subject Index